Contents

THE WESTSIDE BARBELL BOOK OF METHODS

by Louie Simmons

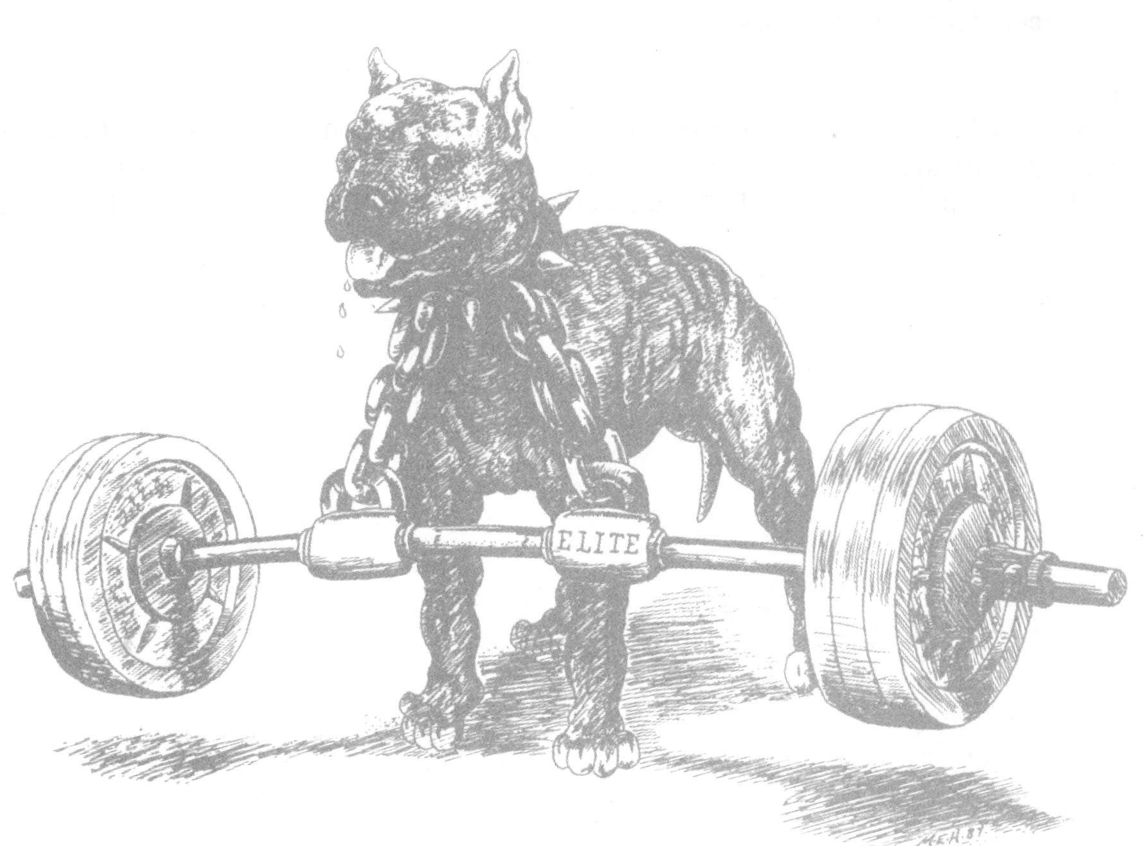

WESTSIDE BARBELL™

THE WESTSIDE BARBELL BOOK OF METHODS - By Louie Simmons

Writer:	Louie Simmons
Editor:	Sakari Selkäinaho
Photographs:	Sakari Selkäinaho, Scott DePanfilis
Covers:	Ville Turkkinen, VPT Productions, Finland
Printer:	Action Printing

Disclaimer

The author and publisher of this material are not responsible in any manner whatsoever for any injury that may occur through following the instructions contained in this material. The activities may be too strenuous or dangerous for some people. The readers should always consult a physician before engaging in them.

Part 1

Foreword

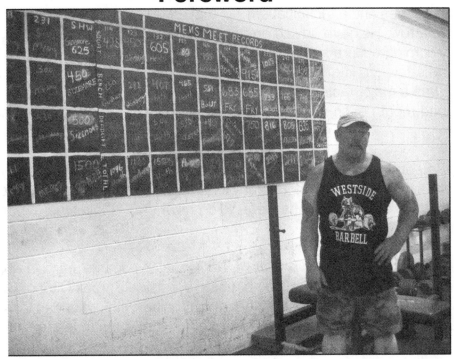

Lou in front of record board

My powerlifting memories start in 1966, just one month before my induction into the army. I feel like Captain Ahab with his obsession with Moby Dick. I am strapped to powerlifting, knowing I will be pulled to my chalky death by it eventually, but I can't stop. All my memories and all my friends are involved in powerlifting, so I am drawn to it even more today than ever. This is my story as I remember it.

My first exposure to powerlifting was at a power meet in Dayton, Ohio, late in 1966. I had Olympic lifted since I was 12 and competed at 14, doing a 175 snatch and a 260 clean/jerk at a body weight of about 155. I really thought I was a strong guy until that first power meet. There were 11 men in the 165s, and I got tenth place, beating only a 55-year-old dude.

This was an eye opener for me. I never Olympic lifted again. My Olympic lifting training partners should have worn signs saying, "I lift weights" because if they were brought into court for it, the case would be thrown out for lack of evidence. However, the powerlifters I saw were not only strong but looked like they were strong.

One of these men was Milt McKinney, a future world champion in the 132s. George Crawford was amazing at 165, trying a 525 world record squat with legs like tree trunks. He later squatted 650 at 165 with no gear back when 500 was good. George was the first to assist me with my squat form. He was always helpful at meets. His son came to visit years later, and it was my honor to help him. Vince Anello was in the meet as well, showing signs of his deadlift prowess even then. Vince told me once that anything made his deadlift go up. He was doing the conjugate system without knowing it. I just saw Vince at the 2004 IPF World Bench Championships in Cleveland, Ohio. He still looks great.

That meet in 1966 was my introduction to Larry Pacifico. He would become one of the greatest lifters I had ever seen. There was nothing I did not do to try to beat him. However, I never did, nor did anyone else until injuries and a technical error in the 1980 Senior Nationals cost him his chance to win ten Worlds in a row. He gave advice on benching, which was to gain weight and work triceps. Larry's son is becoming quite a shot putter, throwing 60 feet as a ninth grader. This group, along with Ed Matz and a few top lifters around the world, had a network of training knowledge at their disposal, which was a major factor in their success. Today we have the internet, but unfortunately, many use it to bad mouth each other, cry about their training partners, or, worse, be a legend in their own mind.

After that power meet, I went into the army. The next month I was in the infantry but did not go to Vietnam. Instead, I was sent to Berlin, I think, because of my father's untimely death in1968. Now, I could train fairly regularly, but my lifts were going nowhere. At this time, no one knew anything about powerlifting.

One day I picked up a *Muscle Power Builder*, which later became *Muscle and Fitness*. In that magazine, there was a powerlifting article about the Westside Barbell Club of Culver City, California. It was about box squatting. I had never heard of this, but with nothing to lose, I gave it a try. To my amazement, the box squats worked to the point that I later made top ten squats in five weight classes.

Through those articles, Bill West, George Frenn, and the guys got me started on the right foot. I was never able to visit Westside in Culver City due to work, which I regret to this day. After getting out of the army in 1969, I built a power rack, got some weights, and started training full- time using what I learned from the articles. They were my only training partners. After Bill West died, I referred to my place as Westside Barbell but never publicly until 1986. Westside Barbell is a trademarked name (and so is Louie Simmons).

I often wondered if I was on the right track with my training. Roger Estep was doing a 1600 total in the early 1970s. Then, out of nowhere, he made an 1800 total. I asked him how he jumped 200 lbs so quickly. He said he went out to Westside in Culver City, and the rest WAS history. Chuckie Dunbar, Jack Wilson, Luke Iams, Paul Sutphin, and some others were known as the Wild Bunch and were a very strong team. They proved to me that I was on the right track. My problem, unfortunately, was that I had no training partners. When I went to meets, I asked lifters who excelled in each lift for tips on that lift. When it came to benching, Larry Pacifico was always telling me to train my triceps and lats.

I was lifting in Indiana and met Bill Seno. This dude was huge. He had won best chest in many Mr. American contests but was also the American record holder in the bench press. I asked Bill how to get my bench up to a top ten lift (at the time there was only a top ten). First, he stared at me. Then, he grabbed me by the arms and said I needed to do illegally wide benches for a six rep max. He told me when progress stopped to go up to eight reps and then to ten reps with one to failure. I hated the higher reps, but the sixes pushed my lousy 340 at 181 to 445 at 198, and finally, 480 at 220 and a top eight bench. Bill was a close-grip bencher, and he was telling me to bench extra wide? What gives?

In the end, he knew what he was talking about. Bill was training with Ernie Frantz. Ernie was 12 or 13 years older than me. A former bodybuilder turned powerlifter, Ernie was old by my standards but not old-fashioned. He was and still is on the cutting edge with power gear— denim shirts and canvas squat suits, which are still some of the best today. For years, he was a top 181, 198, and 220. He also formed the APF and WPC to lift some of the restrictions of the IFF. His wife, Diane, was also a top lifter in the1980s. There were top lifters such as: Jack Barnes, who could out-squat everyone at 181 and 198 and John Kanter at 242 with a 2000 total. The heavyweights were always in the limelight—John Kuc; Jim Williams, one of the greatest benchers of all time; and Jon Cole, who made a 2370 total at 286 with no gear.

Larry Pacifico was not only lifting big but was putting on the greatest power meets ever. I lifted in the 1977 Junior Nationals in Lincoln, Nebraska. It was the first time I saw Fred Hatfield. He would become a squatting machine, maybe the greatest pure squatter of all time. I met a kid there who told me he was going to break the world record in the bench at 148. His name was Mike Bridges. He did break the record. I never saw such a lifting machine. He was and is the strongest man under 200 lbs whom I have ever seen. If he would choose to use the best gear of today, it would be crazy. My friend, Arnold Coleman, broke Mike's and Gene Bell's total record at the 2005 Arnold Classic. I was amazed to see Arnold break these records. It was unexpected, but the unexpected is commonplace today.

Sam Mangialardi, Dennis Reed, and Henry Waters were making big noise as well as Clyde Wright, Larry Kidney, and Paul Wrenn, who at super heavyweight sure could squat deep. I was now a 198. Estep, Jones, Cash, and my new training partner, Gary Sanger, were doing big lifts. In 1978, I was strong again; I was fourth in the squat, seventh in the deadlift with 710, and fifth in the total at 1825. I wanted to go to 220 but had a hard time gaining weight. I thought my injuries were behind me, so I went to the 1979 Senior Nationals. Bridges was killing then, but Ricky Crain was right there. Walter Thomas was at the top of his game, too. I was there to beat Pacifico like everyone else. I did everything I could to beat him, but—of course—I didn't, and neither could anyone else.

The 1979 Seniors was known as the Meltdown in Mississippi for good reason. Bill Kazmaier was making a name for himself and had planned to dominate the meet. I was sitting poolside with some lifters when Bill said, "Beam me up, Scotty." His luck got worse when he bombed out with an 804 deadlift. He would have won by over 100 lbs. It was very humid, which caused many missed deadlifts. I weighed only 212 and made a 733 PR squat and a PR bench of 462.

My opener of 677 would have placed me second behind Larry Pacifico. I pulled the weight easy, but as I locked it out, my grip slipped a little. The head referee was looking at my hand, and then my bicep tore loose, causing me to drop the bar. My second place quickly became no place. What a meet. Only two made a total—Larry and Dr. Steve Miller. To this day, people ask me, "Where's your bicep?" I reply, "Bay St. Louis, Mississippi."

Two surgeons recommended surgery, but one said no, and that's the way I went. Many people asked if I was going to lift again. I said, "Hell yes." Six months later, in January 1980, at the Y Nationals, I was back. I squatted 765, benched 480 (my first top ten bench), and deadlifted 705 to total 1950. It was the third best total ever for a short time. That's the good news. The bad news was that I had hurt my groin and lower abs. I was in extreme pain, but I was getting to like pain, maybe a little too much.

Next stop, the 1980 Senior Nationals in Wisconsin. I opened with 722 but failed. I made my second attempt but with a lot of pain and a popping sound. For the first time, I used my head and passed the rest of the meet. Ernie Hackett, a world record holder and physical therapist, looked at me and said I had torn tendons of the pelvic bone and some lower ab muscles. He was right, and I was out for a while.

Meanwhile, Larry Pacifico had won his ninth world championship at the 1979 Worlds in his hometown of Dayton, Ohio. Japan, England, and Canada had world champs along with the United States. At the 1979 Worlds, Lamar Gant beat Precious McKenzie at 123 by pulling a 617 deadlift.

The world record was 551, and Lamar made 617 to a standing ovation; this was the only one I have ever seen. With the existence of only one federation, my main goal was to do top ten lifts in my third weight class. I had some time to think about training. I knew I was doing something wrong because I was stronger in training than at the meets. After breaking my fifth lumbar vertebra for the second time in 1983, I sought medical advice. The doctor wanted to remove two disks, fuse my back, and remove bone spurs. I said, "No way, Jose." Larry's string of Worlds stopped at nine after jumping 2.2 k's on his second attempt, negating a third. Dan Wohleber pulled the first 900 deadlift. Dave Waddington squatted the first 1000 squat. Mike McDonald got a 512 bench press at 181 body weight. Remember, no shirts!

While I was recovering from my back injuries, I found every book on training methodologies from the old Eastern Bloc that I could. I was determined to outlast my rivals. There were many bright stars, but the brightest stars seem to burn out fast. I found that my new methods were working well. I decided to lift at 242 body weight just to obtain my fourth USPF Elite total. After that, I found a meet in Toledo and decided to try for my fifth Elite total at 275 body weight. The problem was that I only weighed 234. Ten miles outside of Toledo, I started drinking Gatorades. Chuck Vogelpohl kept handing me can after can, but I was still 238 when I stepped on the scale. The official said, "You're good." I retorted, "I'm lifting at 275."

I stayed and drank Gatorades until I went over the 242 limit and officially made the 275 class. I made my fifth Elite exactly where I made my first Elite. I squatted 800 lbs., benched 520, and did a 650 deadlift just to total that fifth Elite. By the way, they were all done with IPF or USPF judges. I was now wearing a bench shirt. They weren't much, a bit better than nothing. Shirts came about in 1984 or early 1985. I have lifted in every era of powerlifting. Things change and so must lifters.

I am one of a few to bench a top ten bench of 480 in 1980 without a shirt and sixth at 575 at a body weight of 220 in 2002 with a shirt at 54 years of age. Everyone asked me about Anthony Clark's benches. Were they good? I always said, "Yes". Now, Gene Rychalk, Jr., is the center of controversy. I saw Gene from the head judges chair do a perfect 1005 bench, which was letter perfect.

I'm sure if some serious cash was thrown at Gene, he would shut the mouths of those who criticize him. My hat goes off to Gene just like Jim Williams, Mike McDonald, Ted Arcidi, Ken Lane, and all the other great lifters throughout the decades. Don't take powerlifting backward. It could end up like United States' weightlifting, whose road is a dead-end street. There are pretenders, but they know who they are. Lifters must respect each other.

In 1970, I was weighing in, and George Crawford and Jerry Bell, the first 700 deadlifter at 165 body weight, were escorting a little kid at the meet. I asked, "Who's this?" Jerry replied, "This kid will be famous someday." His name was Bob Wahl, and he got a 661 squat at 148 body weight in 1983. To this day, I respect every lifter, young or old, who is brave enough to step on the platform.

My old friends Paul Sutphin, Mark Dimiduk, Jay Rosciglione, and many others like Steve Wilson and John Black of Black's Health World of Cleveland were all doing remarkable things. I lifted at the 1987 YMCA Nationals with 2033 at a light 242 and got fourth place. Steve Goggins was already a superstar, just like today. My good friend, Matt Dimel, had squatted 1010 at SHW and was totaling 2300. It was a great loss to Westside when Matt died. Gary Sanger was moving to LSU to teach, Bill Whitaker was going to Pennsylvania to start a vet clinic, and because of medical problems, Dr. Tom Paulucci had to retire. Doug Heath was going strong. Bob Coe, who showed up at my door 25 years ago, is still at Westside.

My knee had been hurting for some time, about five years to be exact. I was going to the APF Nationals and was taking a low hassock record when three-quarters of the way up, I snapped my left patella tendon in half. I had heard a few snaps but never thought I would hear my own. Then, it happened. My kneecap was now on the inside of my leg. The emergency squad showed up in ten minutes. They looked at my leg and told me they thought I had dislocated my knee. I told them, "No way, Jack." Because I am very allergic to anesthesia and have a spinal block, I was awake during my surgery.

All went well, and 14 weeks later, I went back with my friend, Diane Black, to have the wires removed. They gave me a shot to calm me for surgery. That shot put me to sleep, and they proceeded to give me anesthesia. I stopped breathing for four minutes, so they trached me and then inserted chest tubes when my lungs collapsed. I woke up two days later with holes in my chest and throat but no knee surgery! WOW, that really helped! I didn't know that Dr. Howard and Dr. Fine were working on me. Well, they inserted an air tube through my nose and finished the job. After seven days in intensive care to do a four-hour procedure, I was home.

I thought I was never going to compete again, but Kenny Patterson said something to me that brought me out of retirement immediately. That was 1996, and powerlifting hadn't gotten out of hand, yet. I lifted seven times in 11 months and became the first over 50-year-old to bench 550 and the first to bench 600, which was in a closed-back shirt. I had made a top ten bench again. I heard people say that I wasn't built to bench, squat, or deadlift. If I made top ten lifting in all categories, then almost anybody can, except for you lazy bastards who have some excuse why you can't!

Powerlifting comes in eras—no gear, some gear, better gear, and what I refer to as gangster gear, or legal through loopholes. Get used to it; it is here to stay. It makes relative newcomers superstars fast. Big squats, big benches, and most of the time, a poor deadlift! This shows the true strength of a person. The USPF was kicked out of the IPF. I told Peter Thorne we should pull out of the IPF, instead of getting pushed out. Remember folks, there are drug-tested meets but no drug-free meets. Get it straight because that is the way it is. Brother Bennett had a good idea, but unfortunately, there will always be those who bend the rules. This has been the way since the beginning of sports. There was the ADFPA and the USPF. Of course, both seemed power hungry, so Ernie

Frantz started the APF and the world body WPC. Until the USPF (before the IPF started), I had lifted AAU when the bench was performed first, then the squat, and then the deadlift. I believe, it should still be that way, but we had to make concessions with England 30 years ago about, believe it or not, gear.

This is my point. I never made the rules, but I have always followed them. When I dropped out of the USPF, they sent a questionnaire out asking what I would change. It was a little late for that, and I never filled it out. I always wondered how I killed myself to make Elite totals, suffering injuries and thousands of hours in the gym, when a judge could simply study a book, take a test, and become an IPF judge in weeks and not be a class one lifter. Big men are hard to judge in the squat. Lifters are penalized for not breaking parallel in the squat, which is very tough to do with the super strong suits we can wear by the rules. In the bench, we are rewarded by one pound of 700 touching the chest. It doesn't make sense. Bench meets have become the thing.

Countless bench pressers can be seen on the cover of PLUSA. I thought it was called POWERLIFTING USA, not BENCH PRESSING USA. This shows how popular bench pressing is. Even at Westside where we push the squat, we have made only three all-time world records, with five over 1000. Matt Smith's 1124 is the highest, and there are ten 800 deadlifters. We have made over 20 all-time world bench records, 15 over 700, and one at 825, showing what I know.

It's the year 2000, and I'm doing pretty well with an 860 squat at 242 and a 580 bench. I believe I was third with a 920 squat and fourth in a total with 2100 at 235 bodyweight. With the WPO on the scene with some money, it's amazing how money can bring people together. Kieran Kidder has also brought the best lifters together for the first time since Gus Rethwich's Hawaii Record Breaker meet, where unheard of weights were being lifted. The WPO format pits the greatest lifters in the top of each money division.

The 165s are unbelievable with Ron Palmer, who is fairly new to powerlifting, winning most of the time. The kingpin in the 165s is Tony Conyers with an 832 squat and a 1978 total. The guy must use mirrors. He's also one of the nicest guys you will ever meet. He's been at the top for years. My friend, Angelo Berardinelli, has also been at the top for years, starting at the famous Black's Health World. He's over 800 in the squat and 1900 in the total and still moving up. Angelo is a bulldog. Another young lion is Nick Hatch at 148, training at Rick Hussey's Big Iron gym. I saw him squat an unreal 788 at the ARNOLD CLASSIC at 19–years-old.

The second group is the 181 through 220. At the 181, Arnold Coleman broke Gene Bell's all -time total record of 2116. Maybe the meet will be renamed the Arnold Coleman Classic. Consequently, Phil Harrington was not at the WPO but squats 900 at 181. Where will it end? Then, there's a new star, Mike Cartinian, who is aiming at Jesse Kellum's 198 total. Mike trains with Angelo Berardinelli and Kenny Patterson. Speaking of Jesse, I think, he's taking it easy back in the swamps of Louisiana, training with some bad ass gators. I must say, Jesse is not only one of the strongest men in many weight classes but very smart about training. I believe, Jesse and Chuck Vogelpohl are twin brothers from different mothers. At 220, Chuck Vogelpohl has owned the squat record at 1025, but he has worn out his welcome at 220. Travis Mash has risen to the top at 220, breaking Eddie Coan's total record not once but twice.

The WPO has a 48-hour weigh in, which I have had doctors say is no advantage, but it sounds bad. The 242 and 275 world record holder, Steve Goggins, only weighed 264 when he squatted 1102 and totaled 2535. He weighed light at 242 and totaled 2481 with a world record squat of 1043. Steve trains in Atlanta with Phil Harrington, the world record holder at 181 with an unreal 900 squat, and also John Groves, a veteran lifter who has been around a long time. It's important to have a group of strong experienced lifters. Not to be left out of this group is Kara Bohigian who is extremely strong and very knowledgeable about training.

Mark "Spud" Bartley, who trained with Donny Thompson at Maximus Barbell in South Carolina, is really on the rise. At the 2005 WPO Super Open in Columbus, Ohio, he made a huge 2463 total and took second place. It proves a point that the most important thing in a gym is training partners. You can tell who has got balls and who pretends to have a set. How? It takes guts to lift with the strongest men in the world. Kieran has assembled the strongest and summons them to one platform.

A few years ago, 2400 would have won the SHW class. Then, it was 2500. Now, Matt Smith made 2601 and only took third place. And let's not forget Gary Franks! He made the first 2500, 2600, 2700, and 2800. With Beau Moore, Andy Bolton and I hope for the return of Brent Mikesell, one of the best SHW squatters around, but Moore and Bolton could claim it soon.

Beau Moore and Tony Conyers bought a reverse hyper from us some time back, and both have made unbelievable progress ever since. Matt Smith wants me to repossess it from Beau, not for nonpayment but because he's getting to be so strong. All these men are gentlemen and have nothing but good things to say about the competition. It's always been that way with the strongest lifters. The strongest men never bad mouth a beginner or those who are not strong. However, nowadays, there are many on the web being disrespectful to the strongest men and women in the world. Why? What have they done? Oh yeah, nothing! These people are constantly on the web when the men who they are criticizing are training, writing articles, and doing seminars. They are also going to meets and cheering on their competition, or they are backstage helping to put on bench shirts or spotting someone's warm ups. No one in my humble opinion should belittle Andy Bolton's deadlift, Brett Mikesell's squat, Gene Rychak, Jr.'s bench press, or Gary Frank's total lifts.

Are those who critique prepared to train beside men like these for even a year and see what they go through? Then and only then would someone appreciate the work and sacrifice that these lifters make. My goal has been to share what I have been taught and what I teach through my videos and seminars. In addition, my goal has been to share the work of my friends such as: college and NFL strength coach, Buddy Morris; college and NFL player and now coach, Tommy Myslinski; and my friends and training partners Dave Tate, Jim Wendler, George Halbert, and now Chuck Vogelpohl. All of them are giving back to their sport through their time to help lifters and coaches alike learn a similar system that works for everyone.

After moving to Columbus and training at Westside, Dave started Elite Fitness Systems. He is now not only my training partner, but we compete every day in the gym. We are also in competition in business with internet sales on my web site www.westside-barbell.com.

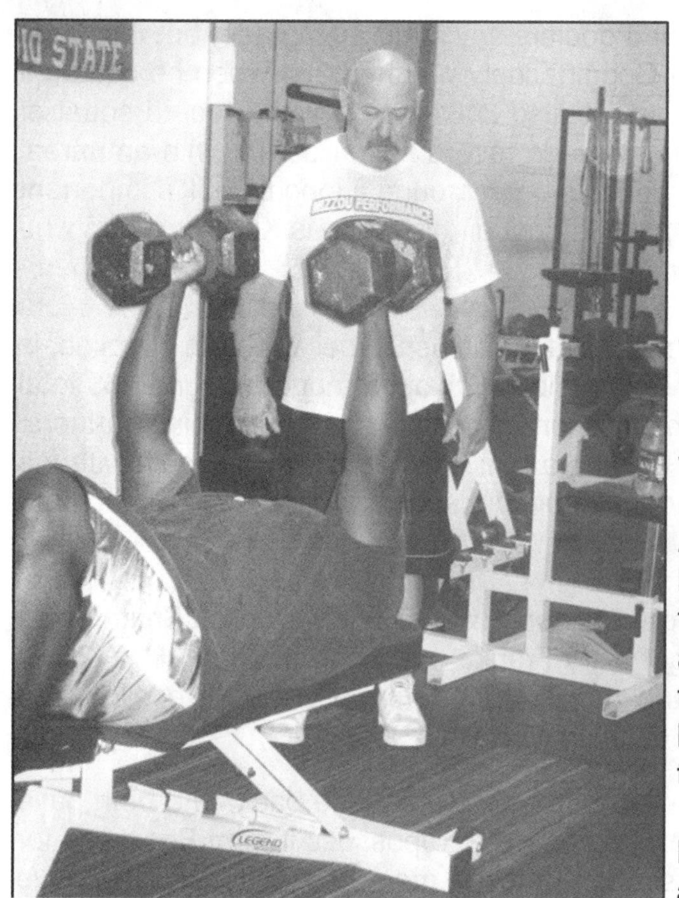

I can't forget Paul Childers, who performs in my workout tapes. He has contributed much to Westside Barbell through his own experiences with the Westside system. Also, my Finnish friend, Sakari Selkainaho, has helped elevate the system. I want to thank my training partners most of all, but I can't thank everyone or mention their names. There are just too many, but they know who they are—my friends from the Ukraine, Finland, Brazil, Japan, Ireland, Germany, Australia, New Zealand, South Africa, Canada, and everywhere else.

All NFL players, track athletes, MMA fighters, the late Dr. Mel Siff, and all the old Soviet Union authors who brought my attention to an advanced and sophisticated training system. Pavel, the kettlebell master, has backed us for years. I support him and his team of instructors for their relentless teaching.

Powerlifters, please band together. I respect all federations, their motives, and the direction they're heading, but we must travel together to achieve true success. I would like to thank the three Westside Barbell team doctors who work relentlessly to keep us healthy—Dr. Dave Beversdorf, Dr. Bill Nucklos, and Dr. Eric Serrano. With three more surgeries under my belt, powerlifting is about to pull me down, maybe for the last Time. However, as a man once wrote, I won't go slowly into the night, but I will rage on into the dying of the light.

Did you know that Westside has only two men on its staff: John "Chester" Stafford and Matt Wenning? John talks about nutrition on his website. I believe, he has the biggest push-pull for a 275 pounder. He also has a 733 bench, an 832 deadlift, and a 2502 total. Matt Wenning is a graduate of Ball State University with a Master's degree in biomechanics. He has already made a 1050 squat, a 650 bench, and a 770 deadlift at 275. These two people, along with me, are the only qualified people to talk about the real truth of what goes on at Westside.

We see the evolution of strength training every day, and every day it changes for the better for our lifters. By following our articles and talking to me occasionally, you know that the experiments we conduct are performed on our top men at two or three major meets to prove that the tested methods work. I don't write B.S. I write about what I see at Westside.

Some things work and some don't. We put forth a lot of effort to help our lifts, and I hope yours, too.

I appreciate how cooperative and loyal our lifters are, young and old. Some have been at Westside for years; for example, Bob Coe has been here over 20 years. Chuck Vogelpohl, Amy Weisberger, and Jimmy Richie have been at Westside for 20 years.

Did you know that Westside contributes to the development of many sports?

A former top soccer player from Manchester United stayed at Westside for more than a month to learn our system.

After returning home, Ben Plevey opened up a training facility to pass on the system to young athletes in his home country. Four rugby coaches from all over the world spent considerable time at Westside, and the results have been quite favorable to say the least. Many professional football players come to Westside and have made great strides. Football players never ask me to make them faster but to make them stronger. Making them stronger, in turn, makes them faster. Also, many major universities have adapted the Westside system to fit their needs.

There would not be a Westside if not for the likes of Huge Iron, Donny Thompson, Spud Barcley, Paul Childress, Andy Bolton (with his 1003 deadlift), and Jeff Lewis (with his 1200 plus squat). Because of them and many like them, we never miss a workout for fear that some of you dudes are working on a secret of your own.

I am proud to be associated with powerlifting, and I hope you are, too.

Loiue Simmons

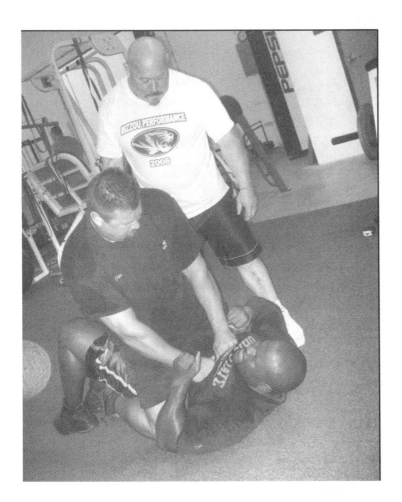

FOREWORD FROM THE EDITOR

I have been involved with weight training since my early teens. Now, after more than 30 years, I have learned a lot about the great sport of powerlifting and strength training. I have always tried to get my hands on any type of training information that I could. I read books, watched DVDs, and talked to lifters. Today, email and instant messenger helps a lot. Many top lifters are easy to approach and offer their advice and opinions. I think that's unique to powerlifting. In my rank, one source of information is above all others. Louie Simmons has helped me greatly, as he has helped so many other lifters and coaches regardless of sport or federation. No one, not even Louie, knows more than all others together, but he will teach you to think.

I first trained using the Westside method back in 1996, and my bench jumped 17.5 kilos (38 lbs) in six months. That convinced me. Before that, I would try anything I could get my hands on. Russian- and Bulgarian-based training routines gave me the best results, but nothing beat Westside, especially because the results are measured by long-term progress. Both systems are still utilized in Westside training.

Today, Westside training has introduced many new techniques and methods in strength training. The most important is the conjugate method, which is what the entire system is built on. The methods and exercises utilized by Westside, such as squatting with a box and utilizing bands, are now used worldwide.

The Westside system uses many principles that were developed many decades ago. Those principles still stand today. Many times people don't understand the idea of Westside. Reading one article or even ten may not clear the picture.

This book is based on Louie's articles over the years. You will notice changes and differences in percents and some other things while others have stayed the same. The main purpose is to outline the information so that the system is easier to figure out. You can study the theory behind the methods or just learn how to bench press. This book is meant for coaches and lifters and will teach you to analyze training so that you can coach yourself and others.

I want to thank Louie for being such a great friend and for his patience and trust on this project. We all know he reads a lot, and it's about time for him to have a book of his own!

Sakari Selkäinaho

World Strength and Power

In Bulgaria where many of the greatest lifters come from, the system is straightforward. Anyone who wants to reach the top (juniors and seniors) must go through the main training facility. Though few exercises are executed, one must be ideally built to succeed and have a particular body structure and muscle type. An individual also has to possess a high work capacity with near limit weights. As many as six training sessions are used per day. This was a proven system and was used for more than 20 years. Only the strongest survived. This system produced high results as well as a high burn-out ratio.

Bulgaria is a small country, economically depressed country. Sport was a way out of poverty. This meant that everyone tried his best for himself and his country. For every lifter who makes it, many go back home denied entrance. The Bulgarian training system was designed to produce one goal—an Olympic medal run. They succeeded through the process of selection of bodystructure to progress with a small number of exercises: the snatch, clean and jerk, power snatch, power clean and jerk, and front and back squats. The athletes had to have the ability to lift maximum weight in more than one workout a day with a 30-minute break between workouts. The second workout was completed with less time on warm ups. The junior and senior teams trained together. Obviously, there had to be top coaches. Normally, there were three involved with the top 20 lifters. Their national coach was Ivan Abadjiev. Because he was the top coach, little variation in the system occurred.

Another super power was the former Soviet Union. Their system was very thought out. They sought to develop top lifters with an assortment of means. The former Soviet system was vast, consisting of many thousands of lifters and a large number of coaches, who were former highly ranked lifters. With so many coaches, a multitude of combinations of training evolved, consisting of different loading schemes, exercises, tapering methods, and restoration. Because of the various types of body structures, it became clear that the same exercises would not work for everyone. In 1972, the Dynamo Club experimented with a system of exercises that were constantly revolved. A group of 72 lifters, all masters or international masters of sport, used 20–45 different exercises. At the end of the experiment, only one lifter was satisfied with the number of exercises. The rest wanted more. This was the conjugate method. Much research was brought to the United States after the fall of the Iron Curtain.

Who were the first Soviets were to participate in the Olympics? They were not sportsmen but camera men, biomechanics experts, and coaches.

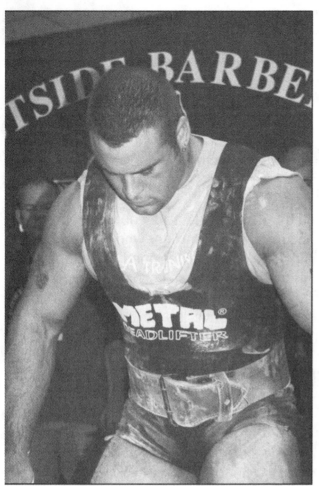

They studied the best athletes from all over the world and at first copied them. Later, however, they introduced new innovations in training. This is exactly what Westside has done. With so much training data, their own coaches could not access it all. Nevertheless, they had hard proof of what works and what doesn't. Many of their coaches were top lifters, training along with other lifters. The very best were on the national or military teams. They were proud of their heritage and defended it fiercely. Their training methods spread to other communist countries. Templates had been created to examine the strength and weaknesses of all athletes. Here is an example for a 110 kg lifter (from *Weight Lifting Fitness for All Sports*).

To be superior, a 110 kg (242) had to be capable of the following—power snatch 396 lbs, power clean 484 lbs, front squat 573 lbs, back squat 639 lbs, and close-grip bench 418 lbs. Does the U.S. weightlifting team do this? Hell, no. This could be the difference between progression and regression.

I have used the methods of many Russians. I have thanked some of them before, but I can't possibly thank all of them or mention all their names. Here are some of them. V. Zatsiorsky's book, *Science and Practice of Strength Training*, confirms that Westside is on the right track. YV Verkhoshansky was the father of the shock system of training. Medvedyev, with his insight into training and restoration, brought my attention to the importance of changing volume and intensity during different phases of training. As Prilepin's research in determining the optimal training loads by intensity zone and number of lifts per workout is the foundation of training at Westside.

Another super power is the Chinese. They have made great strides in all sports, but weightlifting is in the forefront. The Chinese have always been proficient in weightlifting. They have thousands of candidates to choose from. They have always led the way in acupuncture, acupressure, Tai Chi, and meditative methods. Their system was strengthened by adding former Soviet coaches. They have raised high volume training to new heights. In a video filmed in a world championship training hall, I saw a 14-year-old boy squat 370, snatch grip deadlift 330, and clean and jerk 242. This was at a body weight of 110 lbs! The Chinese select a group a lifters whose bodies can withstand the maximum loads required to reach the Olympics. They have barracks after barracks of lifters to choose from. It's a way out of poverty. They pick the best coaches and then assemble the best lifters. They already had perhaps the best psychological and physiological methods. Add all this up and you have a juggernaut. It's quite simple really.

They break training down into separate units to make a whole. This is an example of the conjugate method. In addition to the Russian method, now we have the Chinese method to learn from. However, will we?

With similar methods taught by the Russian coaches but with a higher work capacity, there seems to be no limit. I have talked about three powerhouse countries. What about the fourth— Westside Barbell? Many people compare the world's best lifters to ours. Some say, "Hey, Louie, those Russian lifters are some of the greatest and they don't follow your methods." They also bring up names such as: Ed Coan, Steve Goggins, Beca Swanson, and Gary Frank, who is the strongest man I've ever seen. They say, "Why don't your guys squat as much as Brent Mikesell or bench like Gene Rychlak? What about Andy Bolton's deadlift?" Well, these lifters are spectacular to say the least, and they have my admiration and respect. They make a lift that seems unbreakable but then manage to break it. Nowhere else is there a stronger collection of lifters than at Westside.

Our top six guys rival those from any other nation. Take a look at the Westside all-time ranking lists and clubs later in this book. The best totals and lifts are mostly made within the last 12 months. In addition, we have more back up than an NWA concert. Amy Weisberger has more than ten times her body weight total at 132.

We had the youngest 700 bencher, Kenny Patterson, at 22-years-old in 1995. In his time, Kenny was also the lightest to bench 700 (701) at 238. Back in 1995, we had three teens bench over 600. Anthony Clark was the first to bench 600 as a teen. Then, it was Westside's Andre Henry (605), Tim Harrold (615), and Mike Brown, who as of April made 670 easily at barely 19-years- old. At the same meet, JL Holdsworth made 775 at 284, and another lifter, Paul Keys, who may not be so familiar, hit 750 at 286. The last two hit 800 on third attempts but got them turned down. At the time of this writing, Tim Harrold became the youngest man at 20-years-old (2/4/84) to bench 700 and the youngest to total 2400.

No gym has totals like Westside. We have had four men break the all-time bench record— Doug Heath, Kenn Patterson, George Halbert, and Rob Fusner. These men have accumulated 20 all-time records. A few years ago, we dropped the 500 bench club at Westside. We felt that having 63 members on the list over the years took some luster off it. Now we calculate only 550 and up. We have 43 on this list. Chuck Vogelpohl is the lightest lifter to squat 1000. At 220 body weight, he has made 1025. His best lifts add up to 2419.

I wrote this book for all of you. As Roy Jones, Jr., says, take a look at the Westside record lists and clubs. Some of our own lifters don't know our history, and I just wanted to inform our fans and anyone else who would listen.

The Organisation of Training

When planning training, one must not plan for the next meet but rather the next year or even longer. The effectiveness of training is based on many considerations. The following are some issues to consider:

- Weight gain or loss
- Improving form on competitive lifts or special exercises
- Raising work capacity and improving general fitness
- Gaining general training knowledge
- Testing character and courage
- Learning how to use legal equipment

Weight gain or loss:
First, it is imperative to be in the correct weight class. If a lifter is six feet tall and weighs 180 lbs, he needs to gain weight. Someone like this should increase his protein and caloric intake, or he cannot compete with the top 181s of the world. To solve the problem, on max effort day do max 3s up to max 6s. This builds extra muscle mass while also building absolute strength.

At Westside, we recommend doing only a total of four exercises per workout. To gain weight, add two exercises to add muscle mass. After gaining up to the proper weight class, drop back to the original four exercises not counting abs. As far as food intake, skip the chocolate milk and cookies and learn about proper nutrition. Buy a book or two and read and learn. If an athlete's deadlift falls backwards, he has gained too much. His waistline will get too big, and his hands will get too fat. I know because this happened to me. Discipline is essential. Keep in mind, it might take five years of hard training to build up to the right weight class.

Improving form:
Improving form is a necessity, but it is sometimes difficult. At Westside, we have people who are very good in all lifts. To teach a new lifter, we place them in one of our groups. By interacting with that group, the lifter is taught good form through watching and listening. We never criticize but rather analyze. We always tell the truth to each other, especially visitors because many don't have the luxury of great training partners to watch over them. Special exercises play a large role in perfecting top form in all three lifts by doing exercises for whatever muscle group is lagging. This in itself helps perfect form. It only stands to reason if there is a weakness in a muscle group, it can destroy form. A word of caution: If you are starting out, start out right. Matt Dimel always had a tricep problem. Year after year, he would gain little by little and his poorest lift, the bench press, would increase. After rupturing both patella tendons, he eventually won the APF Seniors again. His improved bench press helped. A champion will become a champion by becoming better at his worst lift.

Raising work capacity and general fitness:
Why is this so important? First, we all need to work on our weaknesses, which could be the ability to train at a fast pace. During a workout, energy levels can drop quickly; some experts say within 45 minutes. Therefore, a lifter must train at a fast pace, ensuring that the most important work is completed in 45 minutes. This involves lactic acid tolerance training, which means a pump in the hips and lower back can occur while squatting and doing back work. To think that an individual must fully rest between sets is old thinking to say the least. If a lifter does a work task and fully recovers and then repeats the same work, he uses the very same muscle fiber. Nothing is gained by training this way. However, by enlisting shorter and shorter rest intervals between work sets (i.e. the interval method), the work becomes far more intense, involving more muscle fiber.

The last half of speed sets is the most explosive of all. When lactic acid is produced so is the growth hormone. If an individual has a high work capacity, a high volume, high intensity workout is not as tiring for him as it would be for someone out of shape. This enables him to train a little heavier and longer as well as a little faster than his enemies. This requires small, roughly 20-minute workouts during the week. The workouts are directed toward any particular weakness the individual has. It could be a muscle group, flexibility, conditioning, or even concentration. It may take years to increase general fitness to a higher degree. A lifter's goal should be to raise his classification ranking from class four to USPF standard Elite.

At Westside, we have developed 56 Elite lifters, who started out with nothing. Some have achieved all-time record performances such as: Chuck Vogelpohl, Kenny Patterson, and Rob Fusner to mention a few. They continually raised their work capacity. As they became stronger, their ability to recuperate, perfect form, concentrate, and raise volume increased. Chuck and I do about 14 workouts a week. We complete a couple sets of dumbbell presses to failure or timed sets with some lat and ab work before squatting. We may also do sled work and glute ham raises before a bench workout. Sled work or the reverse hyper machine can be performed before a squat or deadlift workout with no adverse effects when a lifter is in top condition. By executing a large volume of sled work, work capacity greatly improves.

On max effort day, the heaviest sled work is performed. It may involve pulling up to six, 45 lb plates on a flat, steel sled. The sled is pulled in two ways—with the strap hooked to the back of the belt or holding the strap in your hands between your legs with an upright posture with straight arms. The amount of weight is reduced throughout the week until possibly a weight of roughly 60 lbs is used. The weight is lowered, but the length of pulling is greater—600 feet for the heaviest work and up to 2000 feet for light work. For upper body work, I have dragged for two miles nonstop. I sometimes do a lot of box jumps as a replacement for some of the sled pulling. Light fireman's carries can also be done. We throw a medicine ball for a set time, usually 3–15 minutes with a ball weighing 10–40 lbs. Light power cleans are also very beneficial for conditioning. Do them in one of two ways. First, drop to a hang clean and do power cleans with the interval method; a set can be done every 60, 45, or 30 seconds depending on your level of fitness.

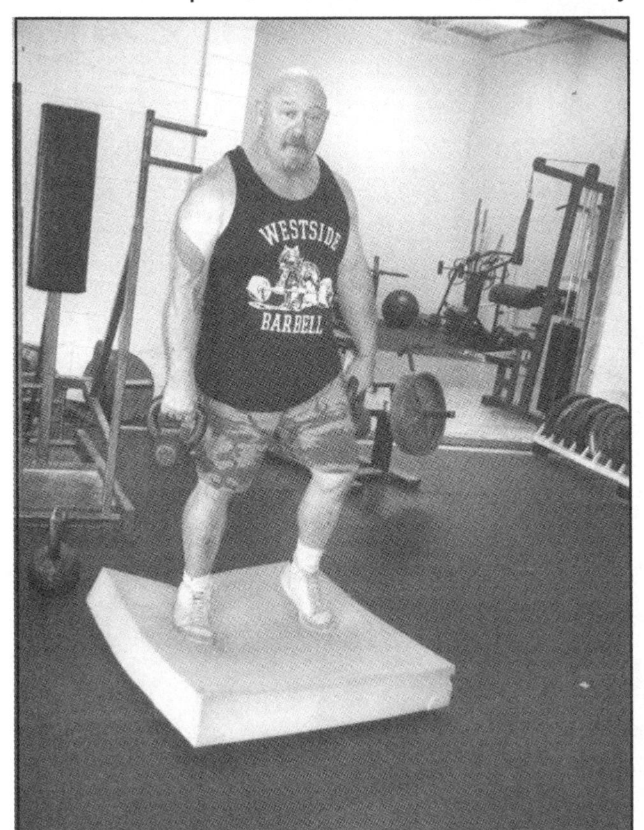

A second variety is to add a push jerk or push press with each set. The sets should last 5–20 minutes. This is a tough one. Dumbbells can be done in a very slow fashion for up to eight minutes. Use the shortest time, two minutes, with the heaviest bells. For example, use 50-lb dumbbells continuously for five minutes, keeping track of the reps.Walking lunges can also be done. Whatever exercise is completed, it should slowly increase in intensity and volume as the years pass. Ease into the work but always aim to increase the amount of work. The better condition an individual is in, the faster new records will come.

There is much to learn if success if the objective, and it takes time. A lifter must gain mentally, technically, and physically. Be patient; it will come.

Testing character and courage:
I am a huge fan of most sports, but when I watch basketball, I frequently hear the announcer say the player passed up an open shot to another player because he did not have the confidence to shoot the ball himself. Or during a football game, the announcer will say that a certain player is a natural leader. What are the other ten players? Natural-born followers? I hope not, but who knows? Why can't the other ten teammates step up and take over? Angelo Berardinelli said it best: "They are two types of people—the prey and the predator." Which are you? And don't stroke your ego. I watched Angelo try to break the world middle-weight squat record for years.

He was always close but was never able to break it. The record kept going up from 766 to 771 to 773. Finally, at the WPO in York, Pennsylvania, in June 2002 he made 777. Now, Angelo has that world record, and he dares anyone to take it away from him. The top middle-weights this year are all predators. When I hear someone tell me what place he got in a meet rather than what his numbers were or if he got a personal record, I know his ego will hold him back. The real contest is with one's self. A trophy proves only what has been done but has no bearing on what will happen next. You must always do better and better. That's the real world. You can be the greatest powerlifter in the world, but the day you retire, you're forgotten. If you quit one time, you're a quitter. You may go for a year or two without progress before coming out of a slump. Training knowledge as well as technology can make it possible progress for a very long time if you want to. Powerlifting is a tough sport. No one said it wasn't. As far as training partners go, if you run with the lame, you will develop a limp. Only train with those who have the same goals as your own. Everyone can't be a world champ, but we can all be better.

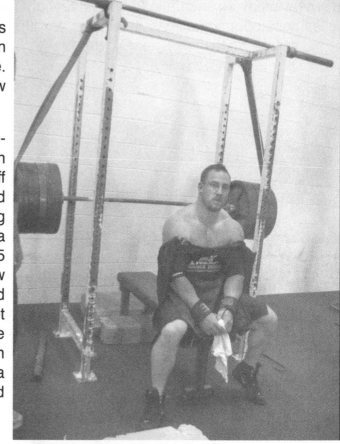

At Westside, we have many in-house contests mostly on max effort day. They usually happen without notice, and most often, that's the case. I recall pulling a heavy sled on a Monday a few years ago.

I was minding my own business when Chuck Vogelpoh yelled out the door, "Get your old ass in here. We're going to have a deadlift contest off pin one in the power rack." Well, I was dead tired from pulling the sled, but someone was running his mouth as usual. Now, I was being pulled into a contest on something I had not broken a PR in 15 years. I was obligated to take part, and somehow I broke my record. How? I guess, I was so pissed off at those nitwits that the only way I could get even was to get a PR. When I lose, I use my age (54) as an excuse. If I win, I rub it in. It's been said, "Show me a good loser, and I'll show you a loser." Thank goodness we have some very bad losers at Westside.

If someone refuses to engage in a spontaneous contest, we throw challenges at him when he least expects it. If someone regularly backs out, we boot him out of the club. We know by experience that if a lifter will not take a challenge in friendly surroundings, he will fall apart in a real meet. Our training in general is designed to build confidence year round by doing so many different exercises. We are always breaking records. Remember, a lifter must raise his mental and emotional limits , or he won't raise his weights. It may take years to learn to focus on training let alone meets. Some of us are late bloomers while others start fast but fade just as quickly. Many times the brighter star burns out the fastest. Westside loves to see successful teams like Donny Thompson's Maximus team advance. The LA Lifting Club is moving up fast as well thanks to Joe's pushing and pulling with the help of his wife, Nance. There is also my Finnish friend, Sakari Selkainaho, who lifts and coaches his teammates Jarmo, Ano, Mikko, and the rest. I love to see teams or individuals gaining momentum to see how the guys at Westside react to it.

Just remember, if you're a betting man and two lifters are coming out to squat and one's psyching up to DMX and the other one is listening to Patsy Cline's "I Fall to Pieces", which one are you going to put your money on? Why do some lifters put limitations on themselves? What I'm talking about is all the "world champs" and "world record holders" I talk to daily.

Now, wait a minute. There's only one world record in each lifting category and one world champ per weight class. That person holds the biggest total of the present year or of all-time in his weight class. Yes, I'm talking to you master and teen lifters. You may think I'm an asshole for saying this, but you are selling yourself short, my man. If you get in a fight and you're a master, do you get to throw the first three punches? Hell, no. When there's a hottie in the lounge, us old guys are always hitting on the young babes, right? Why limit yourself by age? Just do the best you can, and you are a champ.

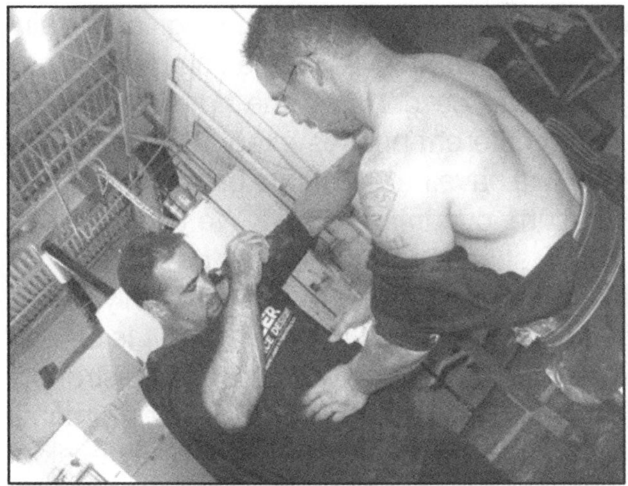

Using equipment:
For example, why don't all federations use monolifts? Or a bar for each event? Not only is it stupid not to do so, it is dangerous. Don't be stuck in the past. If NASCAR kept the same pace as powerlifting, the cars would be much slower because of tire restrictions and other safety factors. How many times do you have to walk out before disaster strikes someone? Some federations are held together by one or two great lifters. Please don't get them hurt because your backward thinking has you on the verge of extinction.

Just look at your membership totals, slipping lower and lower. If there's only one top 100 list, make all things equal—suits, shirts, weigh ins, etc. It's not the gear, drugs, or equipment that make the list. As Vince McMahon says, "It's the size of your grapefruits." You are paying card members, so speak up. Take control of your own destiny.

Gaining general training knowledge:
I hate to say this, but at Westside, we have lifters who don't even read Powerlifting USA let alone some of the books I frequently mention such as those I'm about to describe. Michael Yessis published The Soviet Sports Review. There was some valuable information in those articles translated from mostly Russian sports scientists in a quarterly magazine. It covered many sports but was invaluable to me at the time. The first book that made me a believer was The Managing of the Weight Lifter by Laputin and Oleshko. In this book, they showed a table that explained how to regulate volume by intensity zones. Writings such as Verkhoshansky's *Fundamentals of Special Strength Training in Sports* and Mel Siff's *Supertraining* are valuable books. A highly respected author is Medvedyev, who wrote *A Program of Multi-year Training in Weightlifting.* Of course, there are several other highly accomplished authors including PV Komi, Thomas Kurz, Tamas Ajan, and Tudor Bompa. Lazar Baroga's book *Weightlifting Fitness for All Sports* is a must read. Zatsiorsky is particularly valuable to anyone who participates in sports or weightlifting. Also, try *Science and Practice of Strength Training* . I enjoy Starzynski and Sozanski for information on explosive power training and Pavel Tsatsouline for stretching and ab work. Without these men who have dedicated their lives to the promotion of sports science used in a practical environment, I would have ended my lifting career in 1983. The results worldwide speak for themselves. I wish I could thank each of these men personally. Thank goodness I have had the opportunity to speak with Dr. Siff and participate in a few seminars with him, so I can play a small role in the development of others.

The Regulation of Training

One must consider how many lifts to do in one particular workout and calculate what percent is best used for explosive and accelerating strength. It is also important to establish the number of lifts for the development of an individual's absolute strength. This is a major factor if an athlete wants to reach his top potential.

Also, keep in mind all the components of training—physical, technical, and psychological. If training is regulated correctly, then all of the above can be accomplished while increasing hypertrophy and building general physical preparedness (GPP). This can be done at one time without the use of periodization where one breaks up the training into different phases every 3–4 weeks. By closely following the rep/set recommendations of Prilepin, we have had 18 lifters bench 550 or better here at Westside. This method is commonly known as the dynamic method. We use 60% of a no-shirt best bench for 8–10 sets of three reps. This is how speed-strength is best developed. Siff and Verkhoshansky used a force plate machine to determine the maximum effort a highly skilled weight lifter could display. This lifter generated 264 lbs of force on a 154 lb bar. The 154 is 58% of 264. This demonstrates the optimal relationship between force and velocity where speed-strength is best developed. For the bench, we do roughly 120 lifts at 60% of a no-shirt max in a one-month time period (ten sets of three reps equals 30 lifts per workout times four workouts) for the development of starting and accelerating strength. By using a weight that is 60% of a one rep max, a 600 lb bencher can train along with a 400 lb bencher without one overloading or one underloading. How?

The 600 lb bencher would use 360 for his sets, and the 400 lb bencher would use 240 for his sets. The workload is regulated to one's strength limits. If the 400 lb bencher uses more than 240, his bar speed is compromised, thus destroying the optimal relationship between force and velocity.

You may ask, how does a 400 lb bencher eventually bench 600? The answer lies in the improvement in and development of special exercises. When the 400 lb bencher has brought up his extensions, delt raises, back and lat work to that of a 600 lb bencher, he has grown to be a 600 lb bencher as well. The bench press itself is not used for muscle hypertrophy (growth). The special exercises serve two critical purposes—the development of strength in individual muscle groups and an increase in muscular size, which helps increase leverage in the bench and squat. Prilepin's recommendations for weights above 90% (done on the max effort day) are 4–10 lifts. Here, we are referring to classical lifts or major bar exercises such as: good mornings, box or rack pulls, and of course, a variety of squats.

Prilepin's Table: Number of reps for percentage training

Percent	Reps per set	Optimal	Range
55–65	3–6	24	18–30
70–75	3–6	18	12–24
80–85	2–4	15	10–20
above 90	1–2	7	4–10

Like Medvedyev and other sports scientists, we have discovered that too many weights above 90% can cause deterioration in coordination, which initiates deterioration in form. When training with weights that are over 90% of your current one rep max for 4–5 weeks, negative effects occur to the central nervous system (CNS) and progress can decrease. Yet, one must train with very heavy weights to make gains in absolute strength. So, what's the answer? Train a bar exercise for only two weeks and switch. For example, do bent over good mornings for two weeks, safety power squat bar for two weeks, rack pulls for two weeks, and front squats for two weeks. These are just a few exercises from which to choose. Always max out on this day for one rep in squatting exercises or pulls, such as rack pulls, high pulls, pulls off a box, snatches, or cleans. Do a three rep max in good mornings. The max effort day occurs three days after the dynamic day.

We have adjusted the number of 90% and above lifts in one workout to 3–5 lifts. The reasoning behind this is that the special exercises for powerlifting are much heavier compared to the Olympic lifts that Prilepin's data had been based. To become very strong, many lifts must be performed in limited movement exercises such as: board presses for bench pressing, rack pulls for the deadlift, and above parallel box squatting for the squat. We have discovered it is best to do a single in most cases instead of a triple. Why? A 500lb single equals 500 lbs of work. A 500 triple is 1500 lbs of work, which is much too demanding on the CNS. However, three reps can produce muscle tension. It is advised that the more massive lifters do 3s instead of ls to achieve adequate muscle tension. Extra body mass can reduce the range of motion in many lifters. We usually do a 90% weight as a last warm up, working toward a record over 100% and possibly two or three PRs. We invariably go until we miss a weight. This is the best way to achieve a true max effort.

Let's look at the ratio of the dynamic day to the max effort day. Dynamic day—120 lifts per month. Max effort day—12–20 lifts per month. This is how we are able to train heavy throughout the year—by rotating exercises on max effort day.

Remember, do one type of training per workout day: speed bench, Sunday; speed squat, Friday; max effort for bench, Wednesday; and max effort for squat and deadlift, Monday (the exercises for the squat and deadlift are the same). You can't and should never do two types of strength training in one workout. Your brain will not know what to do when asked to do two completely different tasks in one training session.

This can be best illustrated by watching a professional boxing match. In the early rounds, up to six, is when most knockouts occur. This is where explosive strength is demonstrated. Endurance plays little role in the early rounds. After six rounds, the explosive strength diminishes, strength endurance is dominant, and fewer knockouts occur. Not only is it best to do only one type of special strength training per session, but while doing the dynamic method using only one weight (after a warm up), your CNS can accommodate the task it is asked to perform.

To summarize, change the core exercise on max effort day every week. Use 3–5 special exercises to complement the core exercise. Train speed bench press at 45–50% of your max bench without a shirt. Train speed squat in waves of 50–60%, jumping 2.5% each week and then start over with 50%. The box squats on dynamic day are done with a pair of groove briefs or a suit with the straps down. Never wear knee wraps but wear a belt.

Speed work is done on one day and max effort work is done on another, 72 hours apart. Friday is our speed day, and Monday is our max effort day. Speed day is designed for explosive strength and acceleration for the development of force; whereas, max effort day develops absolute strength. Chuck Vogelpohl, who has won everything from the Y Nationals to the Worlds, simply says it is most important to push up the special work and concentrate on bar speed for squatting and deadlifting. Just remember to push the special core exercises that work best for you closest to the meet.

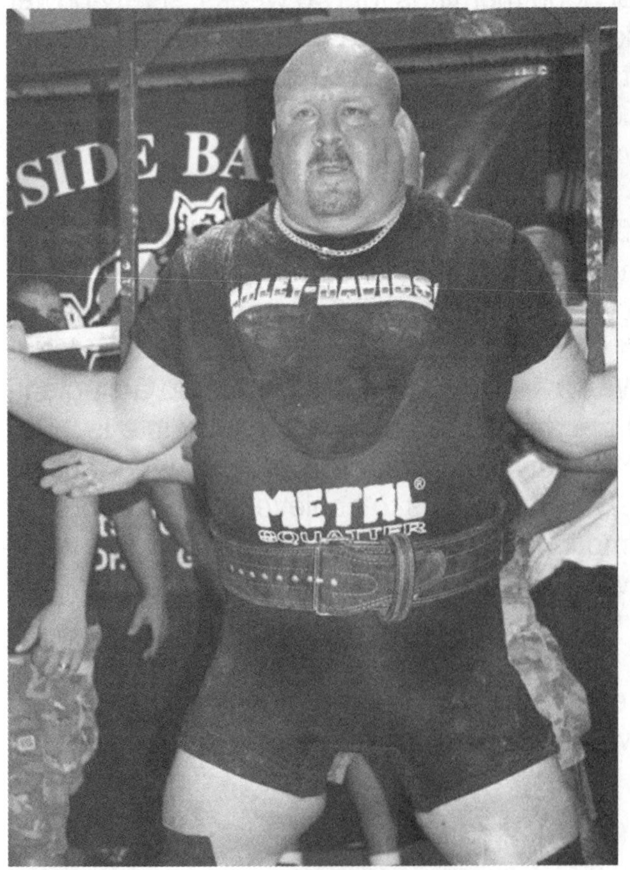

For the bench press, two workouts are done per week—one for speed and acceleration and one for the development of reversal strength. Yes, reversal strength can be stored for the pause rule. Sunday is the dynamic method day. Always train at 60% of a no-shirt max (240 for a 400-lb bench, 270 for a 450 bench, 300 for a 500 bench, and so on). Don't wave the weights in the bench, and remember to train at 60%, 8–10 sets of three reps. Use close and moderately close grips, with the little finger inside the narrow rings on the bar. Lower the bar as quickly as possible. Reverse it as quickly as possible and accelerate to lockout. Always use chains or light flex bands on these sets. After the 8–10 sets, train the triceps very hard. New records should be attempted in a bar or dumbbell extension. JM presses or any other triceps exercise works fine. Triceps are most important.

Lats are next, followed by delt raises, upper back, and forearms. All this should be completed in less than an hour.

Three days later, Wednesday, is max effort day. On max effort day, you must max out (but not in a regular squat, bench, or deadlift). Execute a one or three rep max in exercises such as: the board press, floor press, incline, decline, or seated press, or rack lockouts. Records can be achieved with added chains or bands. Make as many combinations as possible. This is known as the conjugate method. When training a particular exercise maximally for even three weeks in a row, growth hormone production is greatly reduced. That is why special core exercises must be implemented and rotated every two weeks. Sometimes we even modify a special core exercise slightly each week.

Remember to pursue greater bar speed in all lifts. Push up special exercises and rotate as often as necessary to maintain progress. Stay with short rest periods on dynamic day. For squats, rest 45 seconds and for the bench, rest one minute. Any faster and the CNS may be negatively affected. The short rest between sets causes lactic acid to accumulate. By working through the lactic acid, growth hormone production increases greatly. Don't be a wimp. This pain pays. Don't take openers. If you are worried about your opener, what are you going to do with your second and third attempts? Pick the exercises that work best for you closest to meet time.

Percent Training

In the squat, what is considered too heavy and too light to train with? In Russia, much research revealed that 65–82.5% of a one rep max is best to build strength in the squat. They suggest 2–6 reps per set. At Westside Barbell, we do sets of two for two important reasons. One reason is that more than two reps tend to cause bicipital tendonitis and shoulder discomfort. This pain is commonly felt while benching but, in fact, comes from squatting. The bar shifts to some degree, causing damage. Having your hands spaced too close together on the bar may also be the culprit. The second reason is that in a power meet, lifters don't do reps. If you do 12 sets of two reps, you are getting 12 first reps per workout. If you do four sets of six reps, then you get only four first reps.

The velocity-force curve shows that weights can actually move too quickly or too slowly. By staying within this percent range, a lifter is continuously working with poundages that provide both adequate velocity and force to produce record breaking squats. The multi-set system with submaximal weights is referred to as the dynamic method. It produces maximum explosive force as well as maximum velocity. It is one thing to be quite strong and quite another thing to display it. This is important to sports teams if the weight room is to be compatible with the sport.

Let me clarify one important aspect of our training. On our squat/deadlift special exercise day, we train with a revolving system of exercises that are switched every two weeks. We work up to a top single (100% +) in a particular lift such as: the box squat below or above parallel with the safety squat bar. After breaking a record or two, we switch to rack pulls. By continually revolving special exercises and training at 100% +, we apply max force throughout the cycle.

Therefore, as one can see, we have a velocity day and a max force day in the same week. This max force day is referred to as the maximum effort day. This enables us to maintain both maximum force and maximum velocity at the same time. We are able to train heavier and longer than with any other system. The volume of weights by percent makes a lifter stronger throughout the year.

By training the squat with sub-maximal weights with maximal velocity and by rotating exercises that closely resemble the squat on a second day, a lifter can stay within the boundaries of the force-velocity curve. When rotating special exercises such as: good mornings, rack pulls, or Manta Ray squats, anxiety and high blood pressure can be eliminated, which accompanies the competition and can be present when trying heavy training weights in the squat. For most, training with heavy weights in the squat can be so stressful that adrenaline levels drop drastically.

Another negative aspect of progressive overload is that you must always drop assistance work at the end of the cycle even though these are the exercises that made you strong in the first place. When you stop doing special exercises, their effect is lost in a few weeks and sometimes in a few days. For the most part, they must be maintained as closely to contest time as possible. Large muscle groups recover in roughly 72 hours and small muscles in 24 hours.

We do our heavy squat and deadlift work on Monday. It never has a negative effect on our Friday squat workout. Therefore, there is no reason to reduce the work done on Monday when the contest is, in fact, a day or two later than our regular squat day. As far as deadlifting goes, we seldom do it, but when we do, multiple singles are completed with very short rest periods (30 seconds). We start with 60% for 15 singles. During the mini-cycle, the number of lifts decreases as the percentage increases. Use only one weight per workout. The top percent is roughly 85%, and the lifts are reduced to 6–8 singles. If you do this type of training, jump about 5% each week. I recommend that only lifters built to deadlift do this cycle, being very explosive on each lift.

For example, if you pull a max 700 lbs and are using 70%, or 490, you must exert 700 lbs or more of force when pulling the weight. Yes, with sub-maximal weight, you can exert more force than is actually on the bar. This is not possible when you do a max triple of 670 when your max is 700. If there was a force meter on the bar with 670, it may surprise you that not one rep would equal 700 lbs.This also explains why a particular lifter can perform two reps with 800, yet can do only 800 at a contest. His body can maintain 800 lbs of force for a period that allows two reps.

However, because of the slow bar movement, there is a lack of adequate velocity to lift the additional 30–40 lbs on the bar at the meet. Box squatting on squat day works because of the velocity day for the deadlift. On deadlift day, we do a combination of max singles and max reps on a variety of exercises such as: four types of good mornings, five types of squats, five methods of pulls, and an array of exercises for the low back and abs. We may also do static work and isokinetic work. Special exercises with unique devices allow maximum speed at the beginning of the lift and maximum overload at the top portion.

Time in Strength Training

Has it ever occurred to you how fast you can start a barbell moving or how quickly you can move light weights (50–60%) or maximum weights? What about the weights in between? Some athletes are very fast, and others are very strong. Remember two important points. First, be very explosive and accelerate throughout the movement. Second, there is only so much time to complete a max lift or a work set. Then, time runs out and your muscles don't last under the load anymore. You will fail. A common misconception is that the weaker lifter is moving the bar faster than his stronger, more powerful counterpart.

A solution is concentrating on bar velocity, which consists of an acceleration phase and deceleration phase. The latter can be greatly produced by placing bands and chains on the bar. Many think of resistance as the amount of weight on the bar, but every lift is related to time. For example, if a lifter can exert maximal force for only 3.5 seconds and the course of the bar is not completed in that amount of time, he will fail. Learn to build acceleration. Bar speed is critical.

Through many experiments I have performed at Westside, a time effect became apparent. I performed 35 fast reps with 315 in the full range deadlift. This was an all-out effort to say the least. This endeavor took roughly 60 seconds. I have performed 26 reps with 315 in the full deadlift, using a slower, more deliberate style. I was completely fatigued in the same 60-second period even though the effort exerted was influenced by different rates of speed. I was limited by a time of 60 seconds. I couldn't go beyond this time regardless of the number of reps.

In a different experiment, I did 58 push-ups with my feet on a box and with a 100lb plate on my back. This took roughly 60 seconds. At the same level of fitness, I was able to perform only 60 reps without a plate on my back, going to total fatigue, which occurred in 60 seconds. This, of course, is strength endurance. This time element is an important factor.

Many of our all-time world record bench pressers and large 900 plus squatters were timed, and the same time factors occurred. For example, the max bench press effort took 3.25 seconds. This told us that we should be doing max effort exercises that take at least 3.25 seconds in full range movements. We would fail if the max lift was not completed in this timeframe. The time elapsed during strength efforts is dependent on the length of time each individual can exert maximally. This is true regardless of the magnitude of the load. Strength is measured in time and should be controlled by the coach for each athlete.

Importance of Volume

How important is controlling volume? What about the range of intensity? These are issues seldom addressed by today's lifters. I found out the hard way that the volume at a particular intensity range must be closely adhered to not only for the total number of lifts but also for the number of lifts per set. They should be calculated. This was brought to my attention through Prilepin's research in 1974. His recommendations were as follows. If the number of lifts deviates significantly from optimal, a decrease in training effect occurs. This information is found in Managing the Training of Weightlifters by Laputin and Oleshko. Let's look at a simple example. The number of lifts should be performed on one of two training days. The light percents are for the development of explosive or speed strength. A few years ago, we were using between 50–60% of a contest max in the squat. Three lifters used 400 for 12 sets of two reps, equaling 9600 lbs of work at 50% of an 800 squat. At 60%, the lifts were reduced to 20. It was broken down to ten sets of two reps at 60%, representing 480 lbs for ten sets of two reps or 9600 lbs. All three lifters squatted 804.

The training volume must greatly differ from workout to workout, meaning total volume as well as intensity zone. Ben Tabachnik, inventor of the track parachute, said, "To never adapt to training is to adapt to training." Consequently, this is our philosophy also. There are 35 men who have totaled 2400 or more. At Westside, we have 25 members and five of them total over 2400. They have accomplished this by not falling into the trap of accommodation. You must plan for specificity or whatever will raise a particular lift. It is seldom possible to just do the lift. I believe that is why powerlifters are the most successful of all weight sports. Just think for a minute how many special training devices powerlifters use for each lift. There must be 20 for each.

Example #1:

A 700lb squatter would use 350 (50%) for 12 sets of two reps, which is 8400 lbs of volume. At 60%, ten sets of two reps are performed or 420 lbs for 20 lifts, which equals 8400.

Example #2:

A 500lb squatter would use 250 for 12 sets of two reps, which equals 6000 lbs of work. At 60%, ten sets of two reps are performed or 300 lbs for 20 lifts, which equals 6000.

I hope you can understand how important controlling the number of lifts at a certain intensity can be. The squats were done off a parallel box with 40 lbs of chain at the top.

On max effort day, three days later, we used the conjugate method where we perform core exercises similar to the classical lifts. We employ good mornings of many types, special squat bars, and other apparatus, but we never do a regular squat. Start increasing the bar weight after a good warm up. Do a lift of about 90%, try for a personal record and maybe one more, and then do your assistance work.

If you observe at both days, it looks like this—80 lifts for explosive and speed-strength and 12 lifts for strength-speed and absolute strength per month. Remember, this represents training only the classic lifts. It is easy to see, however, a direct correlation between a contest max and volume trained at the correct intensity zones.

A very important factor is special exercises. The coach, who is many times the lifter himself, must find weaknesses (i.e. a lagging muscle group). For squatting or deadlifting, the posterior chain must be developed. This includes the hamstrings, glutes, all back muscles, and hips. At Westside, this means the total work is distributed like this—40% special exercises for strength, 40% barbell lifts, and 20% restoration and flexibility.

This amounts to 14 workouts per week. Close to contest time, we do fewer barbell lifts and raise special work where needed. If your squat is stalled, more squatting won't help. You may need more back work or more ham and glute work. In the real world, a squat does not distribute the work evenly. If it did, injury would seldom occur. When reaching your highest potential, doing more classical lifts will only disturb good form.

The same holds true for deadlifting with even less deadlifting being performed. Training with a barbell held in the hands taxes the CNS heavily, leading to a negative training result. This is why we complement the deadlift with many variations of squatting and good mornings. Deadlifting is done with no more than 70% and only for singles. The intensity is raised by using short rest periods between sets, usually about 30 seconds when doing 6–10 total lifts.
Learn the difference between training and testing the deadlift or squat. Obtain a box squat PR with added bands that represents your contest squat. A low box squat with the safety squat bar is a real indicator of absolute strength for squatting and deadlifting. This is done on our max effort day. Remember, if you squat 300 lbs, use 150–180 lbs on a box; start at 50% in a three-week wave and end at 60%. In weeks one and two, do 12 sets of two reps; then, in the third week, reduce the sets to ten. The bar volume is always the same, 3600, but the total volume increases during the three weeks by adjusting to new special exercises. With a little math, regardless of what you squat, the volume is customized for your top lift. At the same time, you are perfecting y form, raising work capacity, and bringing up lagging muscle groups.

In 1995, Zatsiorsky stated three methods of inducing maximal muscle tension:
(1) Overcoming maximal resistance that causes maximal or near maximal muscle tension (maximal effort method),
(2) Using considerably less than maximal resistance until fatigue causes one to fail (repetition method), and
(3) Using submaximal weights accompanied by maximal speed (dynamic method).

All three must be monitored at all times during the year. This explanation may seem simple to some or possibly too complicated for others. The keys to success are as follows:

1. Volume with correct intensity (refer to Prilepin's intensity chart)
2. Use a max effort day and, 72 hours later, a dynamic method day
3. Raise work capacity

I have often been asked why high work capacity is so important. If you are in shape, the heavy weights and the high-volume training will have little negative effect on the lifter. If you are physically fragile, the training will affect you mentally as well as physically.

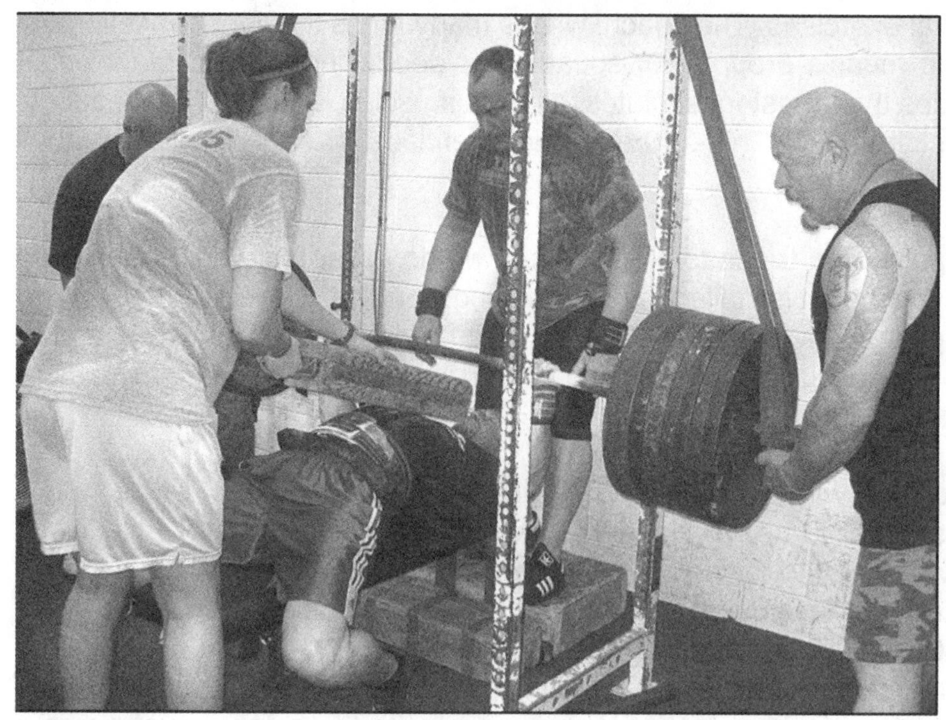

To calculate volume on max effort workouts, there are two methods to consider. The first is when the objective is to increase muscle mass in order to move into a higher weight class (e.g. 6–8 lifts in the 90% range). The second method is 3–4 sets of two reps, the second at 90% and then the next one or two a PR. We prefer the second method from a psychological point of view.

Regardless of how close it is to a meet or right after, try a record. A record is a process of time under tension. That is most important here. How long it takes to complete a max lift must be duplicated with special core exercises such as: good mornings or deadlifts. For ball players or Olympic lifters, the percent for squatting is 65–80% for dynamic day. The same procedure for max effort is used as explained earlier because we don't wear supportive gear on this day. For benching on dynamic day, the percent of a meet max with a shirt is roughly 40% plus chains. If no chains or bands are added, use 50% of a shirtless max. If your max is 300, do eight sets of three reps, using 150 lbs That's 450 per set for a total of 3600 lbs of volume. With a 500 max, do eight sets of three reps with 250. That's 750 per set times eight sets equals 6000 lbs of barbell volume. Remember, this is a no-shirt bench. Regardless of your bench max, the percent and the number of lifts stay the same, but the volume is constantly increasing. We don't record the volume of special exercises, but it must be constantly increasing in sets and top weight. Train special exercises in the correct sequence. For the deadlift and squat, work low back, hams and glutes, and abs in that order. Don't move on to the next exercise until the muscles are thoroughly worked. For the bench, do triceps, lats, upper back, and rear and side delts. The most essential muscle group must be the strongest or injuries can occur.

For bench max effort work, the same principles apply as for the squat and deadlift. On max effort day, the conjugate method must be used (i.e. using exercises that are mechanically similar to the classical lifts). Rotate to a different exercise each week. This allows am individual to lift 100% plus each week.

TRAINING METHODS

There is much talk about training philosophies, methods, and methodologies. It seems everyone has his own, which is devised on the basis of personal experience. These individuals recommend such strategies as doing reps to failure to eliminate assistance work and doing only the squat, bench press, and deadlift. Have you ever wondered what the author has accomplished as a lifter, a trainer, or a scientist? Did they ever total Elite or field a team of Elites at a national meet? Did they ever make a top ten lift in one or more categories? Or is what they are doing a personal philosophy with no proven results?

It has been asked what philosophy Westside adheres to. The answer is none. We use training methodologies and the science of methods. Everything we do is based on a scientific principle. We cannot be so arrogant as to form a personal philosophy. At Westside, we are responsible not only for our own training but for the training of our loyal readers. Many of our "extended members" have become national, world, and European champions.

Training is not as simple as doing five sets of five reps, five sets of ten reps, or any combination of sets and reps. Each lifter must plan to obtain certain objectives. Increases in speed, explosive strength, absolute strength, and stamina are equally important. It has been known and discussed in Weightlifting for All Sports by Ajan and Baroga that a greater training result can be obtained over a greater length of time by using special exercises rather than by doing the classical lifts. Performing the same exercises repeatedly can rapidly decrease coordination. There are many reasons for this. Our observation is that very few lifters can increase their abilities without special exercises.

How do we train heavy continuously? The answer is to pick several special barbell exercises for a particular lift (e.g. the deadlift). The good morning is very similar in motion to deadlifting. A conventional deadlifter will no doubt bend over. Therefore, bent over good mornings will increase the deadlift. When executing the good morning, you must duplicate the action of your deadlift precisely in your brain. It is not so important to raise your good morning as it is to raise your deadlift by performing the good morning. We do many types of good mornings such as one with a safety squat bar suspended from chains. Remember to use the same body mechanics as you do in the deadlift.

Conjugate Method

A question that should be addressed is, when handling max lifts, how do you recover? How do you at the same time increase muscle mass? The conjugate method is the answer. This is a complex method of rotating special exercises that are close in nature, in our case, to the power lifts. This method also increases special strength qualities and perfects coordination, which can help advance technical skill. First, and most important, is to properly select exercises that address particular problems. It could be an exercise that builds up a lagging muscle group or a special strength such as: starting, eccentric, or accelerating strength.

Many methods are combined and rotated in the conjugate system. Combining the speed and max effort days, five elements of strength are trained:

1. quickness
2. explosiveness
4. speed-strength
5. strength-speed
6. absolute strength

This is much like a five-speed transmission in a car. We all know what happens if you miss a gear or take off in the wrong gear. Your car doesn't run very efficiently and neither will you. One must learn many methods to develop special strength and when to use them. You must also know your sports' goals. In some sports, speed is foremost and absolute strength is secondary. Both are more closely related than you think.

When lifters repeatedly use the same simple method of training to raise their strength level, they will eventually stall. Like the scholar who must utilize many sources of information to achieve a higher level of knowledge, the lifter must incorporate new and more difficult exercises to raise their standards. Many have the theory that to squat, bench, or deadlift more, you simply have to do the three lifts. If it were that simple, no one would need special exercises, machines, or systems of training. We know this is not true.

Because lifters have different body types, they may excel at one lift but struggle with another. The great Lamar Gant was the only lifter I have known who held the world record deadlift and bench at the same time. There are men who hold three world records in the deadlift, yet can't make the top ten bench list. Their muscles in the upper body are, I'm sure, as strong as anyone's, but they are limited by body structure (e.g. short torso, long arms). Many of us are affected by this. Is there an answer?

In the early 1970s, the Dynamo Club in the former Soviet Union had 70 highly skilled Olympic lifters. They were introduced to a system of 20–45 special exercises grouped into 2–4 exercises per workout and were rotated as often as necessary to make continuous progress They soon found out that as the squat, good morning, back raise, glute ham raise, or special pulls got stronger, so did their Olympic lifts. When asked about the system, only one lifter was satisfied with the number of special lifts. The rest wanted more to choose from; therefore, the conjugate system was originated.

When you have a body type that lacks say the muscles that squat and yet you squat on a regular basis, then a coupling of special exercises for the glutes, hamstrings, hips, and lower back are needed to fortify those areas. These special exercises enable you to raise your squat once more. Think about it. If you read only one book, you can only learn so much no matter how many times you read it. If you only squat, you can get only so strong because no new stimulusis introduced. This may not happen in the early stages of training, but as you become more advanced, you will need a more strenuous method of training. This training assists your motor potential and helps perfect technical skill.

Before I present some examples of conjugate training, think about this. How much could you bench press the first time you tried? 200? Maybe 300? Now, how did you achieve that level of strength without ever having benched before? You did it through simplified training such as push-ups and pull-ups. Those of you who could bench 300 the first time will never double that amount without doing specialized work to raise your strength, right?

Here are some examples of the conjugate method. Glen Chabot bench presses only twice a month. Both times, he uses a close-grip style; he can do 405 for reps in the low teens. His best single close grip is 635 without a shirt. In between each workout, he rotates heavy dumbbell work on a flat or incline bench or very heavy bodybuilding exercises for lats, delts, pecs, and triceps. This linking of special exercises has given Glen a 705 bench press at 275. Glen does not arch when he benches and has fairly long arms. He realized that he needed a special program to fortify his pressing muscles. This is a simple but very effective training program.

Kenny Patterson had a more complex system. He did floor presses, chain presses, board presses, incline presses, and overhead presses, just to name a few. He rotated a different exercise each max effort day. On dynamic day, Kenny used three different grips on the bench press and used 60% of his no-shirt max for eight sets of three reps. He added many triceps extensions with dumbbells or the barbell, rows (one-arm, two-arm, chest-supported), pulldowns, delt raises, and forearm work. This is a more complex system than Glen's, but it suited Kenny's needs. Kenny was a legitimate 700 bencher, having done it several times across the country.

Back in 2001, Mike Ruggiera and I made 900 squats. It was a 50 lb increase for him and a 40 lb increase for me, yet we did not do a single regular squat between meets. We did box squats on speed days, implementing a large amount of bands and weight. We also used the reverse hyper machine and did glute ham raises, pull-throughs, and abs. I pulled a weighted sled before my squat workouts. On max effort day, we did good mornings (five varieties), belt squats, speed deadlifts (60% for 6–8 singles), and safety power squat bar squats to different box heights. Mike also pulled his first 800 deadlift without having performed any conventional squats or big deadlifts. After squatting, he did deadlifts for singles with 60% for speed, and three days later, he maxed out on special work. This is the conjugate method.

To push up a squat, heavy good mornings or squatting with different bars is done on max effort day. The variety of bars make squatting very awkward and extremely difficult to do, much harder than a regular squat. (The same is true of box squats. They are harder than competition squats.) On max effort day, we may do a type of squat in week one, a good morning in week two, and a front squat in week three. Each exercise contributes to the next week's exercise, which in turn builds a bigger squat by strengthening the weaker muscle group and perfecting form.

The training is linked together, enabling a lifter to raise his total. For instance, to build the glute and hamstring area, push up your reverse hyperextensions as hard as possible until your progress slows. Move on to pull-throughs for a week or two until progress in these slows as well. Then, go to glute ham raises and again push as fast and hard as possible. Pull a sled walking forward to build the glutes and hamstrings. It is possible to continuously gain strength in any body part by changing special exercises. As the effectiveness of the exercise decreases, switch to another one. By training in this manner, it is possible to raise all types of strength throughout the year.

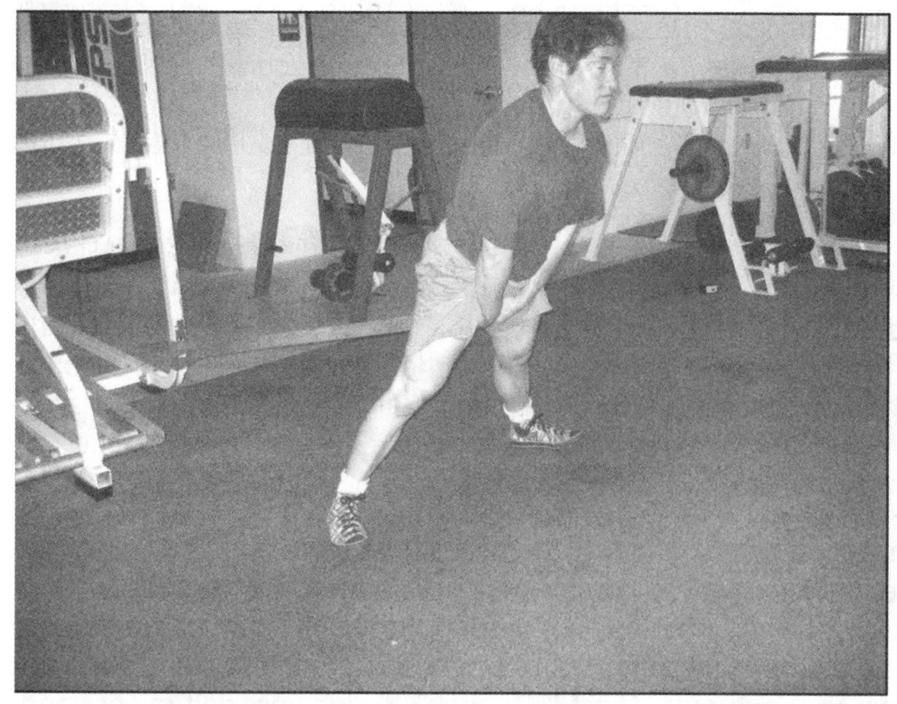

On max effort day, the entire volume consists of unidirectional loading, and one training workout contributes to the next. If an athlete trains a lift at 90% or more for more than three weeks, his central nervous system is negatively affected, and his progress will go backward.

When alternating weekly exercises (for the high level lifter), the order doesn't matter as long as the load is maximal. The time it takes to do a maximal effort (i.e. a low box squat with a Manta Ray) lift is at least the same amount of time it takes to do a max deadlift or squat, which is known as "time under tension."

The conjugate method also improves special physical preparedness (SPP) (e.g. speed deadlifts, plyometrics) and general physical preparedness (GPP) (e.g. sled dragging). This is the most effective method to gain strength continuously throughout the year with no ridiculous off-season. No one can afford to take time off. By maintaining the speed work for the three lifts and increasing general wonk (e.g. upper and lower body sled work, lats, abs, triceps), you won't go backward. There are many methods of training, but by incorporating the conjugate method, you can't miss.

A popular special exercise for the deadlift is squatting off a very low box. Angelo Berardinelli does his off a six-inch box. At this depth, Angelo's back is in a position similar to his sumo deadlift style. We frequently use a safety squat bar. When rising out of a squat or deadlift, the shoulders should move first. The five-inch camber on the safety squat bar teaches a lifter to raise the head and shoulders first. Otherwise, there is a tendency to buckle over forward. To summarize, pick a core lift with a barbell and try to duplicate the same motion of the lift that you're trying to increase. Pick 4–5 core exercises that work for you and rotate one of them every two weeks. Do a max single for a 2-3 rep max, but no more.

For example, you could do bent over good mornings, safety squat bar squats, Zercher squats, or very low box squats and then finish with two weeks of rack pulls. This represents a ten-week cycle, rotating each of the above exercises in two-week mini-cycles. It is important to end with the most productive exercise for you leading into the meet. After your selection of a core barbell exercise, pick 3–5 special exercises. Your workout should last less than 60 minutes, picking a few special exercises and do them very intensely.

If your form is good, then your lower back may be holding you back. Again, select four exercises for the lower back such as: back raises, straight leg deadlifts off a platform, pull- throughs with the legs straight, and reverse hyperextensions. Rotate them when necessary. For weak hamstrings, do heavy reverse hyperextensions, squatting pull-throughs, glute ham raises, and sled pulling with your hands behind your back or below your knees while holding onto a strap.

For weak glutes, do heavy reverse hyperextensions, low belt squats, high rep deadlifts (two sets of 20 with back arched, glutes pushed out to rear, shoulder-width stance, hands outside shoulder-width; after the first rep, drop the bar to just below the knees, and catch and raise it as quickly as possible for the entire 20 reps), and glute ham raises. If the abs are weak, do side bends with a cable bar or dumbbell, leg raises, standing lat machine curl-overs, and strict sit-ups. Again, pick one exercise for each muscle group, using it until it becomes ineffective and then switch.

For the bench press, you could perform board presses, floor presses, inclines, declines, or rack lockouts for singles. Rotate each every two weeks. Do ultra wide bench presses for a 6RM or three sets to failure with dumbbells with a two-minute rest between sets for singles and a 5–6-minute rest for high reps. Then, pick some type of triceps extensions with a bar or dumbbells, some type of lat work, and raises for the front, side, and rear delts.

There are many types of exercises for each muscle group. Just change when one stops working, and your lifts should continue to increase all year long. By training with this system, a lifter can max out every week of the year while working continuously on speed and building muscle mass. It works for us, and it will work for you. It is the most effective form of training we have ever tried, and in the past 36 years, Westside lifters have tried them all.

Just remember, it's the selection that counts. You must pick a lift or exercise that builds your particular weakness. Don't get caught up in doing an exercise that your friends like but that does little for you. George Halbert has special exercises he uses for his bench. Chuck Vogelpohl does things that no one does, but they help his squat and deadlift. Amy Weisberger did front and overhead squats to help her squat.

Maximal Effort Method

The entire volume consists of unidirectional loading on max effort day. Each training workout contributes to the next. If an individual trains a lift at 90% or more for more than three weeks, the central nervous system is negatively affected and progress will go backward. By switching exercises each week, 100% and more can be used each week. As long as the load is maximal, the sequence of exercises employed does not matter. Time under tension is the time it takes to do a maximal effort (i.e. a low box squat with a Manta Ray) lift is at least the same amount of time that it takes to do a max deadlift or squat.

Time under tension is the key for max effort work. Conventional squats or deadlifts don't have to be done to improve these lifts. For example, world class throwers throw everything from medicine balls to hammers to long pipes, using objects of different weights. They throw everything except the official implement. This is the conjugate method in combination with the maximum effort method. It improves form as well as building phenomenal strength.

On max effort day, we do good mornings (five varieties), belt squats, speed deadlifts (60% for 6–8 singles), and safety power squat bar squats to different box heights. Mike also pulled his first 800 deadlift without doing any conventional squats or big deadlifts. After squatting, he does deadlifts for singles with 60% for speed, and three days later, he maxes out on special work. This is the conjugate method.

To push up a squat, heavy good mornings or squatting with different bars is done on max effort day. The different bars make squatting very awkward and extremely hard to do, much harder than a regular squat. (The same is true of box squats. They are harder than competition squats.) On max effort day, we may do a type of squat in week one, a good morning in week two, and a front squat in week three. Each exercise contributes to the next week's exercise, which in turn will build a bigger squat by strengthening the weaker muscle groups and perfecting form.

Dynamic Effort Method

The dynamic effort method is used on squat/deadlift day and in the bench press. This method requires that the lifter lift sub-maximal weights as fast as he can. This method should be together with compensatory acceleration. An lifter must apply as much force as possible to the barbell, pushing as hard and as quickly as he can in the concentric phase of the lift. If an individual benches 700 lbs and are training with 350, then he should be applying 700 lbs of force to the barbell in each rep.

The weight used should be non-maximal in the 50–75% range. Many experts, like Siff, Verkershonsky, and Spassev agree that this is the best range for developing explosive strength. This method is for increasing the force output. Many times being fast and strong are more closely related than you think.

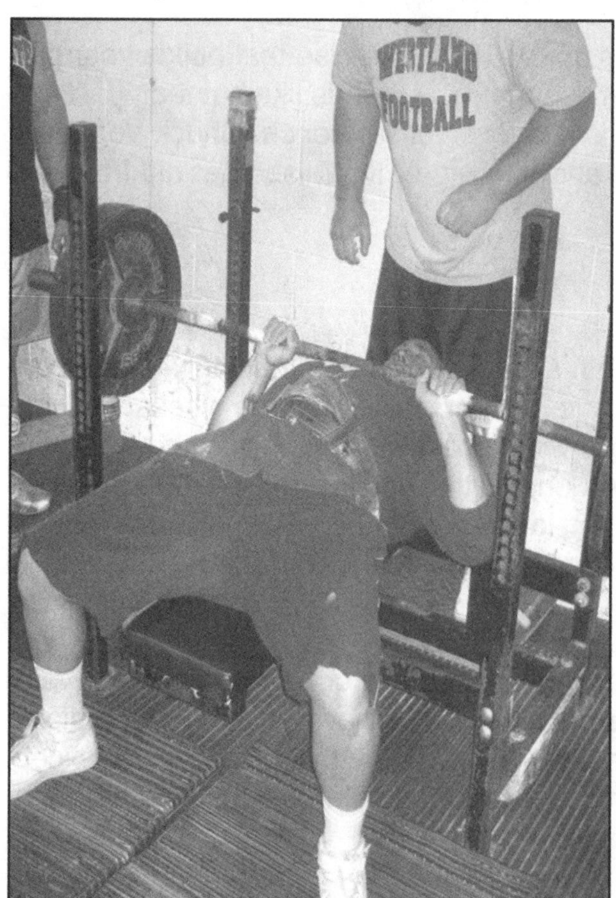

Two methods that develop both explosive and absolute strength are static- overcome-by-dynamic work and relaxed- overcome-by-dynamic work.

Static means isometric, and dynamic can refer to concentric, eccentric, or what I am going to address—reversal strength. Reversal strength is developed, for example, by floor presses, board presses, and box squats. The value of these exercises is also a second means of strength development. When doing the three exercises noted above, both of these methods occur simultaneously. Some muscles and connective tissue are held relaxed while other muscles are held static.

Box squatting is an example. By sitting back, not down, on a box of any height, the squatting muscles are stretched maximally. Relaxing the hip flexors, glutes, and obliques for 30 seconds to one minute and 30 seconds, flexing off the box dynamically in a box squat can also increase a lifter's pulls off the floor. A bar on the floor is static, and this position must be overcome dynamically. A box height that duplicates the position of the second pull relative to the hip position should be used. Rest the bar on the thighs, and execute the second pull.

When executing the floor press, lower the bar until the elbows are in contact with the floor. Relax the triceps and other pressing muscles, flex dynamically, and press upward. For the board press, use 2–3 2x6s attached together. Lower the bar quickly onto the boards, relax, and then explode concentrically.

If a pause squat or bench press is executed, the eccentric speed of the bar will be gradually reduced to zero. By using a box, board, or the floor, the bar has speed as it reaches any level, creating kinetic energy that greatly contributes to the concentric phase. Remember, lower, relax, and then contract dynamically. The stretch reflex should last up to at least two seconds. All this illustrates that at Westside we have combined two proven methods of strength development both used during each week.

Repeated Effort Method

Different methods of training are utilized at Westside. The dynamic method replaces a maximal effort day and builds explosiveness and speed-strength. The maximal effort method builds strength-speed and absolute strength.

Training with weights above 90% for three weeks can cause a negative training effect. To remedy this, the conjugate method is employed. Each week on maximal effort day, we use a different core exercise and max out with 100% or more. It can be a good morning, pull, or special squat for the squat and deadlift or a floor press or board press for the bench press. Think about it, strongman events are really the conjugate method. It's not uncommon for a top Strongman to deadlift 800 or more.

Many don't realize it, but we also use the repetition method to failure, though never in the classical lifts. We do special exercises with dumbbells, belt squats, the reverse hyper, and so forth. I prefer to do repetitions for time in a slow tempo, and I don't bother counting reps.

If this sounds new, it's not. In the 1970s, the great Olympic lifter, Vasili Alexeyev, used a variation of the repetition method for part of his training. He sometimes did power cleans non- stop for 2–3 minutes. He did various hybrid exercises like the front squat, push press, squats with the bar on his back, and drop squats. The bar weight was light but would work every muscle cell. He did a warm up by throwing a 220 lb barbell over his head backward 100 times. Then, after practicing the snatch for over two hours, he spent an hour in the pool, lifting his legs hundreds of times to strengthen his abdomen. He leaped nearly 1000 times and used many exercises to gain great strength in order to raise his work capacity and, of course, his total. This is precisely what Westside is after.

Here are some examples of how the repetition method is used at Westside:

1. For the squat or deadlift, I complete belt squats for 3– 4 sets of three minute sets, 2–3 sets of abs, or the reverse hyper for 1–3 sets of 1–3 minutes each.
2. Another workout consists of band good mornings with a single set sometimes lasting 6–8 minutes depending on band tension. Follow this with light dumbbell presses for 2–4 minutes nonstop.
3. Walking with a sled for up to five minutes with light resistance. Follow with abdominal work.
4. Do light deadlifts for 1–3 minutes followed by abdominal work for at least two minutes.
5. Pick up a barbell and throw it overhead behind you or do the same exercise with medicine balls. This works the entire body. After throwing it, simply walk over to it and do another rep.
6. Do band leg curls for 3–6 minutes followed immediately by band leg extensions.
7. Perform dumbbell power cleans for 1–3 minutes either holding them at your waist, on your shoulders, or, of course, over your head.
8. Do dumbbell pressing on a bench or (my preference) on a stability ball. I use three different weights depending on the day. After the dynamic workout, I use 100s for three minutes. On max effort day, I have done 75s for five minutes. Four or five times a week, I use 40s for a set of 3–10 minutes.

Using weights of roughly 20–30% serve as restoration because they're not heavy enough to stop adequate circulation via strong muscle contraction. To validate some of the findings at Westside, high reps with very light weight are stated as being beneficial in the rep range of 100–200 in Thomas Kurz's Science of Sports Training. Olympic long jumper, Diane Guthrie, had been doing 250 leg curls every day using 10 lb. ankle weights. She noted that when she slacked off the work, she incurred leg injuries.

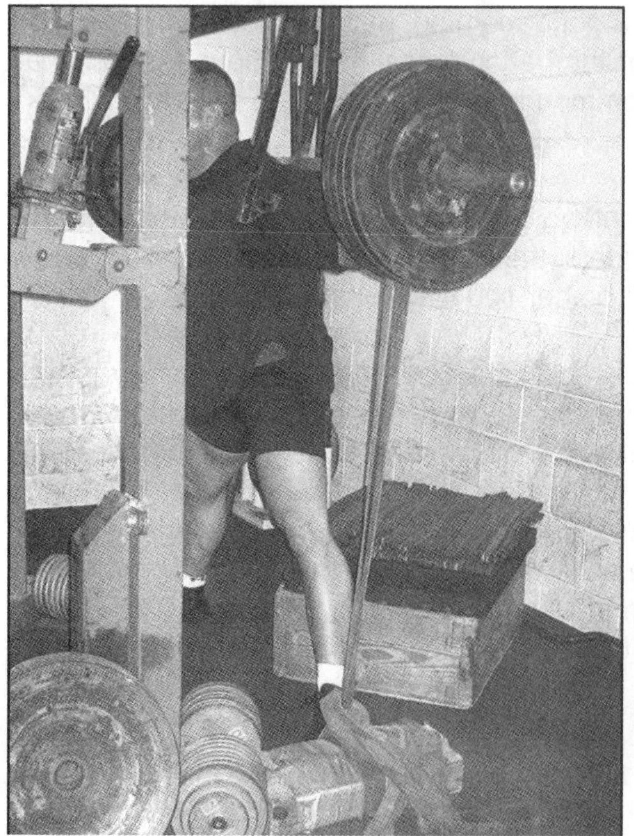

People make a mistake thinking that there is only one method of training. In fact, there are many, and they must coexist in a continuous chain of proven methods. When doing the workouts I have outlined, remember to do them with a slow tempo. This means 6–10 reps per minute, resting between reps while still holding onto the bar or dumbbell. Regardless of where you hold the bar or dumbbell, it works the muscles to their fullest extent.

A great benefit of the repetition method is an increase not only in all strength but also in endurance. This method is also commonly known as lactic acid tolerance training, promoting a high degree of growth hormone production, which can increase size and strength. I suggest that at least two levels of intensity be used—one for strength and one for restoration. The latter should use 30% of the max or less.

As absolute strength increases, all strength qualities increase, too. When I could do 100 lb dumbbells for 40 seconds, I could do 30s for one minute 30 seconds. Later, when I did 100s for three minutes, I did 50s for eight minutes and 75s for five minutes. When top strength goes up, so does strength endurance with less than max weights.

Size strength endurance and restoration can all be gained using this method. It is a simple and effective way to raise work capacity and volume to increase your total as well as your fitness level. This method worked for the greatest Olympic lifter of all time, Vasili Alexeyev, and one of the greatest benchers by formula, George Halbert.

Methods Breakdown in Training

I. Max Effort Day

At Westside, we train with either very light weights or max weights. Very seldom do we use medium weights in the 80% to low-90% range. We prefer to break new ground, continually trying new records in special squats, pulls, good mornings, or benches. Remember, if you train at 90% or higher for more than three weeks, you will fail because of central nervous system fatigue. We max out each week. How? Simply by switching exercises each week. This is the conjugate method.

As Dr. Zatsiorsky states, "Why climb three-quarters up the mountain only to go back down and start back over?" He is, of course, referring to the progressive overload system. This system is a dead-end street. It was obsolete 40 years ago. At Westside, we get faster, stronger, and more muscular all year long. Here's how. Westside Barbell is closed to the public. Members regularly go to meets. Because all 30 members compete, we send about a third of our lifters to a particular meet. This enables some of us to help our teammates. I believe, our success comes from maxing out on maximum effort day even if a lifter isn't going to a meet. This goes on all year long.

Our maximum effort system is much like the Bulgarian model. Regardless of our trainability, we max out. It might not be an all-time record, but it's all the lifter is capable of on that day. This means that lifters who are not close to a meet will not get PRs. The lifters who are approachinga meet should make PRs. Although the Bulgarians use primarily six main exercises, we use countless special exercises designed to build the weakness of each lifter in all three lifts. The system we find most effective is the conjugate system—a wide variety of special exercises are constantly rotated to make training more effective and fun. This system allows for a longer lifting career. If you have a longer career in any sport, you will benefit from new technology such as: tracks, balls, ball fields, and, in our case, supportive gear.

The following illustrates how we use various methods in our training. Let's start with the maximum effort bench day, which occurs 72 hours after the speed bench day. This is because 72 hours should separate extreme workouts, and we max out each week. For example, the floor press can be done with pure weight or with 3–5 sets of chains to accommodate resistance. It can be executed with at least three different band tensions, which also can accommodate resistance but alters the speed of the bar. Because the unexpected can happen at a meet, the weight can seem harder or easier than expected. By alternating the amount of bands or chains, the bar velocity can change, which happens during each attempt. A regular bench can be used while adding weight releasers. This is a pure reactive method. The weight is released on the first rep of each set at the bottom, which causes a contrast effect.

The contrast method is one where the weight is different at the bottom compared to the top of the lift. This method can be used with any style of pressing, including incline, decline, or seated.

In the bench, we lower the bar as fast as possible and then catch it just before it hits the chest, reversing from eccentric to concentric as fast as possible. This ballistic lifting is to be completed with speed-strength weights of 40–60% while doing triples. A word of caution — do not use maximal weights. Although ballistic training is not plyometric, it does ensure a rapid shock loading effect, resulting in a strong myostactic stretch reflex. Consequently, it takes advantage of stored energy of the connective and elastic tissues of the muscle complex during eccentric muscle contraction. Power rack training for developing a fast rate of force enhancement can be done with speed-strength sets off pins or from chains by resting the bar at any point from the chest to lockout and then exploding to lockout. Simply relax the muscles and then contract them concentrically as quickly as possible. Remember to relax after each lowering phase for 3–4 seconds, reducing stored energy before doing additional reps. Avoid overtraining by taking into account the different rates of adaptation to all training systems. Box squatting and floor pressing combine two proven methods of strength development: relaxed-overcome-by-dynamic work and static- overcome-by-dynamic work. Both build explosive and absolute strength.

Box jumps and rebounding on special devices are examples of shock training. To be explosive, this method is necessary. The most extreme work should be performed the day before max effort day. This is to prevent delayed onset of muscular soreness (DOMS), which occurs 48 hours after intense exercise. DOMS can be avoided by doing small restoration workouts 6–12 hours after one of the four major workouts. Small 20-minute workouts for strength gains in particular muscle groups can also be done to develop general physical preparedness (GPP) or special physical preparedness (SPP). A concise workout can be done for flexibility, agility, or balance.

All lifters should do at least 2–10 extra workouts per week. This is especially true for drug-free lifters to provide some form of restoration. There are many methods of training that are used on both max effort and speed day. It is, therefore, very important to change core and special exercises frequently. It is vital to change bar speed by using bands, chains, weight releasers, heavy weight, and light weight. Monitor intensity zones properly. For example, a 400 lb squatter should do proportionally the same amount of work as a 900 lb squatter. Remember that just when your body has all the answers, you have to change the questions.

II. Dynamic Effort Day

While recovering from my second lower back injury (for which doctors recommended removing two disks, taking off a bone spur, and fusing my vertebrae, with no guarantees), I decided that I had to take a new approach to lifting or disappear like everyone else who had lifted in the early 1970s. I called Bud Chamiga in Michigan and asked for several of his books that were translated from Russian. These books contained an abundance of science combined with special strength training.

These materials helped me realize that lifting was a combination of biometrics, physics, and mathematics, unlike what I had previously thought. There was no mention of training with

5s or 3s. I had followed the progressive overload system since my first Olympic lifting meet in 1960. The only period in which I did not compete was from 1966–1969 when I was in the army. In 1983, I was going nowhere with my training. I was stronger but slower. That's where Bud's books were invaluable. They described methods of training and organization that I had never heard of before. Furthermore, no one in the United States used these methods until I started writing about them in Powerlifting USA.

On speed day, sub-maximal weights should be used with maximal speed. This method is implemented to increase the rate of force development and explosive strength, not to build absolute strength. For squatting, do 10–12 sets of two reps; for benching, do 8–9 sets of three reps; and for deadlifting, do 6–10 sets of one rep after squatting.

Contrast and Reactive Methods

Another method for developing explosive strength is weight releasers. Hook chains or bands to the weight releasers (we welded bar attachments to ours) to accommodate resistance while lowering the bar. A key point to remember is not to lower the bar slowly. This diminishes the effect of added kinetic energy production. Weight releasers provide one overload rep on each set. The recommended load on weight releasers is 20% of the barbell load (e.g. 400 lbs on the bar and 80 lbs on the weight releasers). Use chain weight on the weight releasers for best results. Bands are a contrast method. We use only jump stretch bands. Only higher ranked lifters should use bands. For speed-strength, 65% of the total weight should be barbell weight and 35% should be bar tension. For strength-speed or slow strength used with maximal weights, 65% of the total weight needs to be derived from band tension and 35% should be barbell weight.

I will outline some of the more common ones. One reactive method is heavy-light sets. First, lift a heavy barbell for 1–3 reps. Take a short rest of 10–20 seconds, reduce the weight 20%, and repeat for 1–3 reps. The best method is to use two sets of jump stretch bands. Perform a set of bench, squats, or pulls. Rest 10–20 seconds and remove a set of bands. Then, do a second set. Bands work best when used with bar weight. They accomplish several objectives including (1) accommodating resistance, (2) the near elimination of the deceleration phase that exists with bar weight alone, and (3) added kinetic energy by the accelerated eccentric phase, which provides extra elastic excitatory deformation in the muscle and connective tissue. Using the bands to increase the speed considerably in the eccentric phase causes a greater amount of kinetic energy through which a maximal dynamic force is developed quickly. The loads can be made greater by using a combination of bands plus bar weight. If only bar weight is used, it would be too heavy in the bottom. If only bands are used, the weight at the bottom would be too light. By using strong bands to increase the rate of fall or eccentric speed, greater kinetic energy is developed, producing even greater muscular force development at the instant of switching from eccentric to concentric work plus a shorter amortization transition.

While discussing the reactive method, we must also look at the contrast method. Let's move on to two methods that develop explosive and absolute strength. The first is static overcome by dynamic work. Static means isometric, and dynamic refers to concentric, eccentric, or what I'm going to address—reversal strength.

Reversal strength is developed, for example, by floor presses, board presses, and box squats. The value of these exercises is also a second means of strength development—relaxed overcome by dynamic work. When doing the three exercises noted above, both of these methods occur simultaneously. Some muscles and connective tissues are held relaxed while other muscles are held static.

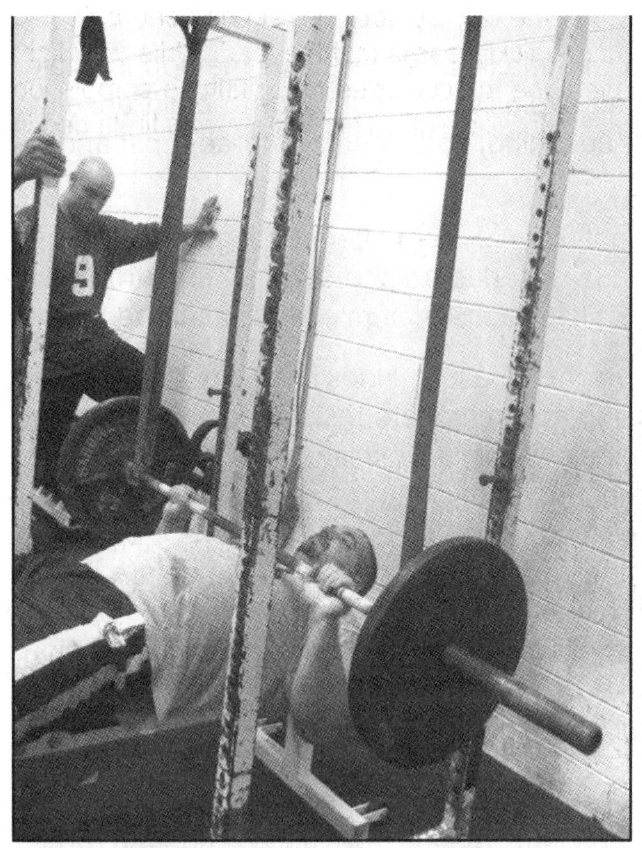

When executing the box squat, sit back, not down, on a box of any height, maximally stretching the squatting muscles. Relax the hip flexors, glutes, and obliques for 30 seconds to one minute and 30 seconds. Flexing off a box dynamically in a box squat increases an individual's pulls off the floor.

By using a box, a board, or the floor, the bar has speed as it reaches any level, creating kinetic energy that greatly contributes to the concentric phase. Remember, lower, relax, and then contract dynamically. It is imperative to stretch reflex lasts up to at least two seconds.

When using barbells for the reactive method effect, it is best to use a large amount of band tension or a large amount of chains on the weight releasers and a small amount of bar weight.

Many strength coaches call me about power and speed training, but very few ask about building absolute strength. If an athlete's reactive strength grows, jumping and running ability also increases. This is why men can outperform women in the 100 meter, shot put, basketball, football, and weightlifting. Most coaches are constantly working on speed and quickness, but that is the trait they recruited. Why constantly work on what they already have? Most stay away from heavy weight training for fear of overtaxing their athletes. However, when running full speed, four, five, and sometimes six times, body weight is produced during foot contact. Still, a 300 lb lineman is lucky to squat twice his body weight. Relative strength is much lower for large men compared with smaller, lighter men. What about lifters and other athletes who aren't very strong? How can they increase their explosive power? They can increase their explosive power by using the reactive method. Here's how.

One reactive method exercise is weight releasers. Extra weight is added to the bar on the eccentric phase by the use of weight releasers. It is common to lower 80% of a lifter's 1RM and raise 60%. This is done by putting 20% of the load on the weight releasers. As they release the load, the body reacts to the sudden reduction of weight and accelerates concentrically to completion. The lifter reacts as if the original 80% was on the bar. This develops maximum acceleration and reversal strength. The eccentric phase should be as fast as possible, preferably five to six-tenths of a second. Lowering slowly builds only muscle size and causes the most muscular soreness. The squats are done for two reps, 6–10 sets. This method is frequently used by Matt Smith and John Stafford.

Basically, the same method is used for bench pressing. We do 6–10 sets of three reps. Of course, only the first rep is a contrast rep because the weight releaser device falls off. This is good because eccentric work causes the most muscle soreness due to muscle spindle damage.

A second method for contrasting a load is the lightened method. At Westside, strong jump stretch bands are attached to our seven-foot power rack at the top. In the bottom of a squat, 135 lbs weighs zero. By adding 90 lbs to the bar, it weighs 90 at the bottom but 225 at the top. By adding a second set of 45 lbs, the weight at the top is 315 and 180 at the bottom. Your brain quickly learns that the load, while very light at the bottom, becomes quite heavy at the top. This teaches one to accelerate maximally to completion and not to decelerate near completion, which occurs with just barbell weight. This system was first used in youth training overseas.

If one could squat only 90 lbs, the load would seem light at the bottom after starting at the top with 225. Unlike the weight releaser system, the total load is reloaded as one stands. An extreme set up would look like this. Fix the bands so there is 250 lbs less at the bottom of a squat. Load the bar to 1000 lbs, and set up with the 1000 lbs.

The weight becomes lighter as one descends to the bottom until it is reduced to 750 lbs. The weight reduction is caused by the bands supporting part of the load. Then, return to the top. As the weight is raised, the bands gradually reload to the original 1000 lbs.
This is a very effective reactive method. One becomes accustomed with a heavy load at the start of the squat while maximizing strength at the bottom and explosively returning to completion.

Westside often uses this method for benching as well. While the deadlift does not require an eccentric phase in contests, we execute deadlifts in a similar fashion. The bar is reduced by 135 lbs on the floor by the support of the jump-stretch bands attached to the top of the power rack. After locking out the deadlift, the entire 135 lbs is lifted out of the bands. This method teaches an explosive start and acceleration to the top.

Let's look at a slightly different method—the heavy-light method. The first system employs bands. For benching on speed day, use two sets of mini-bands with a prescribed amount of barbell weight after a thorough warm up. After doing five sets of triples, take off a set of mini- bands and complete the remaining sets. The bar will feel extremely light.

Fred Boldt does 205 lbs bar weight plus two sets of mini-bands, equaling 170 lbs at the top and 80 at the chest. After four sets of three reps with two sets of bands done with a bar speed of about 0.75 meters/second, Fred takes off a set of mini-bands. Now, the bar speed increases to 0.8 meters/second. Fred's body reacts as if the original two sets of bands were still on the bar.

The contrast between the heavy and light load causes added stimulus to the central nervous system, producing added acceleration. This method can be used for squatting and deadlifting or even Olympic pulls.

If weight releasers or jump-stretch bands are not available, the heavy-light method can be done by first using a weight of roughly 90% for 1–2 reps for 2–3 sets. Then, reduce the bar weight to 40–60% and do 2–3 sets of 2–3 reps. This can be done on all lifts in addition to weighted dips, weighted pull-ups, or box jumps. Reps should be kept low to conserve energy. A note to ball players— it's great to be quick, but quickness is just one component of speed. Quickness is defined as an action of the body not requiring muscular effort or the complex coordination requiring energy (*Soviet Training and Recovery Methods* by Ben Tabachnik).

Lightened Method

By attaching bands to the top of the power rack or Monolift, the total barbell weight can be reduced in the bottom of the lift. The percent reduction can range from 15–25%. This method builds the rate of force development by overcoming a load with a medium to heavy concentric movement. The lightened method is used often at Westside.

Place a set of jump stretch bands over the top of a power rack. Hanging at seven feet, a 155-lb barbell will weigh zero at your chest with blue bands, but after locking it out, it returns to 155. With sub-maximal weight, this does not seem to be productive, but when max or near max weights are used, it teaches one to accelerate to the top. It develops acceleration or strength- speed. If done as recommended, it can duplicate your top bench with a bench shirt. If less band tension is used (purple band), it is very close to your shirtless best. Do pressing without gear; this also works for the overhead press and push jerks.

Use the same process for deadlifting or power cleans. While the bar is on the floor, 135 lbs is deloaded. For squatting, attach the bands to the top of the rack to deload the weight in the bottom. At Westside Barbell, we often use the contrast methods—bands, chains, and, of course, the lightened method. For squatting, we use three different bands: the light band, the monster mini- band, and the mini-band. A light band hanging over the Monolift will reduce the load around 200 lbs in the bottom of the squat. Remember, we always box squat just below parallel. A monster mini-band will reduce the load 110 lbs, and a mini-band will unload the bar about 55 lbs. If the intention is to become stronger, start with the mini-bands. Add weight for three weeks, wave back, and then, start a second three-week wave with the monster mini-bands. Again, wave back and start a new three-week wave with the light bands. The stronger the band creates a greater contrast.

A nine-week wave with a mini-band top would look like this:

Week	Weight	Sets	Reps	Weight at top	Weight at bottom
1	455	8	2	455	400
2	505	8	2	505	450
3	555	6	2	555	505
4	605	8	2	605	495
5	655	8	2	655	545
6	705	6	2	705	595

With a light band at the top:

Week	Weight	Sets	Reps	Weight at top	Weight at bottom
7	755	8	2	755	555
8	805	8	2	805	605
9	855	6	2	855	655

This series of squats is done off a box just below parallel. The rest between sets is one minute and 15 seconds to one minute and 30 seconds.

This system is regularly implemented at Westside. It is less taxing on the body, and it is important to learn acceleration and even more important to change the rate of acceleration. The lightened method is just one way to accomplish this. This method is also used on max effort day as one of our rotations.

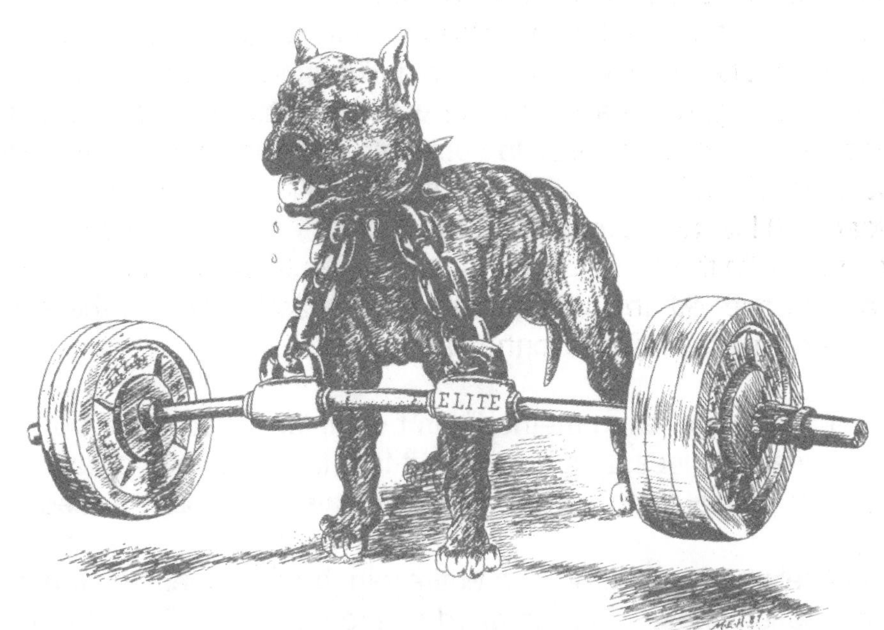

WESTSIDE BARBELL

Harold made a lightened method squat of 1115 at the top and 1000 at the bottom. His best squat is 1005. Matt Smith has used the same method with 1150 at the top and 1035 on the box, which has produced an 1102 squat. Consequently, Tim's effort falls short of Matt's, but this sets a standard to realize a contest potential.

Although this method was used for youth training in the old Soviet Union, Westside uses it in many exercises with great success. It has helped produce two 1100 squats—one at 268 body weight for Chuck Vogelpohl (a world record)—plus five, 1000 squats.

Westside often implements the lightened method in the bench press. For benching, we use four different strength bands. For max effort work, we primarily use the strong bands and the medium bands. The bands are choked at the top of a seven-foot power rack. This reduces the bar weight at the chest by 155 lbs. With 455 lbs on the bar, the weight is reduced to 300 at the chest, but the weight is reloaded progressively until lockout, which is again 455. In a second max effort workout, we would use a medium band to reduce the load 95 lbs at the bottom. After unracking the bar loaded to 455, it reduces to 350 at the chest and returns to 455 at lockout. A light band at the top of the rack reduces the load at the chest by 65 lbs. This time, 455 at the top weighs 390 at the chest.

The greater the band strength results in a greater contrast. This system builds speed or absolute strength depending on band tension. For speed benching, we use a light band or a monster mini-band. A 500lb raw bencher would use a bar weight of 315. Light bands would reduce the bar weight to 250 or 50%, at chest level. This is a good alternative to other speed work; the three most common being bands, chains, and weight releasers.

For pulling, we use a strong band looped over a pin 5'6" off the ground, which will unload the bar at floor level about 135 lbs. Joe Bayles pulled 745 with the lightened method. This resulted in a 775 PR at a meet. This was greater than a 30 lb positive result. Tim Harold pulled 900 and later pulled 855 at a meet, which was a PR but a 45 lb negative result.
Regardless, this gives some guidelines to go by.

This method is also very effective for high pulls as well as increasing the second pull. Kneeling cleans, snatches, and squats are used in the same way.

Use your imagination. The lightened method can be implemented for JM presses, triceps extensions, overhead presses, inclines, and declines. It is a fantastic tool for all sports because it can increase not only your vertical jump and long jump but also your hand speed.

It teaches you to accelerate throughout the entire range of motion. Conventional weight training has a distinct deceleration phase. The lightened method helps eliminate this phenomenon.

With this method, a young ball player can unrack 135 in the squat, but at the bottom, it weighs nothing. Therefore, 225 at the top would be 90 at the bottom and 315 at the top would be 180 in the hole, and so forth. This teaches acceleration. One must take advantage of all training methods to succeed.

People are getting stronger every day and are smart enough to make the most of their equipment. Don't be a hater. Take advantage of everything at your disposal. If the great lifters of the 70s, 80s, and 90s had shirts and suits, you can bet the bank they would have used them. Some of these lifters lasted only five or six years; however, if they had modern day gear, maybe they would still be competing with today's stars.

Ballistic Method

One form of the reactive method is the ballistic method. This is described as a rapid stretching movement. At Westside we use it for bench pressing with sub-maximal weights on speed day. Basically, drop or lower the bar as fast as possible and catch it 1–4 inches off your chest. Reverse to the concentric phase as fast as possible. This is great for building reversal strength. Never, I repeat, never pause the bar on the chest in training. Kinetic energy is lost to some extent. A pause is just a powerlifting rule. The stretch reflex can remain for up to four seconds in highly skilled lifters and two seconds for less skilled athletes as noted by Wilson's studies. Pausing longer than normal reflex time, potential energy is lost. Didn't someone say an object at rest tends to stay at rest? Remember, Newton's first, second, and third laws act in some way during all phases of a lift: eccentric, static, and concentric.

Concentric Method

With the bar suspended by chains or using power rack pins, simply crawl under the bar and raise it concentrically. Going from a relaxed condition to overcoming a stable load with light and medium loads of 50–80% will develop a rapid rate of force development. When loads of 90% and above are used, this causes maximal force rather than the appearance of explosiveness. It may appear somewhat slow because of the massive external resistance. The second method with 90–100% or more should be used on max effort day.

Dynamic Method

For benching or squatting, 20–24 total lifts are standard on dynamic method day. For benching, use 40–50% of a 1RM with a method of accommodating resistance (i.e. bands or chains). For squatting, use 50–60% with a method of accommodating resistance. Bands or chains must always be used to greatly reduce the deceleration phase. A lifter can stand up for a long time with a weight at the top of the squat. However, with a large bar load made up of mostly band tension, he is being pulled back down, causing a force exceeding gravity. Box squats, floor presses, and board presses are good methods for developing a rapid rate of force development after an eccentric phase accompanied by a relaxed phase. Many former college athletes are very explosive but lack a high level of maximal strength.

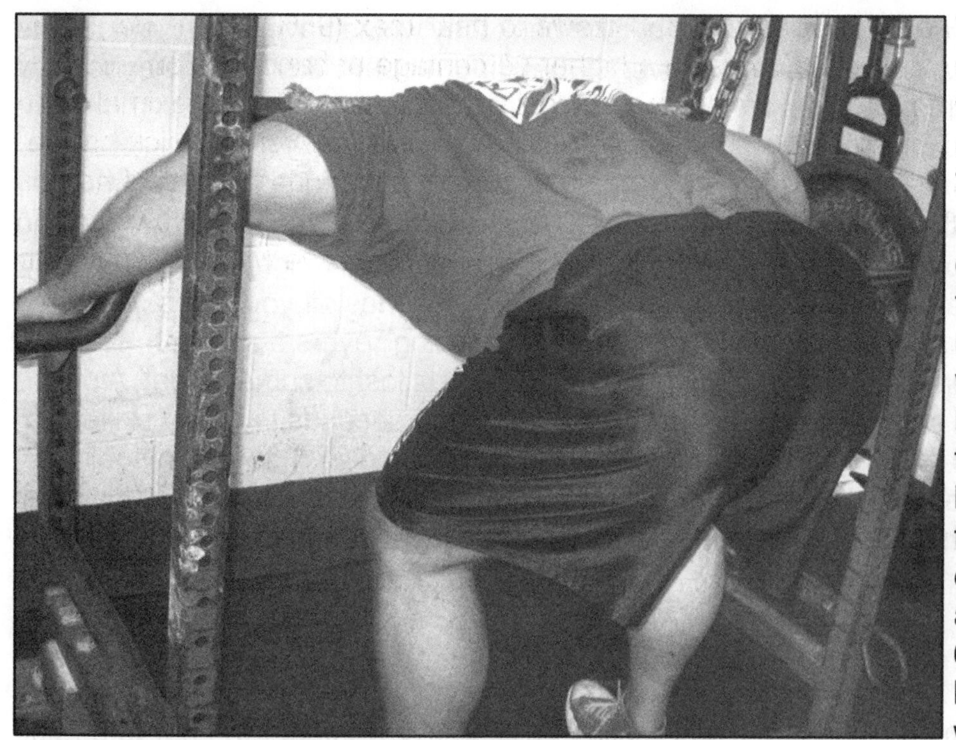

They are very fast with light weight, but as the load grows to near max (95% and higher), they slow considerably. This can be corrected by using a higher percentage of band tension—65% of total bar load. This slows the movement down while developing absolute strength. Maximal force is displayed for 0.3 seconds, which can be prolonged by using bands to prevent a quick bar deceleration. The late Dr. Mel Siff agreed with this. We have a 63-foot shot putter who said he has always been quick with a 363 power clean and a 565 deadlift at 250 bodyweight. However, he could not budge a 600 deadlift. He has zero quickness there. Speed is relative when compared to the amount of resistance.

Pendulum Wave

On dynamic day, use a three-week pendulum wave. For example, for the squat, complete 50% in week one, 55% in week two, 60% in week three, and back to 50% in week four. Change from bands to chains, add weight releasers, use the lightened method of overcoming a rested load, or change grip or stance.

Muscle Priority Sets

Train the most underdeveloped muscle groups or a skill that is lacking first.

Verbal Commands

Always use verbal commands such as: "blast it," "drive it," "speed," "squeeze the bar," "head up," "sit back," and so on.

Conjugate Sequence Method

Always rotate special exercises on speed day. The more inquiring a lifter is (extroverted), the more often he must switch exercises and the fewer exercises he needs. Change is the hardest thing for some lifters. We combine many methods on speed day to fortify our training. If an individual used a single method, it would take forever to utilize them all and they would not be productive. No one can understand the true definition of strength by just reading a book. A person must become strong to recognize a weakness.

They are very fast with light weight, but as the load grows to near max (95% and higher), they slow considerably. This can be corrected by using a higher percentage of band tension—65% of total bar load. This slows the movement down while developing absolute strength. Maximal force is displayed for 0.3 seconds, which can be prolonged by using bands to prevent a quick bar deceleration. The late Dr. Mel Siff agreed with this. We have a 63-foot shot putter who said he has always been quick with a 363 power clean and a 565 deadlift at 250 bodyweight. However, he could not budge a 600 deadlift. He has zero quickness there. Speed is relative when compared to the amount of resistance.

Pendulum Wave

On dynamic day, use a three-week pendulum wave. For example, for the squat, complete 50% in week one, 55% in week two, 60% in week three, and back to 50% in week four. Change from bands to chains, add weight releasers, use the lightened method of overcoming a rested load, or change grip or stance.

Muscle Priority Sets

Train the most underdeveloped muscle groups or a skill that is lacking first.

Verbal Commands

Always use verbal commands such as: "blast it," "drive it," "speed," "squeeze the bar," "head up," "sit back," and so on.

Conjugate Sequence Method

Always rotate special exercises on speed day. The more inquiring a lifter is (extroverted), the more often he must switch exercises and the fewer exercises he needs. Change is the hardest thing for some lifters. We combine many methods on speed day to fortify our training. If an individual used a single method, it would take forever to utilize them all and they would not be productive. No one can understand the true definition of strength by just reading a book. A person must become strong to recognize a weakness.

WESTSIDE SYSTEM INTRODUCTION

To excel at sports, special strength qualities have to be developed that pertain to a particular sport's activities. Don't generalize strength and make it into weak or strong or fast or slow. An individual can, however, be strong and slow or weak and fast. Some believe there is only one way to weight train. They don't recognize that special activities are imperative to increase speed or maximal strength. Many people seem to think that a very strong person lacks endurance or is slower than a man of average strength.

The Westside system uses conjugated periodization. This means that several methods are employed simultaneously to the training system. Unlike the Western method of periodization, which separates these into different periods, the Westside system puts it all together at the same time.

The Westside method is based on three basic methods of achieving maximal muscle contraction:

1. Max effort method
2. Repetition method
3. Dynamic effort method

Overview of the Westside program

The Westside micro-cycle is seven days long. It has two days for the squat, two days for the deadlift, and two days for the bench press. One day is for max effort work in the squat, deadlift, and bench press, and one day is for dynamic effort work in the squat, deadlift, and bench press.

The squat and deadlift are trained on the same day. The speed day should fall 72 hours after the max effort day. This is to allow for enough recovery time.

The training week consists of following days: Monday: Max effort squat and deadlift

1. The max effort exercise:
The max effort exercise should be trained using the maximal effort method. Work up to 1–3 rep max. Sometimes use the repetition method and do reps to failure.

Sample max effort exercise execution:

Reverse band deadlift	Sets	Reps	Weight
	2	5	135
	1	3	225
	1	2	315
	1	1	405
	1	1	455
	1	1	495
	1	1	545 PR
	1	1	575 fail

Max effort work periodization:

	Cycle 1	Cycle 2
Week 1	camber bar good morning	sled work
Week 2	low box safety squat bar	reverse band deadlift
Week 3	rest	sled work
Week 4	take a weight with gear	suspended good morning

This outline is what training can look like after it has been monitored. Do not plan the max effort exercises too far in advance.

2. Supplemental exercises:
This is based on an analysis of the individual lifter. Do an exercise that works glutes and hamstrings, lower back, or abs, depending on what the weakest point is or what adds to the squat and deadlift the most. This can be working up to a heavy set of 5 reps in the 45-degree back extension, doing 3–5 sets of 6–12 reps on the glute ham raise, or doing many sets of curls with bands.

3. Accessory exercises:
These include abdominal exercises such as: standing ab work in the lat machine for 3–4 sets of 8–15 reps and lower back exercises, including reverse hyper extensions for 3–4 sets of 8–15 reps.

4. Other exercises: Do other exercises such as: lat work, grip, or neck training. These can be done for pre-habilitation, added volume, or progressive recovery.

Sample workouts for Monday:

Workout #1:

1 deadlift standing on a block,	working up to max 1
2. glute ham raises	4x6–8
3. weighted leg raises	3x10
4. reverse hypers	3x10
5. neck extensions	2x20

Workout #2:

1. low box safety squat bar	work up to max 1
2. leg curls with bands	3x15
3. reverse hypers	3x15
4. side work with landmine	3–4 sets

Workout #3:

1. reverse hypers	5–8x8–12
2. standing abs on lat machine	5–8x8–12
3. t-bar rows	3–5 sets
4. grip work	3–5 sets

Wednesday: Max effort bench press

1. The max effort exercise: Work up to 1–3 rep max, using the repetition method at times. The max effort exercise should be trained, implementing the maximal effort method. Sometimes the repeated effort method is used.

Sample max effort exercise execution:

2-board press	Sets	Reps	Weight	
	2	5	95	off chest
	1	3	135	off chest
	1	2	185	off chest
	1	1	225	off chest
	1	1	275	add boards from here
	1	1	315	
	1	1	365	
	1	1	415	
	1	1	455	
	1	1	475	PR, stopped here

Max effort work periodization:

	Cycle 1	Cycle 2
Week 1	floor press	dumbbell press for reps
Week 2	reverse band press	3-board press
Week 3	rack lockouts	bench with chains
Week 4	take a weight with shirt	rest

Again, this outline is what your training can look like after it has been monitored. You should not plan the max effort exercises too much in advance.

2. Supplemental exercises: This is based on an analysis of the lifter. In the bench press, this means mostly exercises for triceps strength such as: triceps extensions with dumbbells or a straight bar, 3- or 6-board presses, JM presses, or close grip presses.

3. Accessory exercises: These include lat and upper back work such as: lat pull-downs or upright rows done for 3–4 sets of 8–15 reps and shoulder and chest exercises, including dumbbell presses or delt raises.

4. Other exercises: Do other exercises such as: rotator cuff work, upper body sled work, and forearm training. These can be performed for pre-habilitation, added volume, or progressive recovery.

Sample workouts for Wednesday:

Workout #1:

1. bench with mini-bands work	up to max 1
2. incline triceps extension	5x8
3. chest supported row	3x10–15
4. side delt raises	3x10–15
5. hammer curls	2x20

Workout #2:

1. dumbbell press	max rep sets with 2 weights or 3x8–15
2. straight bar triceps extension	3x5
3. lat pull-downs	4x10
4. upper body sled work	4 trips

Workout #3:

1. 2-board press	work up to max 1
2. 4- or 5-board press	work up to max 5
3. elbows out extensions	3x15
4. one arm rows	3x15
5. face pulls	3x15

Max effort guidelines:

1. Don't prepare mentally or you will burn yourself out.
2. Don't plan the ME exercises too far in advance.
3. The most important things are time under tension and strain (max effort), not the records.
4. Limit the number of lifts over 90% to 2–3. Complete one with 90%, one with 95–98%, and then try for a record. You can also jump from 92–95% straight to a new record.
5. It isn't necessary to do max effort work every week.

Max effort standards:

• Load:	90–100 % +
• ME exercises per workout:	1
• ME exercises per week	1 for the squat/deadlift and 1 for the bench
• Reps	1–3
• Rest	2–5 minutes
• Weeks per ME exercise	1–2

Friday: Dynamic squat and deadlift

1. The box squat: This is the basic format for squat and deadlift training. Perform 6–8x2 at 40–60% of your max, depending on your background and level. The number of sets varies on whether you use chains or bands or straight weight.

- 5–6x2 with bands
- 6–8x2 with chains
- 8–12x2 with straight weight

The most important factor on bar weight and percents is the lifter's level of preparation:

This may sound strange, but the higher your level of preparation, the more force you can put on the bar. Beginners should use only 40% of this strength while top lifters use 70–80% of their potential. Simply put, this is a skill developed through years of training.

Sample dynamic box squat execution:

Box squat	sets	reps	weight
	2	3-5	135
	2	2	185
	1	2	225
	1	2	275
	1	2	315
	8	2	375

2. Speed deadlifts: This means perform explosive singles at 50–70% of your max. These are done after dynamic box squats and are not necessarily performed every week. The usual speed deadlift workout would be 5–6x1 with 50–60% of your best in a meet.

Sample speed deadlift execution:

Deadlift	sets	reps	weight
	1	1	135
	1	1	225
	1	1	315
	5	1	405

3. Accessory exercises: These include abdominal exercises and lower back exercises.

4. Other exercises: Try other exercises such as: lat work, grip, or neck training. These can be implemented for pre-habilitation, added volume, or progressive recovery.

Sample workouts on Friday:

Workout #1:

box squats	6x2x45% using bands
speed deadlifts	5x1x45% with the mini-bands
reverse hypers	4x10
straight leg raises	4x10

Workout #2:

box squats	12x2x55%
sled work	5–6 trips with heavy weight
Russian twist	3x6-8 one leg
reverse hypers	3x6-8
lat pulls to abs	2x15 neck training 2–3 sets

Workout #3:

box squats	8x2x50% using chains
speed deadlifts	6x1x60%
glute ham raises	5x8–12
ab work on a lat machine	3–4 sets
sled work	2–3 trips with very light weight

Sunday: Dynamic bench press

1. The bench press: Work up to eight sets of three reps, using three different grips all inside the rings. The correct training percentage would be 45–50% of a shirtless max for competitive powerlifters and 50–60% for less advantaged lifters.

Sample dynamic bench press workout:

Bench press sets	reps	weight	
	2	5	45
	2	3	95
	1	3	135
	8	3	185

2. Supplemental exercises: Perform tricep work. Try exercises like close grip bench presses, JM presses, and dumbbell or barbell extensions. Sets and reps may vary from 4–6x8–12 to working up to a heavy set of five reps.

3. Accessory exercises: Incorporate other triceps exercises like push-downs or elbows out extensions, lat and upper back work like lat pull-downs or any kind of rows, and shoulder and chest exercises such as delt raises and weighted push-ups.

4. Other exercises: Integrate other exercises such as: rotator cuff work, upper body sled work, and forearm training. These can be done for pre-habilitation, added volume, or progressive recovery.

Sample dynamic bench press workouts:

W orkout #1:

bench press	8x3x45%/raw max using one chain per side
4- or 5-board press	work up to 2–3x5
lat pull downs	3x15
rear delt raises	3x15
upper body sled work	2–3 trips with very light weight

Workout #2:

bench press	10x3x35%/meet best
close grip press	5x5
elbows out extensions	2x20
hammer curls	2x20
reverse hypers	2–3 light sets each for 25–35 reps
ab work	2–3 light sets each for 25–35 reps

Workout #3:

bench press	8x3x45%/raw max, using mini bands
dumbbell extensions	5x12 lying on the floor
chest supported rows	5x12 one arm
side delt raise	2x15
rotator cuff work	4–8 light sets

Dynamic effort guidelines:

1. Bar speed is the most important factor.
2. Percentages are mentioned as a guideline.
3. One set should be performed within a specific timeframe; then, do a max single.
4. Use maximum force no matter what the bar weight is.
5. Do heavier sets occasionally to monitor bar speed.

Dynamic effort standards:

• Load:	40–60%
• DE exercises per workout:	1 (2 when doing deadlifts and box squats)
• DE exercises per week	1–2 for squat/deadlift and 1 for bench
• Reps	2 for squat, 3 for bench, 1 for deadlift
• Rest	30–90 seconds
• Weeks per DE exercise	3–4 week mini-periods

In the other parts of this book, you'll learn how Westside's top lifters train. Also, in part two, you'll discover how many different ways there are to train and how much training can vary.

DEVELOPING SPECIAL STRENGTHS

Having trained Kevin Akins, a 70'10" shot putter, I found that shot putters can be explosive as well as strong. As a freshman at OSU, Kevin was quick, but he was not strong. At 6'4" and weighing 260, he could squat 450, bench 360, deadlift 500, and power clean 275. He also threw 60 feet. As a senior weighing 330, he squatted 825 with no suit, benched 550 with no shirt, deadlifted 710, and power cleaned 420. With his strength and speed development, Kevin made a 70'10" shot. He was good, but was he the very best in the sport?

Udo Beyer of the Democratic Deutsch Republic (DDR) was, to say the least, ungodly strong. Weighing 352, his squat was 992 without equipment. He did a 672 pause bench. Quite possibly his greatest lift was a push jerk from behind the head—660 for ten singles in one workout. His best shot put in 1978 was 72'8" (world record). He was able to make progress up to 1986, making a world record 74'3.5". Udo was a product of great strength with little concern for raising speed. His teammate and prototype of the future was Ulf Timmermann. His strength, however, was not that of Udo's. Ulf had a 727 squat, 352 snatch, and 418 bench. He was the fastest with weights of 50–70%. Ulf's shot put distance was 75'8" (world record). Finding that to succeed, one must become strong and fast; the DDR had arrived.

Vasily Alexeyev, the great former Soviet super heavyweight, was a perfect example of the importance of speed. He was ranked tenth in the late 1960s. At that time, he was required to lose weight until he was able to execute a pull fast enough to satisfy the coaches. Once that was accomplished, he could again gain weight. However, if his pulls slowed, he was not allowed to gain more weight. As time progressed, his strength and size increased along with his speed. The end result was that he produced more world records than any Olympic lifter. Forty years ago, the Soviets knew how important it was to match force and velocity.

Being fast won't do it alone and being strong won't do it alone. We found this philosophy to be true at Westside in 1983. We were constantly getting stronger but not making the big lifts at the meets to correspond to our training lifts. Although we were getting stronger, we were becoming slower. We started using the dynamic method with sub-maximal weights. In 1993, we were working at 72% of our contest best in the bench press. Now in 2001, we are using 45%, and sometimes we go lower. We were already strong in 1993, but now we are much stronger and also much faster. If a lifter is fast, he should not neglect getting stronger.

Remember two important points—be very explosive and accelerate throughout the movement. There is only so much time to complete a max lift or a work set. When time runs out and the muscles being employed no longer work under the load, failure will occur.

Maximal Strength

Maximal strength is the basis of all types of strength. No one can do multiple reps (10–12) with 400 lbs in the squat if his best single is 420. However, if his squat was 550, then 400 for reps would be quite possible. Similarly, a long-distance runner who can squat only 50 lbs for 100 reps can perform better than a long-distance runner who can squat only 50 lbs for 100 reps. It is possible for a stronger person to possess greater endurance, particularly strength endurance.

Strength Endurance

What is strength endurance? Strength endurance is the ability to perform a lengthy display of muscular tension with minimal loss of work capacity. There are two forms of strength endurance—static and dynamic.

To develop strength endurance, the intensity or speed of execution must be considered. Middle-distance runners should do one rep per second for 60 seconds and then rest long enough to bring the pulse rate back to normal; then, repeat. GPP determines how many sets should be executed as well as rest sets. An athlete may feel he has good endurance for running, but he is unable to box for three rounds. The specificity of an exercise must be examined if an athlete is to excel in a particular sport.

Repetitions to failure using sub-maximal weights are one method for building strength endurance. This method is not intended for weights above 75% of a one rep max, which constrains one to develop primarily strength and not endurance. Although hypertrophy is a by-product of strength training, the repetition to failure method can raise volume. However, it can lower intensity levels and add muscle mass, which may or may not be desirable, depending on if the objective is to maintain a weight class or move up. It is imperative to adhere to the correct percentages. For sports using strength in conditions of speed, the weight percent to failure is 30–50%. For weight lifters, it is 50–75%, and for sports where stamina is used, it is 50–80%.

Dr. T. Alan and Professor L. Baroga suggest 9–12 sets per session, which is taxing but fast and efficient. Results also come quickly. Because this method is mentally and physically taxing, we suggest using it for two consecutive weeks at most.

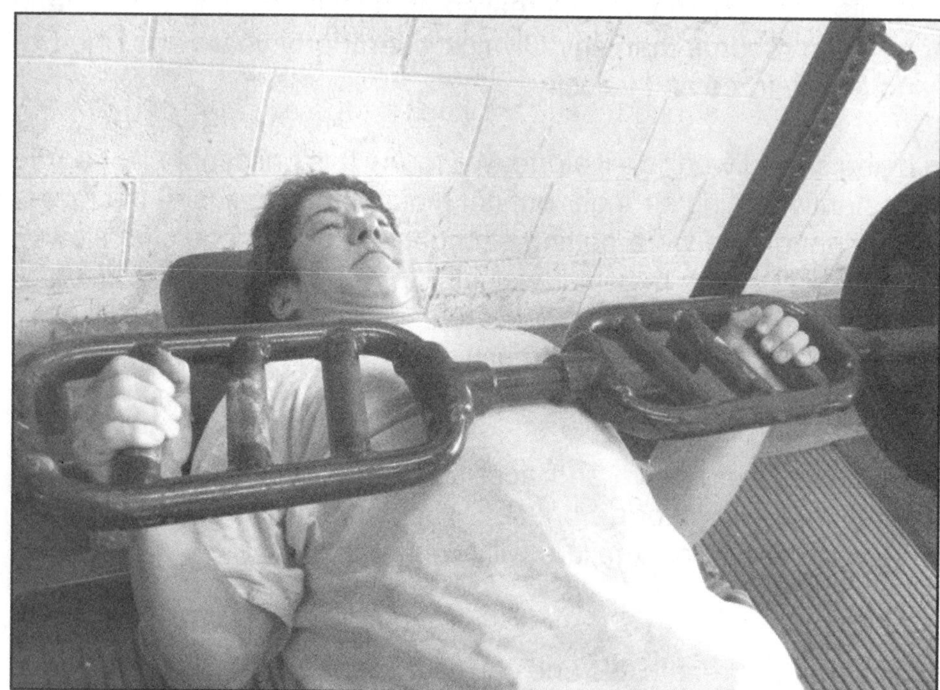

Speed-Strength Powerlifting and weight lifting are speed-strength types of activities. Each requires the execution of a lift at full speed while having the strength to do it. Lifting near limit weights develops quick strength. Two types of training are included to achieve this goal:

- a dynamic day where weight at 40–60% is used to increase force production
- a maximum effort day where very heavy weights are implemented in special exercises

A visitor named Rocco and I were doing strength-speed work. Rocco's best box squat was 415, plus two blues and a green band on both sides. When I was using two blues and a green band, my best meet squat was 900. Rocco's best is 675; in turn, this shows Rocco lacks speed.

The dynamic method employs sub-maximal weights. Although some recommend loads consisting of 66–85% with a rep range of 3–6, we have adjusted the loads for squatting to 50–60%, using two reps per set. At least six sets of two reps should be done by novices, not to exceed 12 sets of two reps with just weight. This is based on a just below parallel box, and the 50–60% max is based on an actual contest max. In the bench press, the training weight is 60% of a one rep max without a bench shirt or eight sets of three reps. Both squat and bench sets should be done every 60 seconds or less, and it is important to use maximum speed.

Strength-Speed

Strength-speed is the ability to move heavy weights as fast as possible. To develop strength-speed, we use the method of maximum effort. On this day, make a maximal effort with weights at 100% plus. When a weight is made over 100%, this is referred to as over maximal. One or two reps are employed. When powerlifting, three lifts work best—one at 90% and one or two lists that are more than the previous max. For weightlifting, use exercises such as: pulls with a snatch or clean grip (4–10 lifts) just as long as the proper height is maintained. How do you know if you lack strength-speed? Chuck Vogelpohl was doing speed work with a visitor named Jack. They both used 405, plus blue bands and both had identical speed. Then, Chuck added 90 lbs for a set. Jack couldn't do the 495, but Chuck worked up to 585 and 635. How? Chuck possesses both speed-strength and strength-speed, and Jack lacks strength-speed. Chuck's top squat is 1000 at 220, and Jack's is 675 at 220.

When using 90% and above for more than three weeks, progress can cease. To avoid this dilemma, switch the maximal effort exercises each week. This is referred to as the conjugate method—using exercises that resemble the classical lift, which is used to perfect technique.

Isometric Strength

How is quasi-isometric strength developed? In powerlifting, a lifter may have to push or pull respectively for a long length of time while locking out a bench or deadlift. However, if thinking in sports terms, this can also occur when two linemen or two wrestlers are in combat. Here, the velocity is extremely slow.

This is different from standard isometrics where the bar or object is motionless or fixed. To develop quasi-isometric strength, use a barbell at the position where problems develop (e.g. the last four inches in the bench press).

Next, apply a large amount of bands to the bar so a slow start is achieved, making the lockout nearly impossible. A second method is to start the bar below the minimax, extending the arms to the precise point where failure occurs with or without the arms locked. This can be completed with any lift, including the snatch and clean. Of course, this can be done in eccentric or concentric fashion. The benefits are that it can build maximal strength and active flexibility, and the cons are that it has no effect on maximal power or speed.

With standard isometrics, strength can be developed not only at the precise angle one exerts from but also in a radius of 15 degrees either way. Here, the velocity is zero. When moving a bar off the chest dynamically, the work at that point is very short. The same would be true when lifting a bar off the floor while executing a second pull. This may occur in only a fraction of a second or the work when is done in a very short amount of time. This can be greatly changed by isometric contraction at those desired positions. In sports where high-speed movements are present, isometric work is less effective. Its main purpose is to develop absolute strength when doing long contractions of 3–5 seconds, but it can also be used to develop explosive strength just as dynamic exercises do by pushing or pulling violently with quick jerks. With pure isometrics, the rise in muscle tension is slow; whereas, with explosive isometrics, the rise in muscle tension is fast. For example, look at a deadlift in simple terms. The rate of movement starts explosively and eventually reaches zero velocity at the top or somewhere near isometric.

Isometric exercises have been around since the 1950s. It was an effective method to develop strength at a particular angle and affordable to most because of the limited amount of equipment needed.

The famous Bob Hoffman of York Barbell fame manufactured an isometric power rack in the 1960s. T. Hettinger and E. Mueller found that a small, daily workout for ten weeks increased strength about 5% per week, which was maintained for a month.

There has always been the question, which is more productive—dynamic or isometric exercises? In my opinion, both must be trained. There are always pros and cons for any type of training. Here are the benefits:

- Isometrics take less time and energy to perform a workout.
- Speed-strength can be maintained while doing isometric training.
- For those wanting to remain in a particular weight class, isometrics won't add muscle mass.
- They fortify technique in crucial positions. A coach can watch to see form breaks at many different angles of the lift.
- Maximal effort can be displayed longer than with dynamic work.

When doing dynamic work, maximal effort is displayed for a fraction of a second at the minimax or sticking point. While doing speed deadlifts, all looks well. The bar is blasted from the floor to lockout. However, with a max effort deadlift, the bar stops at the knee or just before lockout. Hardly any work is done at the minimax; it's just too fast. A three-second isometric hold can be equal to many dynamic contractions.

The work at a particular angle is radiated 15% either above or below the point where the force is applied. It sounds contradictory, but holding your breath can boost endurance.
Remember, a swimmer inhales only once every 3–4 strokes.

The following points are disadvantages of isometrics:

- Isometrics are not to be used before puberty or if one is a novice.
- Isometrics can fatigue the central nervous system.
- If done alone, a loss of some coordination can occur.
- Holding your breath for a long time can have a negative effect on the cardiovascular system.

How are isometrics performed? Here is how Westside does them.
The simplest way is to push or pull against a pin, which can be placed at different positions. For example, if a lifter is weak at the floor, pull on a relaxed bar at that position or just below the knee, at the knee, and possibly at the lockout.

Like all isometric contractions, use submaximal or maximal efforts while exerting on the bar. Also, the duration that a lifter pushes or pulls on the bar can vary from 2–6 seconds per exertion.

Quasi-isometrics is pushing or pulling slowly over a certain range of motion. This can be done by attaching a series of jump stretch bands to the bar. For example, loop a series of bands over a bar placed on the floor, making it possible to lift the bar very slowly through a predetermined range of motion. Adjust the bands to work the part of the lift that needs to be improved.

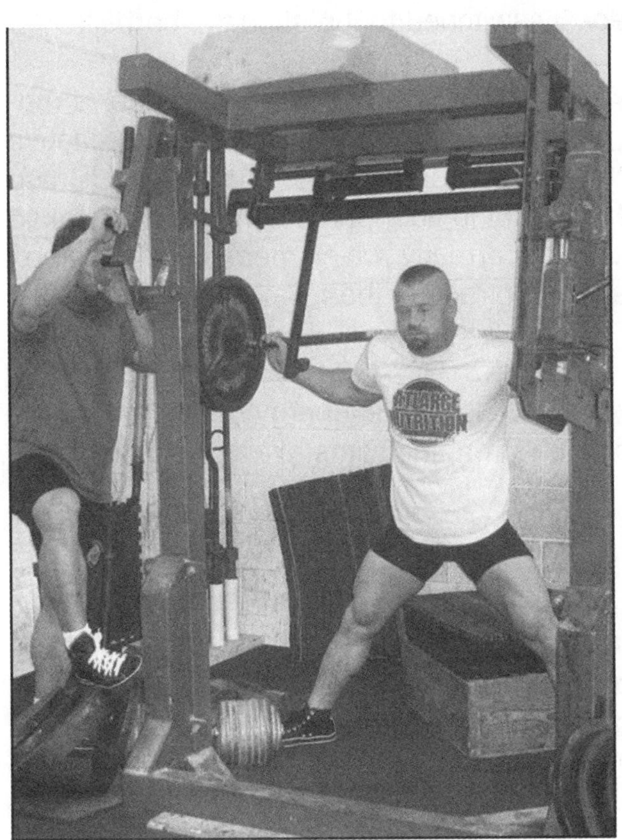

Dynamic isometrics involves pulling or pushing a bar against a pin as fast as possible with a brief contraction. Because of the short contraction, it is possible to do several efforts. However, it is essential to perform the movement as quickly as possible to produce a steep force/time curve like slower isometrics where the contractions are sometimes 3–6 seconds per effort. The dynamic effort can be limited to one second per effort. Three efforts of one second can replace a three- second effort if done dynamically.

Perform 3–5 positions for static work with the work radiating 15 degrees above and below the point being pushed or pulled upon. This satisfies the entire range of motion. Although isometrics are found to develop absolute strength, they also increase dynamic strength. Verkhoshansky found that the time a lifter holds a position isometrically is as important as the intensity of the hold.

I have always preferred the Hoffman method. For example, lift 400 upward for a predetermined distance into a pin. Hold for 3–6 seconds. A weight of 400 would be 75% of a 600 max. It is very hard to calculate how much is truly exerted against a chosen pin. For absolute strength, hold maximal tension. For explosive strength, use maximal speed and exert 70–80% against the pin. The faster you get to 70–80%, the better.

Isometrics are very effective but also very taxing. The faster the lift is performed, the less time the minimax is worked. All training methods must be used during training, and it is up to the coach to know when to utilize a particular training method. For a more detailed explanation of the above, refer to Verkhoshansky (1970) or The Fundamentals of Special Strength-Training in Sport.

Remember, the faster the rate of force development against the pin, the better. The longer the exertion against the bar wields the greater results, even with different intensities. Don't exceed ten minutes of isometric work per workout. Like any training, rotate isometrics throughout the year. For explosive strength, a lifter must produce maximum speed as fast as possible against the pin. The simplest form of isometrics is just tensing the muscles as in a bodybuilding pose, forcefully tensing the agonists and antagonists for every joint. This was advocated by Vorobyev in 1978 and as early as the 1900s by Anokhin and Proshek . I hope just some small part of this awakens your mind to try a new method of training.

Explosive Strength

Explosive strength is the ability to use the muscles and central nervous system, achieving maximum force as quickly as possible after an intense muscular stretch. Research by Frolov and Levshunov (1979) showed that highly skilled weight lifters who had high results in the jerk from the chest performed the half squat quickly and instantaneously switched to thrusting the barbell.

Explosive strength is another strength quality. This type of strength is displayed best after a mechanical stretch, meaning the switch from stretching to active contraction, which is the reactive ability to change directions. When performing pulls, implement hang cleans, and for bench, use the ballistic method, or in other words, the drop and catch, off the floor press done from a relaxed phase overcome by dynamic work. For squatting, box squat correctly, which means sit on the box and release the hips and glutes, holding all other muscles contracted; then, flex.

Explosive strength is developed after a strong stretch that builds kinetic energy during the lowering phase in different forms. Shock training builds explosive strength. Some examples include the following:

- hang cleans or hang snatches
- depth jumps
- push jerks
- box squats or box squats with bands, chains, or weight releasers.
- Two of the best methods to build explosive and absolute strength are:
- static overcome by dynamic work
- relaxed overcome by dynamic work

Box squatting accomplishes both. Some muscles are held statically, and some are relaxed during the movement. Before we move on, I want to address the following—why do many fail to increase their jumping ability while increasing their squat? The most probable reason is that as their squat weight goes up, the bar speed slows. They concentrate only on strength-speed while neglecting speed-strength. Approximately 80 lifts per month must be devoted to explosive and speed-strength and roughly 16 lifts per month for strength-speed. Both should be done during the same week. If working for only quickness, some absolute strength will be lost in two weeks. If the objective is to raise absolute strength, some quickness will be list in two weeks as well. Effective training entails focusing on all types of strength during the week.

Here are some things to contemplate. A boxer fights with eight-ounce gloves. When a boxer goes from 16-ounce gloves to eight-ounce gloves his hand speed increases. This is a contrast effect and an example of explosive strength. Sprinters wear a weighted vest or a parachute when training and remove it for competition. This is also a contrast method.

Whereas depth jumps provide a reactive movement through using the momentum of a falling body, a hang clean or snatch and box squatting enable an individual to direct the body in more favorable angles to pre-stretch the muscles. Regardless of the height of the box, the landing angles stay close to the same in plyometrics. Hang pulls can be done at varying heights to catch the bar before starting the pull. Box squatting can also be executed from many different heights.

Plyometrics are just one type of shock training. Others include maximal eccentrics, forced reps, all contrast methods mentioned above, and anti-restricted range of motions to max (partials).

Accelerating Strength

To ensure the development of accelerating strength, bands or chains should be employed while using a bar or dumbbells. This can prolong the rate of maximal force production during an exertion, which simply means that one is accommodating resistance making barbell training more productive.

Eccentric and Concentric Strength

The powerlifts require many strength qualities. Two of these are the ability to lower and raise weights, which pertains to eccentric and concentric work. In the bench press, there is a pause at the meet, but in training, pausing is not necessary. The stretch reflex is stored internally for most lifters in two seconds and for the highly trained athletes up to four seconds (Wilson,1998).

Concentric Strength

Because the squat and bench require eccentric work followed by concentric work, both must be implemented. The deadlift does not require the ability to lower the weight, only to raise it concentrically. To overcome inertia, an abundant amount of starting strength is required. At Westside, we do good mornings, and half of the good mornings are done concentrically by supporting the bar from heavy duty chains. Chains are used instead of the power rack to allow the bar to swing freely from front to back and left to right, which builds greater stability.

This chain-supported method works well for the bench press, too. With these exercises, inertia must be overcome without the aid of a stretch reflex. Though physically demanding, this type of strength is required in the deadlift. We use different bars, changing the distance between the lower back and the center of the bar. Many different heights are used to ensure strength development through the entire range of motion. This is very awkward and represents only strength work, not technical work. This method of training can overcome a minimax, commonly referred to as a sticking point. Usually the sticking point occurs when the leverages are poorest and the resistance is greatest, causing the lifter to fail at that point.
Momentum is a product of the mass of an object and its velocity. It can carry the bar through the minimax. Training at your minimax is one solution.

Eccentric Strength
What do we really know about eccentric (lowering) work? The eccentric phase causes most muscular soreness or the burn that bodybuilders talk about. When performed slowly, it greatly contributes to muscle hypertrophy (growth). We also know that in an attempt to raise absolute strength, eccentric training alone fails miserably.

In the late 1970s, Mike Bridges experimented with eccentric bench pressing. He told me that the only result he got from eccentrics was a pec injury. This is confirmed by research that shows most injuries occur during the yielding or eccentric phase.

Vince Anello also experimented with eccentric work, performing eccentric deadlifts with as much as 880. When he returned to conventional deadlifts, his deadlift had decreased much to his dismay.

Vince told me that anything can make your deadlift go up, except eccentrics. What does this mean? Are eccentrics a waste? Well, yes and no. Eccentric training alone is a waste. However, a strength-shortening cycle and eccentric training followed by a concentric phase can be very beneficial when done correctly (i.e. with optimal speed).

Training with heavy weights adds strength potential to muscles, and training with light weights with a rapid concentric phase increases speed and explosive strength. It is obvious that without the lowering or eccentric phase, there would be no sudden stretch preceding a voluntary effort.
Kinetic energy is gathered in the eccentric phase, causing a sudden release of elastic energy stored in the tendons and soft tissues of the body. Heavier weight does not add to the rebound phase as effectively as using an overspeed eccentric phase.
How can this be done? Using jump stretch bands can cause a forced overspeed eccentric phase also known as maximal powermetrics. The combination of eccentric and concentric actions forms a natural type of muscle functioning called the stretch-shortening cycle (SSC) (Norman and Komi 1979; Komi, 1984).

In the calculation of kinetic energy, increasing velocity is significantly more important than increasing mass. This is because velocity is squared into the equation KE = (1/2)mv, which explains why the squat- under in Olympic lifting is so important. When the lifter falls under the bar, he is producing kinetic energy for reversing the direction of the bar. This dropping under the bar should not be confused with an eccentric phase. For an eccentric phase to occur, muscle tension must accompany the action. The squat-under has no such muscle tension.

We know that 40–50% more muscle can be used during the eccentric phase, which is where a real problem occurs. As the barbell grows heavier, a lifter tends to lower the bar more slowly. This, in turn, is counterproductive. When slowing down the eccentric motion, the energy that can be stored in the muscles and tendons is emitted. The myostactic reflex occurs when a muscle is stretched by an external force. This causes a stretch reflex, but the faster the eccentric phase, the greater the stretch reflex. This can have a negative effect on the Golgi tendon reflex, which helps prevent extremely high and potentially dangerous loads to the tendon. With overspeed eccentrics, a lifter can try to override this phenomenon. In Science and Practice of Strength Training, Zatsiorsky states that Elite athletes develop very high forces of elastic energy in the tendons rather than the muscles. This should alert an individual to lower the barbell at an optimal speed as the weights grow heavier. If the barbell slows down as the weight grows heavier, the length of the muscle is stretched and the muscle tension increases, which could lead to injury.

Because this myostactic reflex is counterbalanced by the Golgi tendon reflex, an inhibition of muscle action occurs, causing a less than maximal concentric phase. Of course, this limits the potential to overcome heavier loads in training or at meet time.

The answer to this dilemma is to use only enough eccentric muscle tension to control the barbell in the correct path. If in fact a lifter uses 40–50% more muscle tension to lower weights, does it not make sense to use only up to 50% of his eccentric strength when lowering a weight? This will contribute to a stronger concentric phase, producing a better result.

Using the Tendo unit, we found that when performing speed strength work in the bench press and squat, the eccentric phase moves at a rate of 0.7–0.8 meters per second (m/s). This is basically the same as the concentric phase, maximizing the stretch reflex. Basically, this translates to the faster down, the faster up. With near maximal weight, the same trend was observed. The eccentric and concentric phases were both 0.45–0.6 m/s, and band and bar weight were used to achieve these results. When all resistance was from barbell and plate weight, the lowering time was considerably longer. The eccentric phase was 0.4 m/s on the speed squat and bench and 0.6 m/s for the concentric phase. With near maximal weight, the eccentric phase was 0.37 m/s and the concentric phase was 0.40–0.50 m/s. This evidence shows how bands can play a valuable role in increasing the eccentric phase of barbell lifts, teaching an individual to use less eccentric muscle action. As weights grow heavier, the bar speed should find an optimal speed, regardless of external resistance.

The above data was collected using eight 900 plus squatters and eight 600 plus benchers. The results were nearly equal for both phases, with each 600 plus lifter varying less than a tenth of a meter/second eccentrically or concentrically. With circa-max weights, I was the slowest by a small margin during both phases, and Dave Tate was the fastest.

On speed work, the same results were obtained. J. L. Holdsworth was the quickest, and Chuck Vogelpohl was the slowest. Again, only one-tenth of a meter/second separated the eccentric and concentric phase of each lifter. The same results occurred in the bench press. In the above test, all bench subjects benched in T-shirts. All squatters wore standard groove briefs without knee wraps and squatted on a box. All subjects were at the same level of general physical preparedness.

One test was performed on six men who were all national and world champions with squats ranging from 900–975 at the time. First, the bar was loaded to 640 lbs of band tension at the top part of the squat. At the bottom, just below parallel, the band tension was 470. The bands were added slowly as a warm up. Then bar weight was added until the bar had 285 on it, equaling 925 at the top and 755 at the bottom.

All six lifters performed a single rep, which was timed on video camera. Then, 80 lbs of chain was placed on weight releasers. The bar was lowered fairly rapidly at 1.5 seconds. After the 80 lbs of chain was deloaded at the bottom, the lifters recovered quicker concentrically than without the additional chain. The lift represented 1005 at the top, which was deloaded to 755. Again, an additional 80 lbs of chain was added to the weight releasers, making the weight1085 at the top and the original 755 on bottom. The concentric phase was even faster. When 80 lbs of chain was added to 1165 on top and 755 on the bottom, the bar speed increased again.

The key to lifting larger weights is concentrating on the eccentric phase, especially with the overspeed eccentric method, using a large amount of tension. The key is learning to relax to reduce muscle tension in the eccentric phase, preventing inhibiting the stretch reflex. By following these simple steps, a lifter can undoubtedly watch his total go crazy.

Part 2

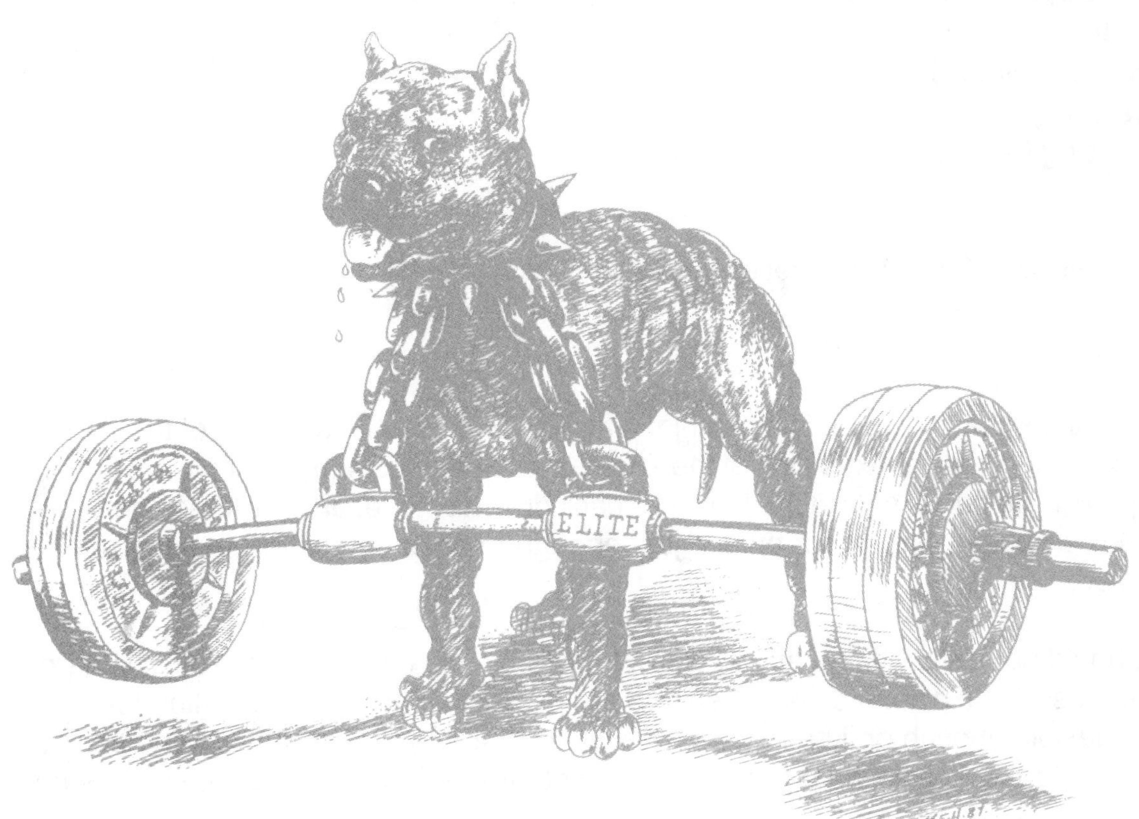

WESTSIDE BARBELL™

TRAINING OF THE POWER LIFTS

A lifter must become faster to become stronger. To become stronger, a lifter must become faster. The special work is what makes an individual bigger. Bigger, faster, and stronger—isn't that what we're after?

Technique

When striving for proper technique, our intensions are to lift the most weight in contest situations. Proper technique is not intended to produce a championship physique but rather a world record performance.

Technique is a tool for a lifter to build the best leverages possible. With good form, an athlete can stress his strong points and eliminate weaknesses. To analyze and build technical skills, the lifts can be divided into smaller segments:

1. setting up
2. unracking the bar
3. ascent
4. reversing direction
5. descent
6. replacing the bar

For the deadlift, parts 2–4 are unnecessary.

Squat

Most people think that the squat is a multi-joint movement. I see it as flexion of the spinal erectors and hip flexors and a slight extension of the knees. Watch a good squat technician; nothing moves but the hip joint. He bends only at the hips. His back doesn't move, and his knees don't go forward. Others push gradually throughout the lift, just enough to accommodate the external force that is being applied.

The feet should point straight out and forward, forcing the hip muscles into play. It is hard to break parallel because the hip flexors and extensors are put into a very strong position for flexion. If the lifter is not flexible enough or if he has a thick waistline and thick upper thighs, he should turn the feet outward slightly. People who walk with their feet turned outward have weak hamstrings.

When squatting, think about pushing the feet out, not down. This ensures that the hip muscles are working correctly. Push the knees out the entire time, starting from the moment the bar is unracked. This movement should be felt in the hips. Next, the glutes should be pushed to the rear as though searching for a chair that is too far behind where the lifter plans to sit. The lower back should be arched hard while keeping the chest and head up. To keep the bar in the center of gravity the lifter should lean as much as possible.

To ensure correct bar placement, raise the chest and pull the shoulder blades together. This creates better leverages by placing the bar as far back as possible. However, if the bar is carried too low, it causes an individual to bend forward and destroys the leverages. The hands should be wide enough to avoid bicep tendonitis, and the elbows need to be pulled forward by contracting the shoulder blades together.

Which stance should be used? Box squats need to be executed with a wide stance. This builds the hip muscles, which is vital. Over 30 years ago, the great Jim Williams said to train as wide as possible and pull the stance in so parallel can be broken in a meet.

While descending, always squat back and not down. If a lifter pushes the glutes back, the knees won't go forward. By forcing the knees apart, this significantly increasing leverages. After breaking parallel, first push against the bar. After all, the bar is what we are trying to raise. Pushing with the feet first is a mistake. This causes the lifter to bend over and most likely to miss the lift.

Breathing is important. First, take air into the abdominal section and chest. Hold the air until the hardest part of the lift is reached; then, exhale when near the top position.

Bench Press

For training, use 3–4 different grips, alternating from the index finger just touching the smooth part of the bar to a grip that is two inches wider than the grip where the little finger is in contact with the power ring. Take the bar out of the rack by yourself, pulling the shoulder blades together and gripping the bar as tight as possible. Next, pull the bar out of the rack as if you were doing a pull- over. This properly activates the lats. Pull the bar straight above the point on the chest where you want to lower it; then, lower the bar quickly in a straight line.

Press the bar straight up and slightly toward the feet. This is the shortest distance to press and eliminates shoulder rotation. Rotating the bar back over the face can cause rotator and pec injuries. Never intentionally push the bar over the face.

Hold your breath for up to five reps because holding the breath defines heavy training. Take as much air in as possible before lifting the bar from the rack. Lower the bar as fast as possible. Stop the bar as quickly as possible and reverse to the concentric phase just as fast. When training, raise the head as the bar is lowered, keeping your eyes on the bar throughout the movement. Use either a thumbless grip or a thumb grip.

During competition technique should be the same as in training with one exception. Use a maximum wide grip with a thumb grip and use a lift off. As the bar is lowered, raise the head first and then the shoulders as if doing a sit-up. This enables you to bring the bar lower on the body without rolling it out of the hands.

Once the press command is given, slam your head and shoulders back down on the bench for stability, keeping your feet out in front of the knees and pressing down on the heels to ensure that your butt stays on the bench. Because a longer torso is more advantageous for bench pressing, avoid shortening the torso by arching the lower back. Consequently, an extreme arch can cause an injury.

Deadlift

When executing the conventional style, center the bar over the joint of the big toe or a little closer. A good distance to start pulling is usually when the bar is 3–4 inches from the shins. Getting too close to the bar, may cause the bar to swing forward when you pull upward, causing difficulties at the lockout. The shoulder joints must be behind or over the bar when starting the pull. Pull slightly toward the center of the body to keep the bar close to the legs and always push the feet out to the sides. For most lifters, pointing the feet out provides a stronger start because of the greater leg drive. This position enables a strong finish because of increased hip rotation.

The back position can vary because of the wide variety of body structures. Most lifters arch their lower back while rounding the upper back at the same time. However, the back should not be rounded too much because it will be difficult to lockout. Though you may get stuck in the knees, it is an advantage as long as the bar stays close to your shins. The head position can vary anywhere from looking straight ahead to looking downward about six feet in front of you.

The most common grip is the standard reverse grip; however, some lifters use an overhand hook grip with the arms hanging in a straight line. As a lifter increases in size, he may have to use a wider grip. When executing the sumo style in deadlifting, the width of the stance implemented depends on flexibility. Longer the legs mean a wider stance. The hips should be kept as high as possible, providing the back is in the proper position. Pull yourself slightly lower than your optimal starting position, and push the hips against the bar and rebound out of the bottom.

Use abdominal breathing while keeping the air out of the lungs. This keeps the torso short for better leverages and builds stability. Remember body structure dictates which style is best for each individual.

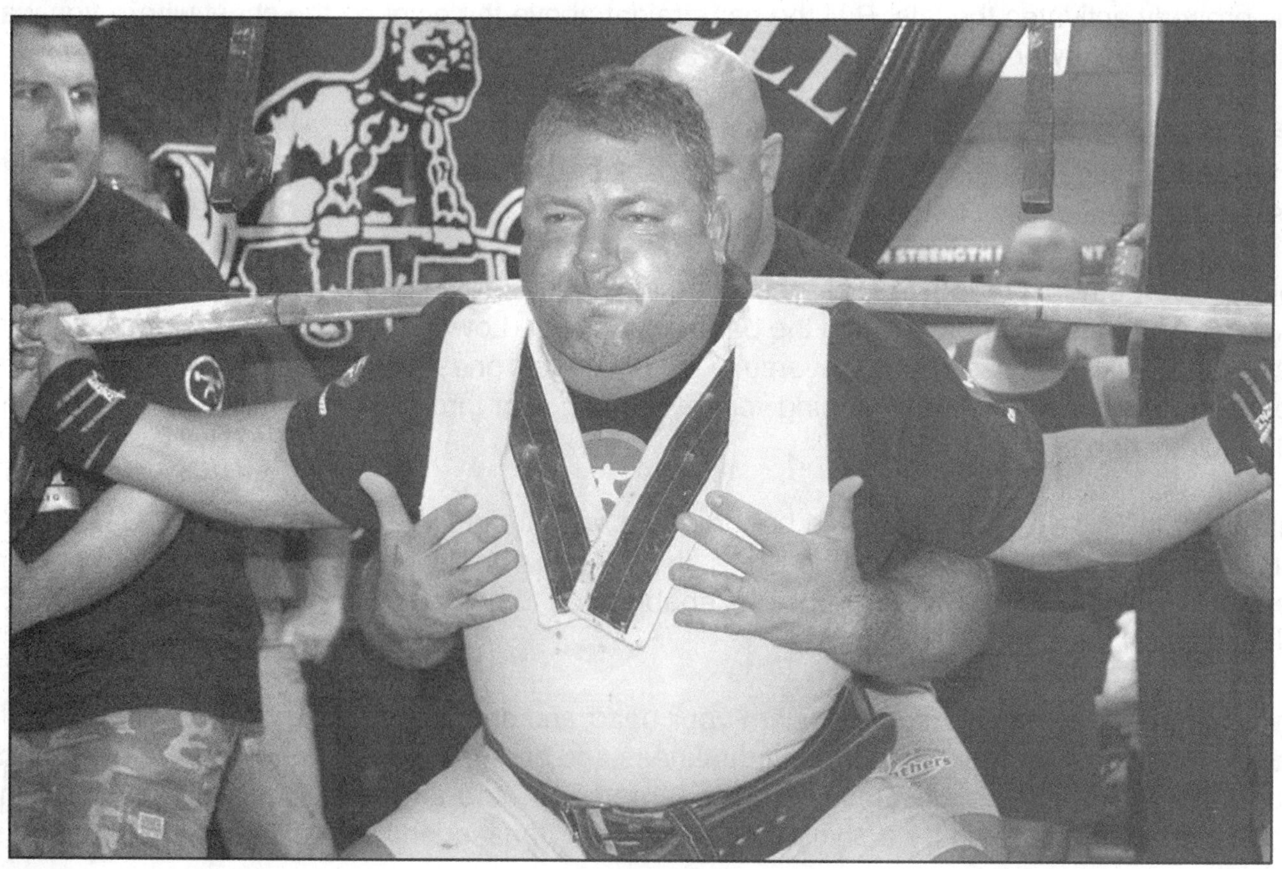

Competition Lift Picture

PERIODIZATION

Periodization simply means the organization of training plans for one year or more into shorter manageable plans (i.e. weekly or monthly). At Westside, a weekly plan is used on max effort day. Each week, the lifter switches a barbell exercise, always working up to a max single in a special squat or box, rack, or band deadlift. This is the maximal effort method. Only good mornings with an eccentric phase preceding a concentric phase are performed for a 3RM, which is the method of heavy efforts. Westside has proven that the max effort method is superior. Why? A new plateau is reached, creating positive physical and psychological effects.

The heavy efforts method raises a problem of high volume but no new, absolute records. A heavy effort means weights above 90% of a 1RM. Lifting weights at 90% or more for three weeks or longer causes a negative effect on the central nervous system. To prevent this phenomenon, we switch the core lift each week. As a lifter's special physical preparedness increases, the training effect decreases. This is why new means of training must be introduced constantly and why exercises are rotated each week. This is the conjugate system—using exercises that are similar to the classic exercise for either weight lifting or powerlifting, which provides unidirectional loading that highly stimulates motor potential and perfects technical skill.

The same holds true for bench pressing. The floor press, board press, rack work, incline, decline, and others are conjugate exercises. To clarify, max effort work is done once a week. For bench pressing, it is implemented 72 hours after speed-strength benching. At Westside, speed bench is on Sunday and max bench is on Wednesday. The speed squat and deadlift are on Friday, and max effort work is on Monday. Extreme workouts can occur every 72 hours. Max effort work is a weekly plan but must be considered into a yearly plan.

Speed-strength work is done for a three-week cycle. The weight with bands, chains, or both is changed each week, normally increasing each week for the three weeks. On the fourth week, the load is decreased or changed, and again, another three-week wave is started. Why do we start again after three weeks? We found that after three weeks, a lifter can't become faster or stronger, which is exactly why a three-week wave is used. Dr. Mel Siff informed me that Vasily Alexeev used a similar wave system for his remarkable training. Remember, he was a weight lifter who did not use gear. It worked because he became physically stronger.

When squatting with different bars, each has a limit weight that has been obtained. For example, I have done 805 with a regular squat bar on a parallel box, 640 with a safety squat bar, and 675 with a 14-inch cambered bar. I mention this because when using a three-week wave with one particular bar, the same percentage is a different amount of weight.

For example:

Squat bar: 50% = 402, 60% = 482
Safety squat bar: 50% = 320, 60% = 384
Cambered bar: 50% = 337, 60% = 405

This must be closely governed. For me, these numbers represent the weight equivalent to my max meet squat of 920. By changing bars each three-week wave, a true max meet squat can be calculated. If an athlete breaks a personal record on, the cambered bar, a new meet record should be expected. The percents are calculated off of the particular bar used as well as the contrast method applied (bands, chains, or both). If weight releasers are used, they also must be taken into consideration. Note: Use weight releasers for only two-week waves because eccentrics are responsible for most muscle soreness due to damaged muscle cells. Speed pulls are done after speed squatting. For a three-week wave, three weight changes, one each week, can be employed. The second method is to introduce three different band tensions, starting with light bands and working up to a stronger tension band for the next two weeks. If a contest is the goal, a reverse wave must be used. Simply start with the strongest tension and reduce band tension each week for three weeks.

The top benchers I have spoken with reduce bar weight or band weight as the meet approaches, building a greater rate of force development. This is part of the delayed transmutation phase, working with the maximal effort work. Remember, each week the bar speed should be changed by altering the amount of chains, bands, or weight releasers, or a combination of all three.

I have covered speed work and max effort work, but what about GPP? For squatting, John "Chester" Stafford rotates box squats with and without added weight. He also does sled pulling for the upper or lower body, the reverse hyper machine, glute ham raises, abdominal work, and band work. For band work, he does 1–2 extra workouts a week. The workouts are 20–30 minutes long. He does band leg curls for about 60 reps in 2–3 sets followed by good mornings (arched or rounded back) for 2–3 sets. Then, he performs pull-throughs for three sets of 15 reps. The combinations are endless, and after 7–10 days, he starts a different complex.

The conjugate system is employed for speed work, max effort work, and extra workouts for strength development or GPP. Subsequently, restoration methods must be included as well. Water therapy, massage, spinal adjustments, acupressure, and acupuncture can be constantly rotated throughout the year and divided into weekly and monthly plans. Seventy percent of the world is covered by water. It is constantly moving in waves. Some are just ripples while others are as large as tsunamis. Yet, somehow they are coordinated together by the seasons just as our training is. It is natural to train in waves if thought about it in a systematic way.

When people come to Westside, they witness all the stages of training for an upcoming meet— the training just preceding a meet and the training months before a meet. They also get to see how a particular type of training is utilized. Anyone training for a meet has undergone some form of periodization. Unfortunately, most have misused a system in order to peak for a meet. Progressive gradual overload, or Western periodization, is based on a hypothetical goal, so at any time the percent of a lifter's contest max may be off by as much as 20%. Many times the lifter is missing weights three weeks from the contest because his expectations are too high or possibly too low.

Training should be calculated by using a formula based on math, not dreams. I suggest everyone read books on periodization by noted authors such as Tudor Bompa or Vladimir Zatsiorsky. These books explain periodization in terms of micro- and mesocycles. After all, periodization refers to the division of training into a yearly plan or even a four-year plan (i.e. an Olympic cycle). This system is used for weight lifting, powerlifting, and track and field, and of course, should be used for all sports requiring the development of power.

The former Soviet Union had so much data on training that they did not know what some top coaches were doing. Mel Siff (Supertraining) asked how I arrived at our three-week pendulum system. It was quite similar to that used by the great Soviet Union SHW champion, Vasily Alexeev. I said that after three weeks we could not become faster or stronger, so we waved back down and started over. Mel said that Alexeev found the same to be true, so with the help of Russian and Bulgarian research and that done at Westside with over 70 Elite powerlifters plus feedback from some of the greatest powerlifters around the world, our loading is based on Prilepin's table.

For benching speed work, we do nine sets of three reps, which is known as the dynamic effort method. Its purpose is to build a fast rate of force development. For squatting, the sets vary from 12 without bands or chains (i.e. a contrast method) to as low as three for the last week of a circa max phase, and the reps are always two. For speed pulls, the reps are one and the sets are 5–8.

The power clean and snatch are commonly used to develop speed-strength in high schools and colleges, but power lifts can be used to achieve the same purpose. For the bench, the bar speed should be a minimum of 0.75 meters/second (m/s) and a maximum of 1.0 m/s. Jeremiah Meyers and John Stafford have pulled 495 at 1.2 m/s for sets.

To find a lifter's total loading volume, multiply the sets by the number of reps. For example, nine sets of three reps for benching with 200 lbs on dynamic day is 5400 lbs. Always use chains or bands to accommodate resistance and help reduce bar deceleration. For squatting, 12 sets of two reps with 500 lbs is12,000 lbs. Only training sets should be calculated. At Westside, we follow the "rule of 60%." An extreme workout should occur every 72 hours, and the max effort day is about 60% of the dynamic day. By adding the weights employed on max effort day using weights of 70% up to max weight lifted, it is surprising to see how low the total volume actually is. We lift about 45–50% on average. The rule of 60% was introduced through Olympic lifting. Powerlifting training requires one to make much larger jumps, making it almost impossible to lift 60% of the total volume on max effort day.

At Westside, we don't follow the method of heavy efforts where two reps of multiple sets are used. By incorporating the conjugate system, we try an all-time max each week on a special core exercise. If the same core exercises are repeated, a lifter will regress if he is training above 90% of a 1RM.

The conjugate system originated at the Dynamo Club in the former Soviet Union. Seventy highly qualified lifters were observed to gather input. At Westside, we have had over 70 Elite powerlifters who have provided data over the years in addition to many highly skilled athletes from all sports just like at the Dynamo Club. The training can't be a flat loading system, meaning the volume can't be the same when the intensity goes from a low of 60–70% to a high of 90–100%. Through years of experience, it has been established that to gain better results, an increase in the training load must take place.

This can be done by increasing the number of workouts, increasing volume, and raising intensity, making the workouts more complex through special exercises.

Periodization plays different roles in training. At Westside, we use a three-week pendulum wave. To execute the wave, go up in bar weight for three weeks, using 8–10 sets with the suit straps down, and base the weight on a contest max. Use 50%, 55%, and 60% over the three weeks; then, wave back to 50% the following week.

Weights are based on a box squat max, using 75%, 80%, and 85%. For a preparatory phase that lasts nine weeks with a safety squat bar max of 640, it should look like this:

First wave: light band, 70 lbs of tension

325	10 sets 2 reps
375	10 sets 2 reps
415	8 sets 2 reps

Second wave: medium band, 140 lbs of tension

325	10 sets 2 reps
375	10 sets 2 reps
415	8 sets 2 reps

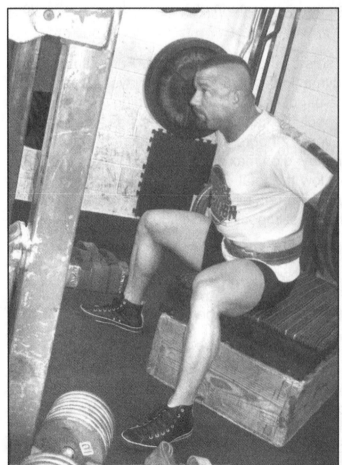

Third wave: strong band, 260 lbs of tension

325	8 sets 2 reps
375	8 sets 2 reps
415	6 sets 2 reps

Bars can be rotated to a 14-inch cambered bar, front squat bar, MantaRay, or a regular squat bar for a three-week wave, increasing bar weight, chain or band weight, or a combination. For the strength-speed cycle, a rule to follow is two weeks. To do this, use about 50% band tension and 50% bar weight. For example, Joe Bayles did a two-week wave for strength- speed with 520 lbs of band tension and 505 lbs of bar weight on a parallel box using four sets of two reps on week one and three sets of two reps on week two with 545 in bar weight and 520 in band tension. Going longer than two weeks for strength-speed is too taxing on the CNS.

For speed-strength, Chuck Vogelpohl had 440 lbs on the bar, plus 110 of band tension on the box and 260 lbs of tension at the top.

This is done for a three-week wave for ten sets in the first two weeks and eight sets the third. The bar weight goes to 480 for week two and 520 for week three. A speed-strength cycle precedes a strength-speed cycle, and a speed-strength cycle should come before a circa max cycle. With two major meets a year, a circa-max wave lasts three weeks. The bar weight is 47.5%, 50%, and 52% of a lifter's contest best with 40–45% band tension.

Week 1: 435 x 5 sets of two reps plus 440 lbs of band tension
Week 2: 485 x 4 sets of two reps plus 440 lbs of band tension
Week 3: Work up to a max single

"Dollar Bill," a 308, and Phil Harrington, a 181, have done 600 lbs plus 375 lbs of band tension to squat 900 and 905, respectively, at a meet. Phil's 905 was a world record at 181. These results are very reliable. The math reveals that a lifter's contest squat is about one-third higher than a box squat max with the suit straps down and no knee wraps. The results can vary about 3% either way. Greg Panora made a box squat with 645 plus 440 lbs of bands to squat 1000 at 238 and total 2485, a world record at 242. The larger the squat, the greater the band tension must be. The band tension must be great on the box as well.

We use a two-week wave for a circa-max cycle if three large totals are attempted in one year. Greg won the 2006 APF Nationals with an improvement from 2255 to 2369. In September, Greg made a 2485 total. For the September meet, he did 505 for two sets of two reps and 555 for two sets of two reps with 440 lbs of band tension on week one. For week two, he worked up to 645 with 440 lbs of band tension. He squatted 1000 lbs at the meet, a 60-lb PR. Good form is imperative on both a box and contest squat, and a lifter needs to be mentally prepared as well as in a highly trainable state.

Training for a meet can take its toll on anyone. A period of 1–2 weeks to download the total volume and intensity must occur. This period is referred to as the delayed transformation phase. Heavy weights should not be taken 1–2 weeks before a meet. All this does is show a lack of confidence. If a lifter is worried about his opener, he must be scared to death to take a third attempt in front of real judges.

For benching on the dynamic method day, every three weeks change the reactive method that is used (e.g. stronger bands for three weeks, more chains each week for three weeks, or added weight to weight releasers each week).The bar weight must stay the same. For speed deadlift pulls, the bar weight is 50% of a max deadlift and 30% band tension at the top. The band tension for deadlifts remains the same, but the bar weight should be raised slightly for three weeks and then return to the original weight. The max effort for improving the squat, bench, or deadlift must be rotated each week. A one-week plan is always used for max effort day. The conjugate system was intended for highly skilled lifters, but at Westside, when we start a new lifter who shows promise, he is placed in one of our groups and trains just like the advanced. This technique has yet to fail.

One-week and three-week cycles are arranged to produce high results at meets where they count. A yearly plan must be divided into one-week and three-week plans to fit a year of competition. It doesn't matter how strong someone is before a meet or after a meet; it only counts on meet day. With 13 lifters with totals above 2300 and five over 2500, our system has served us well.

Intensity Zone Loading

A loading plan is necessary if an athlete intends to reach the top in any sport, including powerlifting. The training plan must be divided into micro-cycles of one week. At Westside, all maximal effort work is done in micro-cycles. This way enables us to do lifts of 100% or more each week simply by switching a core exercise that resembles and contributes to raising the squat, bench, or deadlift. At Westside, we have a speed day for squatting, benching, and deadlifting. This is also referred to as the dynamic method, meaning using submaximal weights with maximal speed. This develops a fast rate of force in minimal time. Dr. Ben Tabachnik has said that it is common for athletes to be adapted to quickness exercises, which must be addressed either by:

- varying intensities
- changing the apparatus you are using

We do both:

- by using a pendulum wave, mostly with 50–55–60%
- changing part of the resistance by adding chains or bands

This is essential to completely developing speed-strength (i.e. starting and accelerating strength).

Controlling Volume

With the progressive overload method, it is virtually impossible to control the volume. If training at the 1% range, it is easily controlled. To squat 600, a total volume of 7200 lbs is needed. This is arrived at by using a top percent of 60% and a lower percent of 50%. For example, 50% of 600 = 300 x 12 sets of 2 reps = 7200 lbs. On week three, the weight is 60% of 600 = 360 x 10 sets of 2 reps = 7200. A volume of 9600 is used to squat 800 so 50% of 800 = 400 x 12 sets of 2 reps = 9600 lbs and 10 sets of 2 reps with 480 (60%) = 9600 lbs. This works for any squat of any weight, which is also called flat loading. During the three-week wave, special exercises are rotated, such as: glute ham raises, pull-throughs, and the reverse hyper. In week one, a lifter is unfamiliar with the exercise that promotes a bigger squat, so the volume is understandably low. By week three, the same lifter has grown familiar with the exercises and the volume grows. Success can't occur by doing only the classical lifts; progress will cease. The greater the lifter becomes the more tasks that are needed to stimulate progress.

Progressive gradual overload accomplishes only one goal at a time while actually detraining the phase just completed in as fast as 2–3 weeks. In addition, after a contest, a lifter must start over exactly where he initially began. The system Westside has adapted from the old Soviet system allows an athlete to build muscle mass, speed, and absolute strength; perfect form; raise GPP; increase flexibility; and practice restoration all year long, year after year. We raise all qualities gradually, never neglecting one for another. I am in no way criticizing the doctorates in the United States. It is, however, the material in the textbooks that is terribly outdated and perpetuates the truth when it leads nowhere, just like my dog Jackie's tail chasing. I suggest reading books such as Supertraining, which contains the ideas of many well-respected foreign experts on strength qualities.

Speed Training

At Westside there is a speed day for squatting, deadlifting, and benching. This is also referred to as the dynamic method, which implements submaximal weights with maximal speed. It is designed to develop a fast rate of force in a minimal time.

Dr. Ben Tabachnik has said that it is common for athletes to become easily adapted to quickness exercises. This must be addressed either by varying intensities or by changing the apparatus used. Westside lifters incorporate both by using a three-week pendulum wave, mostly with weights of 50%, 55%, and 60%. This also entails changing part of the resistance by adding chains or bands, which is essential to completely develop speed-strength (i.e. starting and accelerating strength).

Off-Season Training

I have been asked many times what we do in the off-season; we don't have an off- season. This would waste part of the year's training. We are a private gym and only powerlifters train here, with the exception of NFL prospects or sports teams that come to visit from around the world. The fact is some groups are always training for a meet, meaning their training partners must train with them regardless of their level of preparedness. For our max effort days, I copied the Bulgarian system. Just like the Bulgarians, we like to max out on an exercise that we have established a record on such as: the floor press, safety squat bar, low box squat, or pin two rack deadlift.

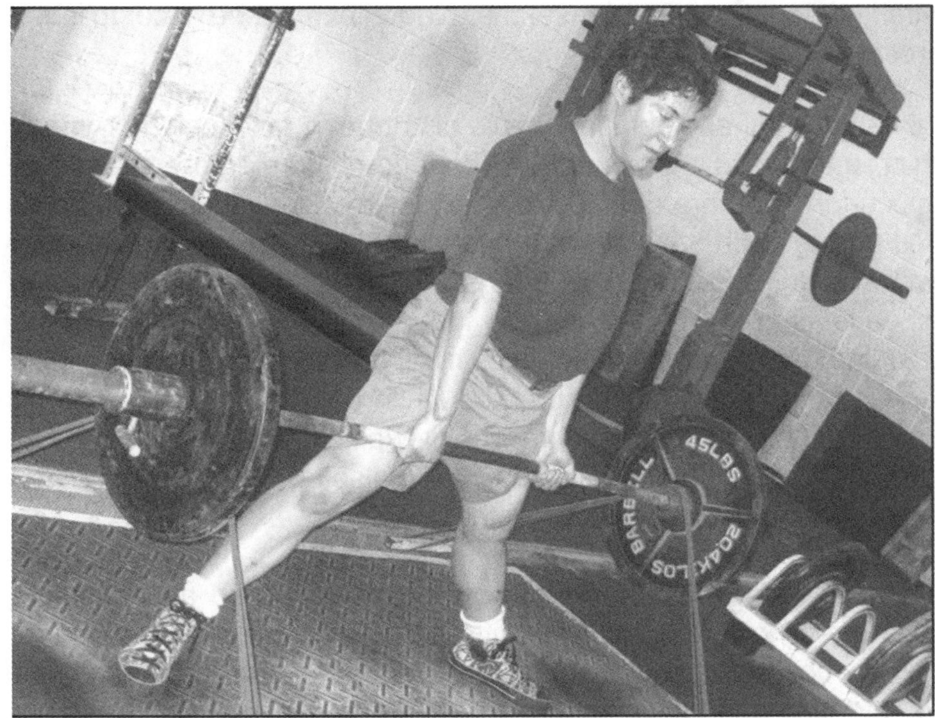

We may not be able to set a new record, but we do as much as we are capable of on that day. If a lifter stops training for two weeks, he could lose 10% of his strength. For example, a 1500 lb total would mean a reduction of 150 lbs. A 2300 total would show a loss of 230 lbs. Who can afford to do that? We can't. Can you?

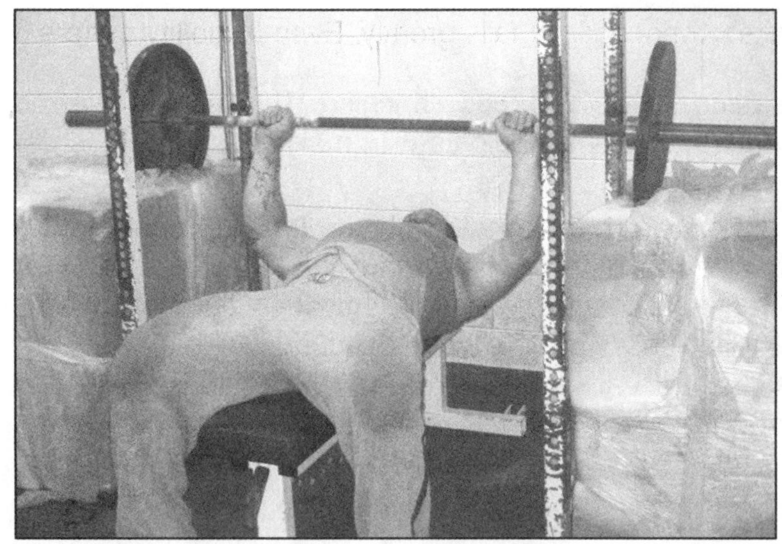

Unlike the top Bulgarians, we perform several exercises.We do squats with various bars (safety squat bar, Buffalo bar, and cambered bars) and with different apparatus (MantaRay, front squat harness, bands, and chains). It's the same process for bencing, implementing the following: three- or five-inch cambered bar, EZ curl bar, dumbbells at different angles, board press with 1- to 5-boards, benching with five different band tensions, full range band press, full range chain press with 3–5 sets of chains, benching with the lightened method, foam box pressing with real weight, and bands over the bar.

Our deadlift training is coupled with our squat training. Rack pulls, band pulls, lightened method deadlifts, and a variety of good mornings are used. Remember, when training with those who are going to meets and going through the circa-max phases, the other training partners must train along with them. The lifters who are not competing sometimes are training harder than those who are because of their level of preparedness. An individual can't be at his best at all times, but he must train as hard as possible all the time, year in and year out.

We must always raise our general physical preparedness. This is must be a priority to reach the top in any sport endeavor. The training must be very dense, meaning a lot must be accomplished in a training session with short rest periods.

Martin Rooney said a pyramid is only as tall as its base. This is also true in any sport. Too many pay attention to special strength preparedness and not enough to general strength preparedness. Because of this, many of our max effort days are devoted to special exercises such as sled pulling. We do a wide variety of sled pulling such as: walking forward with the strap hooked to your power belt, walking backward with the strap hooked to the lifter's power belt, walking forward with the strap held in the hands at knee level or lower, and walking forward with the strap held in the hands doing pressing motions, curling, pec work, or static holds in all positions. Upper body style holds build upper body size because the individual can breathe while holding statically for long time periods. This is great for football or hockey. Another variation is walking backward doing high pulls, upright rows, bent over rows, or external rotation exercises. We also do chins and dips, and we have a machine that reduces body weight while executing these exercises.

We try to build muscle mass all year long as well as work on explosive speed and absolute strength. In addition, we work on perfecting form in all three lifts. In an effective plan, one must increase speed, work capacity, and of course, absolute strength. All this is possible with the conjugate method. There is truly never an off-season when aiming for greatness. If an athlete does not train for two weeks, his strength can drop 10%.

If sled work is not engaged in for two weeks, work capacity falls greatly. Even flexibility suffers if not maintained.

Advanced System for Beginners

I hear all the time that Westside training is for the advanced and only top ten lifters can do the training that is required at Westside. It is true that our training is advanced, but it is also great for beginners. Why start out wrong or start with a program that yields only small results?
Our stats show that we have developed 63 Elite lifters. Many of those received their start at Westside and became world record holders including Heath, Patterson, Fusner, Dimel, Halbert, and Vogelpohl as well as many women. It's true that we have many advanced methods for all ages. It's also true that I totaled Elite in five weight classes, all USPF meets, and had never heard of chains, bands, circa-max, pendulum waves, or delayed transformation; however, I had the commonsense to read and learn.

What Chuck Vogelpohl did to make his first Elite total in 1988 is the basis for what he does today. Because the Westside system is mathematical, it is based on a percent of a lifter's limit strength. It can be used by a 300 squatter or a 900 squatter. They would both train with the same percent and use a three-week pendulum wave. The percents range from 50–60%. A 300 lb squatter would use 150–180 lbs on speed day:

- Week 1, 150 for 12 x 2 reps
- Week 2, 165 for 12 x 2 reps
- Week 3, 180 for 10 x 2 reps

These weights ensure correct form. Using proper form is a must for beginners who are learning how to do power lifts. Speed-strength is built, which is a very important element of total strength development and best taught early in the career. Interjecting short rests (45 seconds) between sets is known as the interval method. The short rest builds general physical preparedness (GPP) and mental toughness. For the novice, building the weak links in the chain is imperative; otherwise, if this is not addressed at an early stage, poor form, or worse, injuries can occur, cutting a career short. Much of the training volume should consist of special exercises. If a lifter's squat stops making progress, more squatting will not help. The lagging muscle group must be targeted.

A novice must have good coaches. Notice that I said "coaches," not "coach." When a lifter reaches a high standard, it does not mean he can coach. At Westside, we have many great lifters who have risen from nothing to greatness. As I taught the Westside training system to our lifters, they were learning what constitutes good form, what volume to use, and what exercise is best for a particular body type. In essence, I taught them to lift as well as to coach. Every lift is thoroughly coached at Westside. We constantly analyze each other before something becomes a problem.

It is important for beginners to learn everything about training. At meets, our new lifters all display good form. This is not the case with most beginners at meets. We insist that beginners squat wide and bench close. This ensures that the correct muscle groups are developed.

For squatting, it's the posterior chain—the hamstrings, glutes, calves, and spinal erectors. An individual with little knowledge will try to build the quads to increase his squat. This, however, reduces hip flexion, resulting in difficulty reaching a parallel position in the squat and destroying the lockout in the deadlift to the point where the lifter can't make the top 100 in the weight class below him.

When we bring a new face in, we don't try to train his squat like Chuck trains today, but rather how he started out plus chains. We update our training continuously. We no longer use a five- week wave but rather a more efficient three-week wave. In Chuck's early stages, he used 50–60% for a three-week wave. For example, when Chuck's squat was 600 at a meet, he would do the following:

- Week 1: 50% (300) for 12 sets of 2 reps, 60 seconds rest
- Week 2: 55% (330) for 12 sets of 2 reps, 60 seconds rest
- Week 3: 60% (360) for 10 sets of 2 reps, 60 seconds rest

On week four, Chuck would start over at 50% and repeat the three-week pendulum wave. As his meet squat increased, his workload would slowly increase. When Chuck squatted 600, his squat volume was 7200 lbs: 300 (50%) for 12 sets of 2 reps = 7200 lbs; 360 (60%) for 10 sets of 2 reps = 7200 lbs. When Chuck's squat was 700, his volume was 8400 lbs: 350 (50%) for 12 sets of 2 reps = 8400 lbs; 385 for 12 sets of 2 reps for week 2; and 420 (60%) for 10 sets of 2 reps = 8400 lbs. It took 1200 lbs of squats to push his squat from 600 to 700.

When Chuck made his first 800 squat, the work load looked like this:

- Week 1: 400 for 12 sets of 2 reps = 9600 lbs
- Week 2: 440 for 12 sets of 2 reps to raise volume
- Week 3: 480 for 10 sets of 2 reps = 9600 lbs

When training at 50–60%, the work is equal for all. Up to this point, Chuck used three sets of 5/8-inch chains placed correctly on the bar (see the reactive methods video). He slowly raised his squat volume systematically, along with other special exercises including the reverse hyper, pull-throughs, back raises, abs, lats, and sled pulling. Chuck's extra workouts went from one a week to four over the course of five years. The extra workouts not only raise work capacity and increase flexibility, mobility, general physical preparedness, they also enhance special physical preparedness (SPP). A beginner should use chains to accommodate resistance. This builds a strong start, enabling a lifter to overcome the additional resistance that the chains provide. Chains also help eliminate bar deceleration. This program is based on percents of 1RM and can be used for someone who squats as little as 100 lbs.

Chuck's squat was 865 when bands were introduced to his training. After a year, his squat jumped to 1000 at 220 lbs, but this was after years of intense training. It's simple; Chuck raised his work capacity through box squats, special exercises, extra workouts, and restoration work. I started Chuck out at the beginning. He was not born squatting 800 but systematically rose to world record status. Someone who does not squat three and a half times his own bodyweight should not do the circa-max phase, nor does he need a three-week delayed transformation phase. At Chuck's first meet (1986), he totaled around 1600 at a light 220. Today, his total is 2319, plus his best lifts consist of 2419 in the same weight class.

This is a portrait of training adaptation. Not only is the volume increased but the training has become more sophisticated, and the form in all lifts is constantly improved.

Because everyone likes the bench, let's look at George Halbert's history at Westside. We saw George bench in Columbus for two years and make zero progress. During this time, he was stalled at 475, which is when we convinced him to join us. Like most beginners, his bench form was terrible. It took a couple of years to correct it, focusing on both with technique and exercises. George's pecs were much stronger than his arms, so we changed his arm position and concentrated on his triceps. After one year, his bench jumped to 628 at 275 bodyweight. George learned from Chuck to watch his diet, lowering his weight to 198, enabling him to set the world record three times in one meet ending with a 683. This was done mostly with chains.

At first, George was taught a lot of exercises. Later on, he began to teach us, much like Chuck did in the squat and deadlift. I have many books about training adaptation, but at Westside, I have watched it as well as participated in it. George began at the lowest level and started over correctly. Like any beginner, he started doing lots of triceps, so he could take the pecs out of the lift. He found out how to push the bar straight up, eliminating pec pulls and shoulder problems.

When following the writing in Powerlifting USA, it becomes evident that the training constantly changes year after year. Though training has become much more complex, it's much easier today than 15 years ago. We have eliminated the useless work, and as we have gathered more information, it is much easier to progress. The poundage barriers have fallen. For example, in our gym, 700 lb benches and 1000 lb squats are common.

It took George Halbert several years to go from a 500 bench to 700, yet Paul Keyes, a newcomer who trains under George, went from a 585 bench to 750 in an astonishing 51 weeks. He's still progressing. Matt Smith came to Westside with a meager 1800 total. In four years, he took that to 2400 by training under our more experienced lifters. Now, Matt has totaled over 2500, and his training made it possible for the astounding progress of SHW Tim Harold. Tim went from 1800 to 2400 in two years. What we learned from working with Matt made it possible to take a novice to prominence at the tender age of 20. This made Tim the youngest to bench 700 and total 2400.

When reading this, I hope it is clear to see that Westside uses an advanced system for the beginner. Why start out incorrectly? Or why do the same program for years just to total the same numbers?

Westside not only teaches correct form, how to raise GPP and SPP, how to raise work capacity, how to teach others, how to know when to wear stronger gear, how to separate different types of training and to know the effect of a particular training load, but also how to find the proportionate training load that matches an individual's maximum strength while organizing training for an annual goal.

We have developed 63 USPF Elites at Westside, many participating in their first meet under Westside's supervision. If only I had the advantage of starting out under Chuck Vogelpohl, George Halbert, Joe Bayles, Matt Smith, Mike Ruggeira, and so on. In the 1970s, it was Tom Paulucci, Doug Heath, Gary Sanger, and Bill Wittaker who helped orchestrate the early Westside system.

Then in the early 1980s, I turned to the top former Soviet sports scientists such as: V. Zatsiorsky, T. Bumpa, A. Medvedev, P. Komi, N. Ozolin, AS Prilepin, R. Roman, and of course, Mel Siff, whose Supertraining manuals have brought much to the United States. Even though we have rivals, we can learn from everyone, including Bill Crawford who has conducted several seminars for our lifters, and Jesse Kellum who has also offered much to use. Along with Crawford and Kellum, Bill Gillespie has voiced his views on benching.

Beginners should first learn form and then add chains and later bands. There should be no circa-max squatting until a lifter can squat three and a half times his body weight. Light equipment should be mastered and then graduate to stronger gear, and lift in positive federations or face the reality of being frozen in time. There is no reason that a beginner should not start with an advanced system, just as everyone sends his son to Bobby Knight's basketball camp. I've seen lots of lifters come and go; don't be one of those. Start right to avoid incurring injuries, failing to make progress, or being forced to stop lifting.

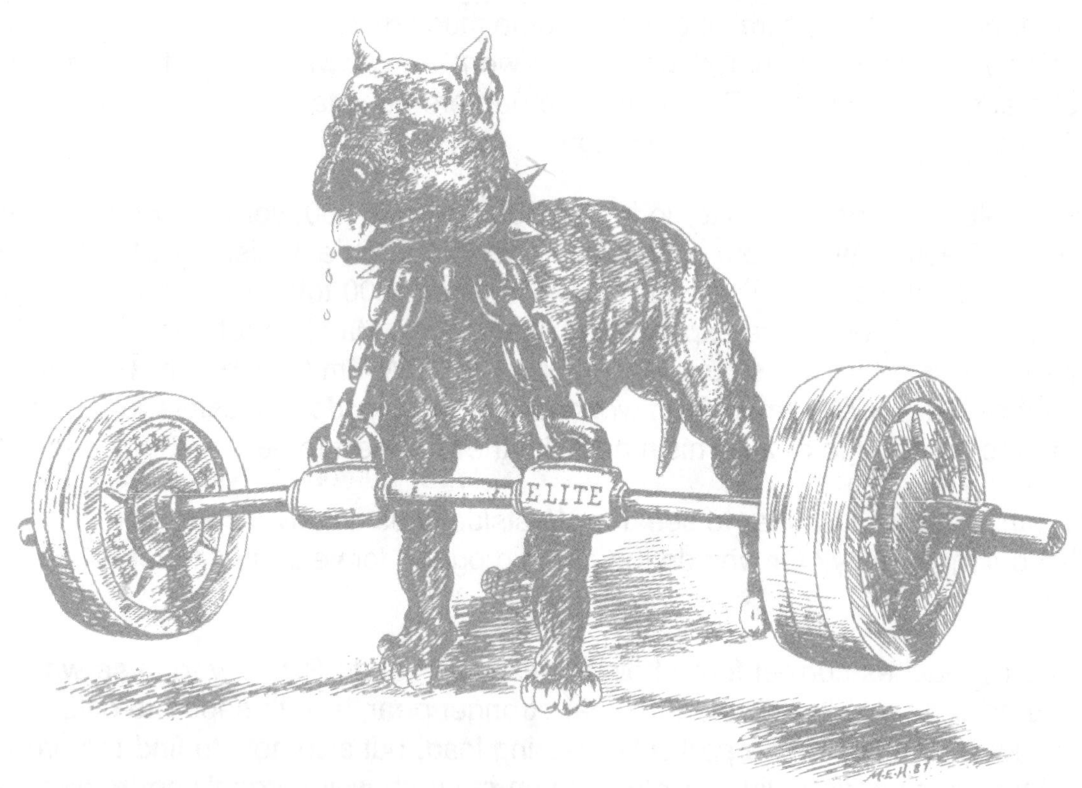

WESTSIDE BARBELL™

WESTSIDE BENCH PRESS TRAINING

Everyone strives for a goal, one may be a 500 bench. The problem is how to achieve it? For me, it was a mystery until I discovered a method of training known as the conjugate method.

Dynamic Effort Day

On Sunday, Westside lifters use the dynamic method. We do 8–10 sets of three reps, and it's best to use three or more grips in a workout. Most of the sets are done with a grip inside the power rings on the bar, or with the little finger inside the ring. Using grips inside the rings aids greatly in triceps and anterior delt development. The reps must be very explosive, so lower the bar quickly but with control. Lowering contributes to raising concentric strength. Lowering a bar slowly builds muscle mass but not strength. Plyometrics is the energy gained by the body dropping and then responding to that dropping with reversal or explosive strength. The bar should be pushed back up in a straight line, not back over the face, which requires strong triceps. This path is a shorter, safer distance and requires no shoulder rotation. The barbell always seeks the strongest muscle group, causing most push the bar over the face because the delts are stronger than the triceps. However, it should be the reverse. Shoulder and pec injuries are prevalent unlike triceps injury. Why? The triceps have not been pushed to their maximum potential. At Westside, we do approximately 20 reps out of 200 above our training weight. We may add only 30–50 lbs to the bar, checking that bar speed remains high. If the bar speed or reversal strength slows, there is a problem.

After bench pressing, immediately follow with triceps work. Basically, 60 total reps are done with dumbbells broken down into five sets of ten reps or possibly seven sets of eight reps. The palms should be facing inward toward the body when dumbbells are used for extensions. When a barbell is used, 40 reps should be done, bringing the bar to the forehead, chin, or throat. We do a lot of JM presses, named after JM Blakely. This is a very effective exercise that is executed with a close grip, lowering the bar 4–5 inches off the chest above the nipples, and holding for a split second, and then, pressing back up.

Following triceps, complete front raises with a bar, plate, or dumbbells. Use heavy weights. Also, do side delts with dumbbells or a cable, rear delts, 4–5 sets of lats, and a few hammer curls. Delt and lat work should be completed by feel but continuously do more adding heavier weight. This workout is executed on Sunday and lasts no longer than one hour and ten minutes.

Here are a few examples:

Speed bench with bands: These should be done for 8–9 sets of three reps. A lifter should use 45% of his 1RM on the floor press. The bands provide 40 lbs of tension on the chest and 85 lbs of tension at the top.

Speed bench off power rack pins: Set the pins at chest level. Lower the bar to the pins, relax for a second, and then, blast the bar to completion. This relaxed state is overcome by dynamic work. Use bands or chains.

Buffalo bar: The same can be done with a Buffalo bar, which has a two-inch camber. Bill Gillespie of the Seattle Seahawks used this method and the previous one and so far has a 782 bench in a single poly to prove it.

Floor press: Chuck Scherza uses the floor press for his dynamic work. His bench has gone from 525 to about 700. Consequently, Chuck had triceps surgery after he did the 525 bench. Incline or decline press: Incline and decline presses can be completed with a bar. Use jump- stretch bands to accommodate resistance and build starting and accelerating strength. Bands can even be used with dumbbells by placing the band around the lifter's back and looping the ends over his palms before picking up the dumbbells like Clay Brandenburg does.

Lightened method: This is done by attaching bands at the top of a power rack or Monolift to reduce the bar weight at the chest. We attach jump-stretch bands at the top of a seven-foot rack. Blue bands reduce the weight by 150 lbs at the chest, green bands by 95 lbs, and purple bands by 65 lbs. Chains can also be used.

Maximum Effort Day

Wednesday's workout is called the maximum effort method day. When using a barbell, do singles. Naturally, work up slowly but always try a new max. We do many exercises on this day, resembling the bench press but are not regular bench presses, which is known as conjugate training. After doing an exercise with weights over 90% for 5–6 weeks, strength regresses. We train at 100% plus all year long by changing a barbell exercise every 2–3 weeks. Westside lifters are constantly going to meets, which are small and primarily in Ohio. Because top lifters should lift in their respective states to entice new talent into the sport, we like to represent Ohio.

Westside lifters also attend the biggest meets such as: the APF Senior Nationals, IPA Nationals, IPA World Cup, WPO Bash for Cash, WPO Show of Strength, and the WPO Finals at the Arnold Classic in Columbus, Ohio, our home base. While the squat used to be a crap shoot, it's now the bench that causes the most bomb-outs lately. Sometimes the shirt is too strong, or the lifter is too weak. Confidence can make an individual a champ while overconfidence can make someone a chump.

Though some prefer to lift "raw," bench shirts are here to stay. If one has a sense of history and remembers names such as: Mike MacDonald, Larry Pacifico, Jeff Magruder, and of course, Jim Williams (675 in 1972 at SHW), the truth is that what people think is that good raw benching today is mostly pretty sad. What does it take to bench a personal record at contest time? The first is methods of training, and there are three standard methods.

Dynamic method:
Submaximal weights with maximum speed are used. This method teaches the lifter to display explosive strength and improve the rate of force development.

Maximum effort method:
This is defined by lifting the heaviest weight possible for one rep with no time limit or without a large emotional stress, meaning a training max not a contest max. At Westside, the above two methods occur 72 hours apart.

Repetition to near failure:
Westside lives on special exercises, but reps are done to near failure for triceps, lats, and delts. Basically, these are the muscle groups used in the three lifts.

The problem today is the popularity of bench shirts, and their ability to raise one's bench considerably. There are some who will only do shirt work, or that is, band pressing with a bench shirt. The lifter sets his shirt to barely touch 3-boards and then adjusts it to touch 2-boards. Finally, the shirt is cranked to maximally work on 1-board. In our gym, George Halbert's group followed this for months only to discover that it didn't work. They became very good on board pressing with a shirt, but they discovered they had no groove, or even worse, the ability to touch their chest. This resulted in a lot of bomb-outs. At our gym, 20 feet away from George's group, a second group tried the same routine and came to the same conclusion. This time, four top lifters had miserable results. Only one out of four made a bench, and it was 70 lbs under his best. Why? Using a bench shirt is not max effort work because the shirt is doing the work, not the lifter. Remember the three main methods of training? The shirt work replaced max effort work but not really. All of a sudden, the lifters couldn't lock out weights that had been easy, and some did not do speed work.

The dynamic method is not intended to raise maximal strength but to teach a lifter to display explosive strength and improve the rate of force development. Zatsiorsky explains this in Science and Practice of Strength Training. I have heard many say that speed is not important; this is incorrect thinking. There is only so much time to complete a max lift. A lifter will fail to lift more weight when his muscles are contracted for a given time limit. The sprinter can only sprint so far before decelerating. The top sprinters accelerate a longer distance than a novice sprinter. The stronger a man or woman is, the shorter period he or she can exert maximal force. This is why speed and acceleration are so important.

When using a shirt in training, it takes a long time to work up to a max. Because testosterone drops rapidly after 45 minutes, dense training is a must. Dense training refers to how much training is done in a particular time limit versus how much rest is taken during the same time limit. When putting a shirt on and taking it off, actual training time is limited, resulting in little time for exercises for the triceps, delts, pecs, and lats to be done. As a lifter learns to use a shirt, he must also learn to touch his chest. Bill Crawford says that the chest must be touched.

Before a lifter board presses with a bench shirt, he should have a shirt that he can touch 450, establishing a max record such as 510 in that shirt. Next, the same lifter should use a shirt that allows him to touch 500 and possibly a max of 570. Finally, the individual should use a shirt that allows 550 and find his max with that shirt, which I'm guessing is maybe 625. A bigger bencher would use three stronger bench shirts, and a lesser bencher, say a 400 max, would do the same with a weaker set of shirts. Today, anybody can achieve a big bench quickly due to the perfection of bench shirts. However, soon after a lifter's bench tops out, he must become physically stronger. If he doesn't, he'll disappear from the power scene. The answer is, of course, to learn how to use a bench shirt while raising natural strength.

George Halbert has set 11 all-time world records in the bench in three weight classes, yet he recently made an all-time gym personal record of 625 without a bench shirt prior to making 746 and 766 at Kieran Kidder's Bash for Cash in Orlando in September 2004 during a hurricane. Fred Boldt, at 181, made 597 in Orlando with George. He also made a 622 world record, which was turned down for a technicality. George and Fred both do shirt work, touching the chest in the gym. As a second and more successful experiment, Joe Bayles, who had a 630 bench, made 700 lbs in a full meet and totaled 2325 at 242. Mike Brown, at 19-years-old, made a 735 bench and totaled

2300 in his first meet at 295 body weight, and Tim Harold hit a 715 bench and totaled 2455 at SHW at 20-years-old. Zach Cole went from a 575 to a 600 bench at 276. This group did shirt work off their chests, and most of the board work was done without a shirt. Joe made a 605 2-board press with no shirt prior to his 700 at the IPA Nationals in 2004. Nowhere have I read that wearing a bench shirt is max effort work. The shirt is doing the work, not the muscular system of the lifter. In fact, a true max strength decreases as we have discovered. Recently, I have seen four lifters break an arm doing a contest bench. I believe this is due to training shortcuts. As one buys a stronger bench shirt, he neglects to train harder to become stronger. Unfortunately, something has to give, and it is the lifter. Therefore, if a lot of cash is going to be spent for a shirt, try spending some time getting stronger. Musashi Miyarnoto has said that to do nothing is worthless.

Floor Presses

To properly execute a floor press, lower the bar until the triceps are completely on the floor and relaxed before pressing the bar up. By relaxing the arms, the eccentric/concentric chain is broken, building explosive strength as well as the bottom part of the bench press.

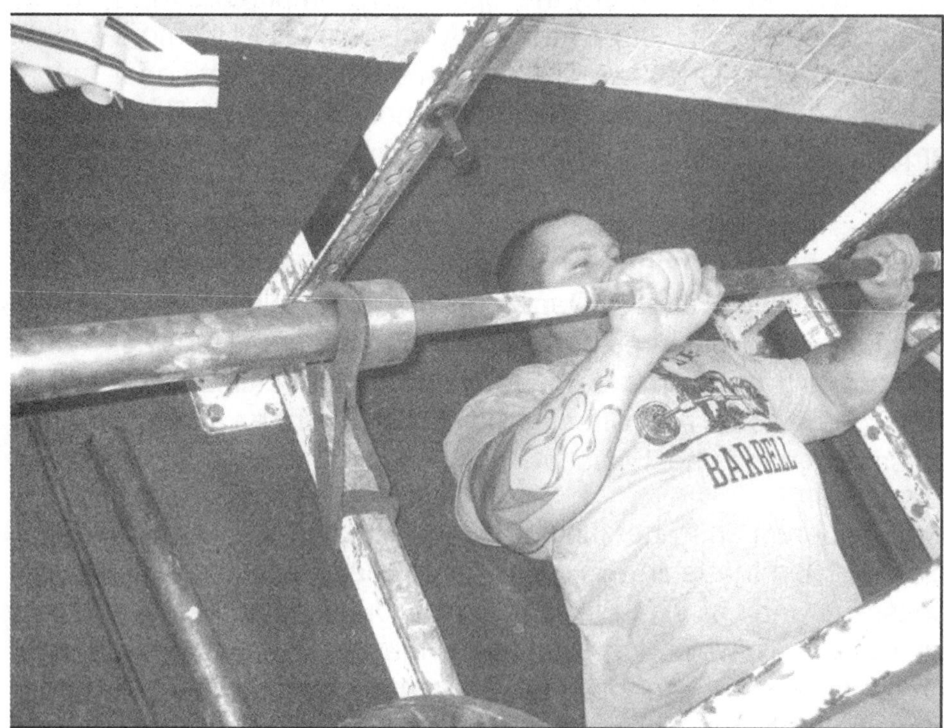

Board Press

Board presses build the middle part of the bench press. Lay 2–3, 2 x 6s on the chest, bring thebar down to the boards, and pressback up. This is much different from a rack press because the weight is transferred on to the chest, shoulders, and arms. When using 3-boards, use a close grip, with the index finger just touching the smooth part of the bar, and with 2-boards, place the little fingers on the power rings.

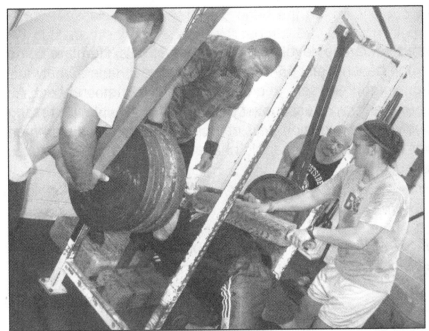

Rack Lockouts

We use many pin positions all at the top.

The bar moves 4–5 inches on the top pin and 10–12 inches on the lowest pin. Always use a close grip. Never lower the weight. Instead, press the bar off the pins concentrically.

When dumbbells are used for incline, decline, floor, seated, or regular presses after a warm up, go to a heavy weight such as 110s, trying a rep record.

The repetition method encompasses a rep range of15–20, and the lifter must go to failure. Weighted push-ups with the feet higher or lower than the hands are done the same way. A lifter should warm up and max out with a 25, 45, or 100 lb plates on the upper back or have a training partner sit on his shoulders, facing the same direction. Dumbbells and push-ups also act as a hypertrophy aid. Illegally wide bench presses, an inch or so outside the power rings, act as a strength and muscle builder when a six rep max is established for a 2–3 week mini-cycle. The elbows must be tucked. Note: A six rep max means the most weight one can get for six reps after a warm up.

One core (above) exercise per week should be implemented followed by a total of 4–5 special exercises for the triceps, delts, upper back, and lats. Always push up special exercises. Key notes: It is not necessary to do a max bench press to develop absolute strength. All that is required is to place the muscles in a situation, involving a strong contraction for a period of time that duplicates the time in which a max bench press is performed. This works best through maximizing a certain portion of the lift (bottom, mid-way, or top) using the maximum effort method. Fast lowering, or the eccentric phase, of a bench press produces momentum that is converted into kinetic energy that aids in raising the bar back to arms' length. Floor presses, like box squatting, builds explosive strength by overcoming a static position through active or dynamic work. Don't pause the bench press in training. This builds mainly static strength. The stretch reflex lasts up to two full seconds, much longer than a legal pause.

However, do pause when doing floor presses and board presses. When doing rack presses, remember to press off a prescribed pin setting. This requires one to overcome inertia. As the triceps get stronger, add chains to the bar for bench pressing. Use 5/8 chains that are five feet long looped through a half-inch chain that is fixed around the Olympic bar sleeve. Half of the 5/8-inch chain should be resting on the floor to start. When the bar is on the chest, all the chain should be on the floor. At this position, have the original 55–60% of the 1RM on the bar; this is critical.

Periodization for the Bench Press

For benching, explosive and speed-strength can be developed by many methods. Here are some guidelines to follow for speed work for the bench. Rest 45–60 seconds between sets and always use proper form. Use bands, chains, or weight releasers to create the reactive method effect. Although there is a pause with the floor press and pin press, never pause on the chest. While resting a bar on the chest, many of the muscles will retain tension. This dampens the stretch reflex. When the bar is resting on pins on the power rack after the eccentric phase, the entire body can relax. Then, explode like a boxer throwing a jab.

Dynamic method:
Do regular benches with 40–55% of the shirtless max. Lower the bar quickly and reverse as quickly as possible to completion. Perform 8–10 sets of three reps.

Ballistic method:
Use the same 45–50% load of a shirtless max. Drop the bar quickly but control it in the descent with the lats, not the triceps. Catch the bar 1–3 inches off the chest, and reverse it concentrically as quickly as possible.

Floor press:
Again, apply the same 45–50% load of a shirtless max. Lie on the floor inside of a power rack, and lower the squat J-hooks to use as bench supports. Lower the bar until the triceps are resting on the floor and the arms are relaxed. Violently contract all the pressing muscles and drive the bar to completion. The floor press, like the box squat, allows the lifter to have some muscles relaxed and some static.

Weight releasers:
This is an explosive eccentric phase. Load the bar to a 50% of a shirtless max. Add weight releasers to the bar with 30% weight of the lifter's best. Lower the bar loaded to 80% at the top, and after stripping the 30% off, press the remaining 50% up as fast as possible. This is a contrast method that really increases a lifter's reactive ability.

Speed-strength:
Attach a 4x4 under each side of the power rack and loop mini-bands underneath it. Stretch both ends of the mini-bands under the bar. Do eight sets of three reps and lower the bar as quickly as possible.

Strength-speed:
Use two mini-bands in the same manner as above. This may sound light, but for the development of strength-speed, bands are much harder than regular bar weight.

Speed bench off power rack pins:
Set the pins at chest level; then, lower the bar to the pins and relax for a second. Blast up to full completion. This is relaxed overcome by dynamics work. Use bands and chains. Arch bar or Buffalo bar: This can be done with the Buffalo bar or the Westside arch bar. It has a two-inch camber. Bill Gillespie of the Seattle Seahawks used this method and the previous method to achieve a 782 bench in a single ply poly.

Incline or decline press:
The incline or decline press with a barbell can also be used. Jump-stretch bands can be implemented to accommodate resistance and build starting and accelerating strength. Bands can even be used with dumbbells by placing the band around the lifter's back and looping the ends over the palms before picking up the dumbbells.

Lightened method:
This is performed by attaching the bands at the top of the power rack or Monolift, reducing the bar weight at the chest. At Westside, we attach the bands on a seven-foot power rack. Blue bands reduce the weight 150 lbs, green bands by 95 lbs, and purple bands by 65 lbs. The lightened method can also be used by using foam, which is very efficient and sports-specific.

Intensity Zone Loading for the Bench Press

The loading for the bench press is similar to that for squatting, but of course, it must be somewhat lighter due to the smaller muscle groups used. It has a dynamic method day, occurring on Saturday or Sunday, and the max effort day is about 72 hours later on Wednesday, which is the amount of time required to recover from extreme workouts. We do a circa-max phase, but the de- loading phase is somewhat differently.

With the dynamic method day, we do nine sets of three reps because we use three different grips on the bench. We do three sets with the index finger just touching the smooth part of the bar, three sets two inches from the smooth part of the bar, and three sets with the little finger on the power ring. These can be done in any sequence.

Increasing bar speed is most important, not raising the bar weight. Remember Fred Boldt? He made a 495 official bench at 165 training with 185 lbs and two sets of 5/8-inch chains or a mini-band. In October 2002, he made a 540 bench, weighing 163 with the same bar weight. How? A faster bar equals more force. Eskil Thomasson at 275 made a 485 bench, and Fred did his 495 and a 550 at the same meet in October. They train together, but most importantly, they use the same bar weight.

In a weekly plan, or a micro-cycle, the bar loading equals 27 lifts per week. In four weeks, or a monthly load or meso-cycle, the number of lifts is 104. The percent may vary slightly, but the main reasons for this day are two-fold:

1. speed strength preparation
2. develop the ability to direct one's movements correctly.

Why three reps? We set the number of reps so the lifter can still do the last, or third, rep of a set at maximal velocity. A fast descent and a fast reversal phase increases reaction time. Not only must a lifter increase coordination and technical skill but also develop a complex manifestation of velocities:

- increasing velocity
- gathering momentum

The training percent with a combination of bar weight and bands looks like this. The bar weight is 33%, the bar and band weight at the bottom is 42%, and the bar and band weight at the top is 50%. The number of lifts per week or per month remains the same when using chains (i.e. 27 per week or 104 per month).

What about max effort day? By our own research, it has been found that lifts above 90% of a 1RM look like this. The last lift before a record attempt is about 90%. After a 90% lift, try a new record and possibly one more lift. This is a total of three lifts. For example, if a 2 board record is 500 lbs, the lifter's 90% weight would be 455, easy to load. Then, do 505 for a personal record followed by 510 or 520. This is all an advanced lifter will achieve.

The number of lifts remains the same regardless if they are full-range or partial. Frequently, I refer to Prilepin's table, but we do somewhat vary the number of lifts. In actuality, Prilepin's table was calculated for the Olympic lifts, not the power lifts; therefore, I calculate the percent on dynamic day on the basis of a contest max, meaning a bench shirt max. No bench shirt is used on max effort day, but the changes in the number of lifts are due to the fact that the pressing muscles can't withstand the work that the pulling or squatting muscle systems can.

How does the two days' loading look? The dynamic day for a microcycle or weekly load is 27 lifts. A meso-cycle, or monthly load, is 104 lifts. Note that 20% of the load should be above the normal percent. However, if the weights are too heavy, this negatively affects max effort day. A microcycle for max effort is three lifts as described earlier. A meso-cycle would be 12 lifts per month. Of course, special work for the triceps, delts, lats, and upper back must follow both workouts.

Loading for Repetition—Work to Failure

For dumbbell work, we do three sets to failure with a set weight such as 100 lbs. First, warm up with lighter dumbbells. Then, do a max set to failure. Rest about five minutes, and follow with a second set to failure. Take five minutes of rest again, and complete a final set. Keep a record of one set and three set maxes. Try records in the seated, flat, incline, and decline presses and presses on a stability ball, which can be done for push-ups as well. When using a barbell, a 6RM works well. Either a close grip, wide grip, or illegally wide grip can be applied.

A dumbbell or barbell rep max should be done every 4–5 weeks for two weeks in a row. A guideline for barbell work is that it should represent about 80% of a 1RM without a shirt. When u dumbbells are employed, simply add the total reps on all three sets. As a lifter's total volume increases with the same dumbbells, his bench should go up. A better bench shirt can be purchased only for so long because eventually, an individual just has to get stronger.

Sample Bench Press Workouts

I am frequently asked to write personal workouts for a fee; however, I don't have the time to do this. Westside makes training tapes on all matters of training, plus I write articles for Powerlifting USA almost monthly. This way Westside can reach a large audience. Besides not having the time to do personal workouts, if I can't see an individual in person, I can't tell his weaknesses, which could be anything from a lagging muscle group to bad form.

Power lifts take years to learn. After 13 years of training, I realized I knew very little about it even after making top ten lifts in all categories from 1972–2002. I was eighth in the bench press in 1980 without a bench shirt, so I know how to raise a raw bench. I was sixth in 2002 with a bench shirt, but I was very weak. Shortly after that, I received a new shoulder socket and had bicep surgery followed by a second shoulder operation. In1993 after 23 years of continuous training, I started to understand bench pressing. Back then, Westside had three, 600 lb benchers who were all juniors. Now, after 25 years, I am beginning to understand more fully how to bench. As of 2005, Westside has produced 16, 700 plus benchers and one, 800 plus bencher in addition to 25, 650 plus benchers with the lightest being Jason Fry, who did 650 at 180 lbs.

The following is a six-week general program that Westside follows. Incidentally, all the men I write about train at Westside. Anyone is welcome to visit; just set up a date with our office because we are not open to the public.

Speed work, or the dynamic method, develops a fast rate of force, and maximal strength comes from special exercises. Speed work should be completed on Saturdays or Sundays. After a good warm up, complete nine sets of three reps. John Stafford's bench is 733 at 275; his weight on the bar is 205–225, which is 45% of his 1RM on the floor press. This formula works for everyone. The grips encompass the following: three sets with the index finger touching the smooth part of the bar, three sets with the thumbs extending from the edge of the smooth part of the bar, and three sets with the little fingers on the power ring. Mini-bands or 2–3 sets of chains Westside style must be employed.

This simple method builds all major muscle groups. The safest way to bench is to press the bar in a straight line, not over the face, remembering the shortest distance between two points is a straight line. Lower the bar as quickly as possible, creating a strong stretch reflex for reversal strength. A lifter's speed with his worse grip should be at least 0.7 meters/second. After benching, choose a bar to complete a triceps exercise such as the JM press, straight bar for triceps extension, or football bar for extensions, consisting of 3–6 reps per set. Work up as heavy as possible on that particular day; then, choose a second triceps exercise with dumbbells (e.g. extensions with elbows out to the sides or roll backs with palms facing), working up in weight or choose a weight and do multiple sets. Dumbbell reps should be in the 6–12 range for 40–70 total reps.

Because the triceps are the prime bench press mover, they must fire first, so they have to be the strongest muscle group. At the first sign of staleness, change the barbell or dumbbell exercise or both, allowing progress to continue throughout the year. Next, do lat work, choosing 1–2 exercises such as: barbell or dumbbell rows, chest supported rows, or lat pull-downs. The lats help place the bar on the chest, helping to lower the bar. As for all exercises, reps and sets are based on an individual's level of preparedness. Lastly, work the side and rear delts, upper back, and biceps with hammer curls. Pre-hab work should be completed for the pecs and rotators.

On max effort day, work up to a max single, which may not be an all-time record, but it must be a current max. Doing sets of 2–3 reps with weights above 90% is known as the method of heavy efforts. The volume is high but the intensity can be higher. If training at 85, 90, or 95%, an athlete is really only using 85, 90, or 95% of his muscle potential, not 100%. Technique must be built by singles, and limit the top lifts after a good warm up to three. The first weight should be at 90% or so, the second near a record or just above, and then, possibly one more single. For example, for a floor press record of 500 lbs, the first attempt might be 450, the second 490, and the last 505. This workout should occur on Wednesday, allowing ten days off heavy weights before meet time. This is also 72 hours from the last extreme bench workout.

Below is an outline of a six-week program. The sequence can change to fit an individual's preferences, adding or replacing the core exercises in this program.

Workout # 1: Do floor press with 200 lbs of chain draped over the sleeve. Next, add weight to the bar until a max on that day results. George Halbert's best is 445 with 200 lbs of chain. For example, here is how George works up to his best:

1. 135 plus chains for 5 reps
2. 225 plus chains for 3 reps
3. 275 plus chains for 3 reps
4. 315 plus chains for 1 rep
5. 365 plus chains for 1 rep
6. 405 plus chains for 1 rep

Try a new max or the most on this day. Then, as on speed day, do triceps, lats, upper back, and rear and side delts. A 300–350 lb raw bencher should use three sets of chains, and a 350–450 lb bencher should use four sets of chains. Although the amount of chain can vary to set a record, a lifter has five workouts to choose from if he uses two different grips with all three chain weights.

Workout #2: Do overhead band presses or the lightened method by attaching a jump-stretch band at the top of a power rack. Reduce the weight at the chest by 155 with a strong set of bands. A medium set reduces the weight at the chest by 95 lbs. A light set reduces the weight by 65 lbs. After warming up, work up to a max single.

My personal records were 580 with strong bands and 520 with medium bands. This coincides with the 60lb difference between the band strengths. In turn, Amy Weisberger has a 370 bench, using mostly the medium and light bands. This is very close to duplicating the value of a bench shirt without using one. Establish a PR with a close grip and a wide grip with three different band strengths and two different grips. This represents five completely different workouts. Always follow with triceps, lats, upper back, and rear and side delts.

Workout #3: Do football bar presses. This bar allows the palms to face each other while taxing the triceps. Westside lifters work up to a new PR for three reps or a 1RM. The bar has different width grips to choose from including close, medium, and wide. We use it by itself or with mini-bands, light bands, or a set(s) of chains. During the workout, at least two grips are used.

Flat, incline, or decline presses follow. The JM press is performed at times also duplicating the groove of a bench press shirt. It is very effective; though, it hits the triceps very hard, too. A lifter must again work extensions with dumbbells with the elbows in or the roll back variety followed by lat work. Always rotate exercises that work the same muscle groups but in a slightly different way. Finally, do upper back, rear and side delts, and hammer curls.

Again, look at the possibilities—two different band tensions, three chain weights, and three grips to choose from adds up to eight different workout PRs to break.

Workout #4: Do illegally wide benching. Take a grip outside the power ring, wider than allowed at a contest. Work up to a max six reps. I got this concept from Bill Seno, a great bencher and bodybuilder from the 1960s through the early 1980s. A lifter can also work up to an 8RM and even a 10RM. This was Bill's intention for me, but I didn't like 8–10 reps because they took too much energy. Sorry, Bill, but those wide 6s gave me a top ten bench in 1980. If an individual never trains for a raw bench, he will never know how to get one. I'm sure Scott Mendelson has some good tips for a raw bench.

On the day after benching, do dumbbells on an incline or decline for several sets. This is primarily a hypertrophy day. Most dumbbell presses are executed with the palms facing each other. A few sets can be completed with the thumbs facing each other because this simulates taking the bar out of the rack. As always, do triceps first, followed by lats, upper back, and rear and side delts. Note: We don't work front delts directly too often due to overtraining. I observed that the guys who do a lot of front delts are not our best benchers. It should be noted that max effort day can be replaced with a repetition day to increase muscle mass. No one method works; all proven methods must be implemented.

Workout #5: Do band presses by attaching bands to the bottom of the rack, building a fast start and a strong lockout. A mini-band attached to the bottom of the power rack (see the Bench Workout DVD) adds 40 lbs at the chest and 85 at the lockout. A monster mini-band adds 50 lbs at the chest and 110 at lockout, and a light band doubled up at the bottom adds 100 lbs at the chest and 200 at the top.

Halbert, Wolf, and Winters, all who bench over 600 raw, use medium and strong bands and even multiple bands. Work up to a single. Full range is mostly used but sometimes we press off power rack pins or boards. Band tension may vary depending on the hook up of the bands. Use two grips—either a wide grip or a close grip. This will result in two PRs. Don't forget to train triceps, lats, and so forth.

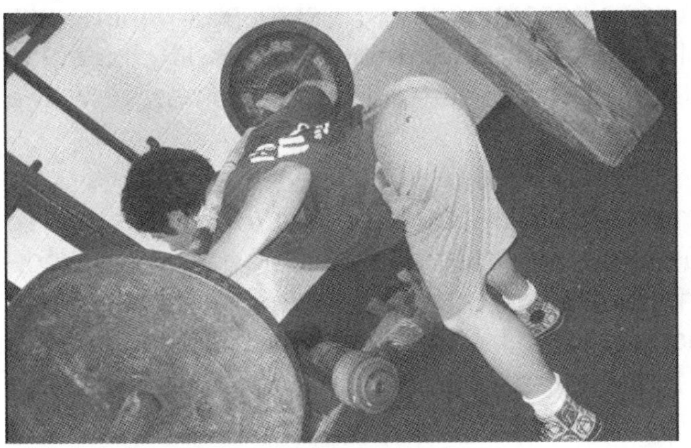

Workout #6: Do board presses. I did board presses in 1970. The Culver City Westside guys were doing them at that time. I got very little out of them. Why? I had weak triceps. Larry Pacifico said I had to work my triceps if I was to have bench big, and he was right. In 1993, Jesse Kellum said I should use board presses again. By this time, we were training our triceps very hard. After our success, everyone was doing board presses, and everyone was an expert.

Here's the truth about board presses. They are not a triceps builder if an individual starts the lift with his pecs. Unfortunately, many do just that. Start the motion with the arms. I watch a lot of people do board presses, thinking that they will build a strong lockout. I saw people do board presses with bench shirts continuously, and two of them lost their lockout at the meet by 60 lbs. The others were not top ten benchers anyway. The bench is a full range motion. Perhaps, this is why so many dump the bar on their belly and don't practice full range motion. The workout is simple. After a warm up, work up to a max single. One-, two-, or three-boards are used at Westside. Four- and five-boards are for isolating the triceps.

There are exercises that build strength and those that test strength. Board presses test strength. Have you ever watched point karate? They always stop the punch just short of the face. I believe the board press does the same thing. I hear what so and so did off a board press only to attend a meet and be unable to touch the chest. I think his name was Curly or Moe. Or maybe it was Larry. But who cares? What a stooge! These workouts give a wide variety to choose from. Mix and match any way you want, I'll see you at the meet.

Westside's Top Benchers' Training

I receive many calls asking how our top benchers train. We have 17 benching over 700. For example, one has done 830 (Mike Wolf), two 198s have done a 683 (George Halbert) and a 655 (Jason Fry), and one 181 (Fred Boldt) has done 628 and is an Arnold Classic winner. Then, there's Nick Winters, who made 650 raw at the New England Strength Spectacular. In 1993, I wrote an article titled "Three of a Kind." We had three guys benching 600; one of whom (Kenn Patterson) went on to become the youngest to bench 700 at 22. His actual lift was 728, a world record at 275. Then, along came Mike Brown. At 19-years-old, he made 735 at 308 and totaled 2300.

Favorite routines and exercises:

First, everyone does speed work, which is known as the dynamic method. This alone will not make a person strong but will rather build a fast rate of force development. Research shows that 154 lbs can develop 264 lbs of force with maximal acceleration. Nine sets are performed—three sets with the index finger on the smooth part of the bar, three sets with a two-inch wide grip, and three sets with the little finger on the power ring. After speed bench, using about 40% of a 1RM on the floor press, Westside lifters do two sets to near failure with one of three dumbbell weights. Fred uses either 155,125, or 100 lb dumbbells; sometimes a barbell is used.

Fred's weights are 365, 315, or 275. Remember, Westside lifters go to near failure. Then, it's triceps, lats, upper back, and rear and side delts. Some hammer curls finish the workout. Speed work can be waved, using two sets of 5/8-inch chains to accommodate resistance or mini-bands, which add 45 lbs in the bottom and 85 at the top of the lift. A monster mini provides 110 lbs at the top and 50 in the bottom. Speed benching can be done off rack pins, in the floor press, or with a cambered bar.

Jay Fry has made incredible progress in a short time, going from 530 to 650 at 181 in less than18 months plus 655 at a body weight of 193. He has become quite a student of the game while working with George Halbert. To raise absolute strength, he uses heavy assistance work such as: kettlebell triceps extensions and JM presses. This teaches him to fire the correct muscles at the right time. Using chains or bands or hanging kettlebells from the bar not only allows the muscles to become stronger but develops muscle coordination for benching. Jay feels this is far more important than just throwing heavy weight around. To test his strength, Jay uses full range band presses, floor presses with chains or bands, or just weight. These records are dependent on the special exercises that are mentioned above. Jay does a lot of upper body sled work, making him stronger and raising his GPP. The sky is the limit for Jay. His potential is very high and with his drive only time will tell.

Jays's teammate, Fred Boldt, has been at Westside for close to five years. Fred's bench went from 400 at 165 to 556 at 165, placing him second to the great Marcus Schick. Fred then won the 2005 WPO semifinals with a 628 over Jay's 622 in Chicago. He went on to win the Arnold Classic in 2006 with 628. It's not easy to win the Arnold with all the chaos that goes along with it. How does Fred do it? To test his bench press max, he tries a max off the floor press with five sets of chains, weighing 200 lbs on the bar. His best is 345 with his little fingers on the power ring of the bar. A second strength test is a full range bench with light jump-stretch bands that add 100 lbs in the bottom and 200 at lockout. His best is 370. This is what Jay has also done, and their bench presses are very close.

Of course, like all Westsiders, Fred uses the conjugate method. He rotates from 4- or 5-boards with bands to a steep incline with a barbell. Fred uses a cambered bar on boards to reduce the camber to one inch. For hypertrophy work, Fred likes dumbbell presses. His one set record is 34 reps with 100 lbs. He rotates three dumbbell weights—100, 125, and 155 lb. His best three set record is 14, 12, and nine reps with 155s. He also has done 104 push-ups with his feet elevated 12 inches. Fred's speed work incorporates 185 or 205 plus mini-bands, adding 85 lbs at lockout or with two sets of 5/8-inch chain; when locked out, this is roughly 60 lbs.

For special work, straight bar extensions and kettlebell extensions are his mainstay. He does lots of lat and upper back work along with rear and side delt work. Fred never misses a workout (nor does anyone at Westside). Fred's motivation is his desire to destroy Jay. I'm sure you will see Fred for a long time to come.

Mike Wolf made rapid progress after coming to Westside. His 585 soon became 825 and then 830. Mike is huge at about 405 lbs. George started working with Mike finding his weaknesses. First, George had Mike push up the triceps work and board press with lots of bands, up to 400 lbs of bands plus weight. Mike also did full range band presses, including flat, incline, and decline.

At Westside, we do a lot of triceps extensions, implementing the straight bar, dumbbells with palms facing in, roll back style, dumbbells with elbows out to the sides, JM presses, and kettlebell extensions. Mike also does a lot of benches with kettlebells, hanging from the bar with doubled up mini- bands.

Mike found his floor press well below our average for his shirt bench, so to raise it, he pushed it up to 515 with 200 lbs of chain. Lots of lat work, pull-downs, bar rows, and dumbbell rows have made it possible for Mike to control the bar placement on his chest. Last is speed work, which entails a fast rate of force development, which is essential to lift heavy weights fast. Let's see if Mike can give Westside its first 900 bench.

George Halbert is our most decorated bencher. He has 11 all-time world records in three different weight classes. George's main view on benching is that speed work is most important. He knows that if he misses a heavy lift, it wasn't too heavy but wasn't lifted fast enough. His speed work consists of chains, bands, and hanging kettlebells from the bar.

For max effort work, it is heavy band presses at all angles. This sometimes includes benching almost upside down, reverse or lightened band presses including flat, incline, or decline, board presses (without shirt), and lots of dumbbells. He also does the repetition method to near failure for 15 reps with hanging kettlebells. George is very innovative in his training. His bench methods are responsible for much of Westside's benching success. He does many workouts a week, just lats or delts or pre-hab work. He is one of only a few men who have made world records in three weight classes, and he's got more up his sleeve than just triceps.

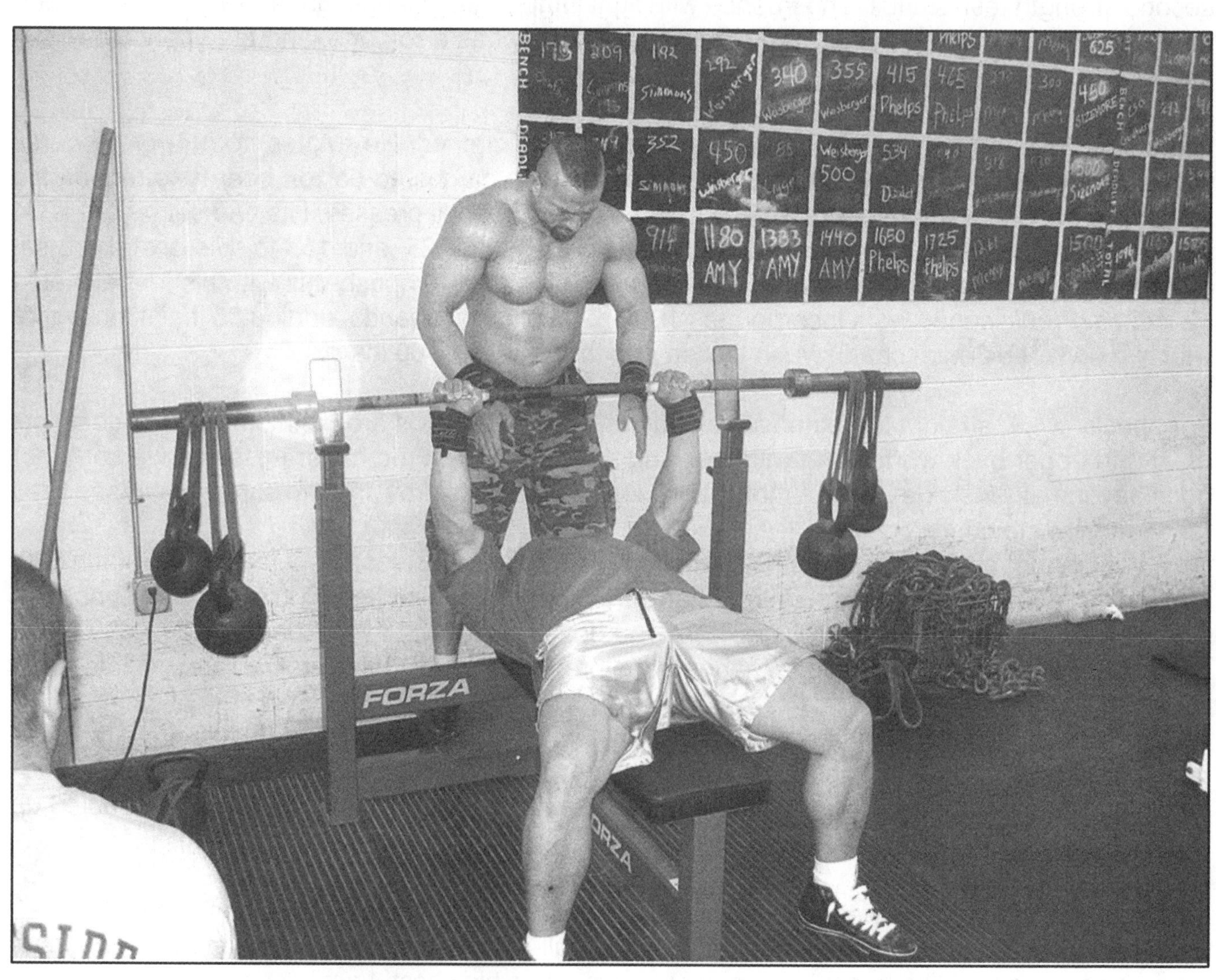

THE SQUAT

Using the Box in the Squat

Box squatting is the most effective method to produce a first rate squat. This is, in my opinion, the safest way to squat because a lifter doesn't use as much weight as he would with a regular squat. Let me say first that, no, box squatting won't hurt the spine. An individual doesn't use 1000 lbs on a 25-inch tall box, and he doesn't rock on the box. Don't touch and go, and there is no need to do regular power squats before a meet. No knee wraps are worn nor are the straps of the suit pulled up.

By doing sets of two reps for at least eight sets with short rest periods, a lifter can get about a 200 lb carryover to his regular squat. Two of our lifters finished their lifting cycle before a meet with eight sets of two reps with 505 lbs off a slightly below parallel box, and both squatted 700 for a meet PR. One was competing in the 242s and the other as a 275. Two years before, in his first meet, our 275 squatted 465. Quite an improvement! There are many advantages to box squatting. One of the most important is recuperation. An individual can train more often on a box than he can doing regular squats. The original Westside boys (Culver City, California) did them three times a week, which I feel is a bit extreme, but they paved the way for this type of training. We do them for the squat part of our workout on Fridays and occasionally on Mondays to build hip and lower back power for deadlifting. The NBA's Utah Jazz do box squats for the same reason—recuperation. Greg Shepherd, their strength coach, is a former member of the Culver City gym.

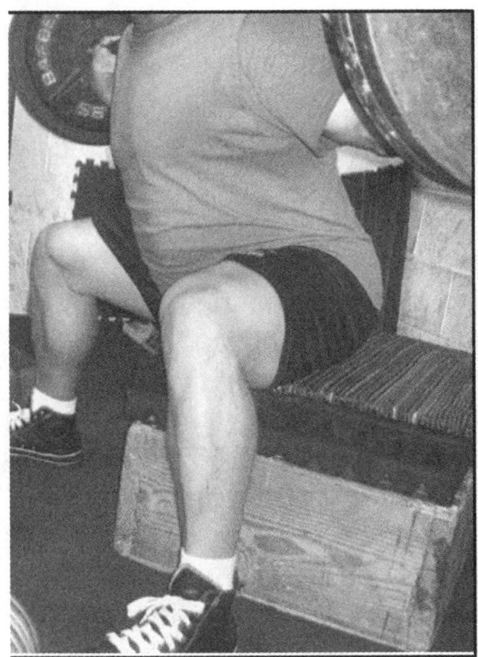

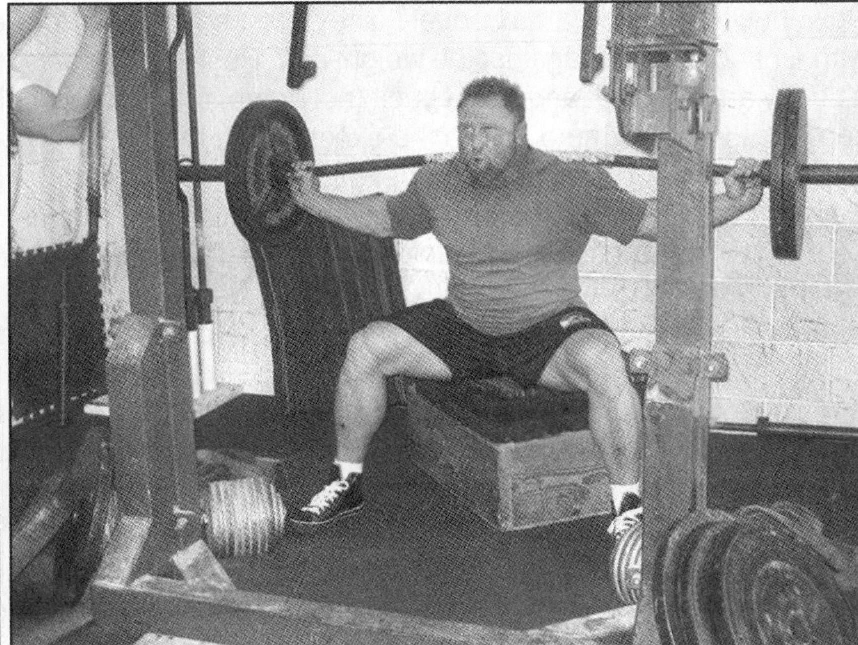

The second reason is equally important. It is generally accepted that an individual should keep his shins perpendicular to the floor when squatting. With box squatting, he can go past this point (that is, an imaginary line drawn from the ankle to the knee, pointing toward the body), which places all the stress on the major squatting muscles—the hips, glutes, lower back, and hamstrings. This is a tremendous advantage.

Thirdly, the lifter shouldn't have to ask anyone if he's parallel. Once the lifter establishes a below parallel height, all of his squats will be just that—below parallel. I have seen it over and over. As the weights get heavier, the squats get higher. This can't happen with box squats.

- If the hips are weak, use a below parallel box and a wide stance.
- If lower back power is needed, use a close stance below parallel.
- If the quads are weak, work on a parallel box.
- If a lifter has a sticking point about two inches above parallel, work on a box that is two inches above parallel.

Our advanced squatters all use below parallel boxes. This builds so much power out of the hole that there will be no sticking points. As an added bonus, box squats build the deadlift as well by overloading the hips and lower back muscles. The ability to explode off the floor will increase greatly.

Now, how do you do a box squat? They are performed just like regular squats. Fill the abdomen with air and push out against the weight belt. Push the knees out as far as possible to the sides with a tightly arched back and squat back (not down) until sitting on the box completely. Every muscle is kept tight while on the box with the exception of the hip flexors. By releasing and then contracting the hip flexors and arching the upper back, jump off the box, building tremendous starting strength. Remember to sit back and down, not straight down. The hamstrings will be strengthened to a high degree, which is essential. Many don't know this, but the hamstrings are hip extensors. Some great squatters have large quads, and some don't, but they all have large hamstrings specifically where the hamstrings tie into the glutes. Remember to sit on the box completely and flex off.

Now, how does a lifter know how much he can full squat if he box squats all the time? Well, let's say he has squatted 600 lbs in a meet and decides to box squat. If the lifter can do 550 off a parallel box, that's a 50 lb carryover. Now, if a lifter is doing only box squats and he takes a weight 4–6 weeks into the cycle, he'll hit a 575 squat, a 25 lb jump on that particular box. This will carry over to his 600 contest best. Following this, expect a 625 at the next meet. Box squats are much harder than full squats! Do 8–12 sets of two reps with a one-minute rest between sets. This is a tough workout! Don't get psyched up to do sets. We have found that two reps are ideal. If a lifter is completing 12 sets, he is doing 12 reps per workout. After all, the first rep is the most important one. This makes the contest squat much better. Our most talented lifters do best on their first rep and then tire quickly; whereas, our lower skilled people perform better after the first rep is completed because they use the first rep as a body awareness tool. As they become more skilled, their first rep becomes their best, too. I know box squatting is not common, mostly because no one knows how do them. After reading this or watching my squat tapes or DVDs, there should be a full awareness to the benefits.

Many great squatters have done box squats, including Marv Phillips, Larry Kidney, Roger Estep, Matt Dimel, and of course, George Fern, who did an 853 squat in track shorts in 1970. If box squats didn't work, we wouldn't do them. I am often asked, why do box squats? We do them to produce world record squats. The late, great Matt Dimel made 1010 in 1985 at SHW. Chuck Vogelpohl pushed the limit of the squat by doing 1025 at 220 lbs, the lightest man to do a grand. I am sure that the original Westside Barbell in Culver City, California, was asked the same questions in the 1960s and early 1970s when Bill West and George Frenn were breaking squats records beyond comprehension. Frenn made 854 in gym trunks at 242 and held a world record in the weight throw.

Later, men such as Larry Kidney and his training partner Marve Phillips broke many world record squats by box squatting. Paul Childress has made 1123 at 308, and I am sure Paul has to defend why he box squats. My friend, Eskil, from Sweden, found a training manual demonstrating the box squat from the 1950s at a Polish weightlifting facility. Today, my friend, Sakari, from Finland, teaches box squatting to his strongest lifters. Lifters from Ireland, Germany, England, Canada, and Sweden are also box squatting. At Westside, in Columbus, Ohio, we have 11 men who squat more than 1000 lbs and a woman, Amy Weisburger, who at 148 has squatted 565. Because I am asked why do box squats, I explain simply and scientifically why we do them and why all lifters should, too.

First, there is only one way to box squat. *Pure Power* had an article on ways to box squat, but there is only one proven way—the Westside way. Here's how. First, push the glutes rearward as far as possible. With a tight back, arch to descend to the box. Push the neck into the traps. Push the knees apart to maximally activate the hips. When sitting on the box, the shins should be straight up and down or even past perpendicular. This places all the work on the hamstrings, glutes, hips, and low back, which are the precise muscle groups that do a very large percent of the squat. After sitting completely on the box, some glute and hip muscles are relaxed somewhat. Then, forcefully flex the abs, hips, and glutes and jump off the box. To ascend correctly, push the traps into the bar first. This flexes the back muscles, the hips and glutes, and finally the legs. If a lifter pushes with the legs first, he will be in a good morning position because the glutes raise first causing the lifter to bend over. Remember that where the head goes, the body will follow. Note: Always push the feet out to the sides, not directly down. Chuck Taylors are the best shoes for squatting; this was tested at Ball State University in lab conditions.

Box squats have tremendous advantages over regular squats because an individual does not get as sore from a box squat workout, and he can recover much faster. If the box being squatted on is below parallel and a thousand squats are executed, they will all be below parallel regardless of the weight. This is important because when many lifters warm up, they can't break parallel with light weight, or as the weight nears a max, many cut depth. However, with a box to sit on, the individual will always break parallel or any depth desired. Box squats can increase flexibility. When monitoring flexibility, a lifter should be able to break parallel with his competition stance.

If this is not possible, he should sit on a box about two inches above parallel. After mastering that height, he needs to reduce the box height by half an inch. The easiest way is to remove a half-inch rubber mat. Then, he can sit on the box at that new height until comfortable, and then, reduce the height half an inch again. A lifter should continue this until he is not only at parallel but below. Start with a shoulder width stance; then, widen the stance by an inch or two each time until a very wide stance is achieved. John Stafford has sat on a six-inch box. Note that he is six feet tall, 285 lbs.

I am always concerned when a coach asks me how low we can squat, referring to Olympic squats. A very close squat stance makes no sense.

Look at a pyramid. The wider the base, the greater the pyramid. I guess, if my only claim to fame was bouncing my ass off my heels with 315, I would ask that question myself. Box squatting with a slow count is a form of proprioceptive neuromuscular facilitation (PNF), commonly used in clinical settings. This type of stretch involves a maximum pre-contraction of the muscle groups to undergo elongation. As the box is lowered to an extreme for an individual's range of motion, a box squat can become a safe ballistic stretch method. This not only increases range of motion in the muscle groups but also increases joint mobility.

Box squats also resemble a form of stretching called contract relax agonist contract (CRAC). This information can be found in Strength and Power in Sport (1991). If a lifter lowers to the box slowly and widens his stance slowly, more muscle flexibility and joint mobility can be achieved. A lighter weight can achieve a bigger squat with box squatting. By training at 50–60% of a 1RM in a three-week wave, a large squat can be developed. For example, three lifters trained with 405–480 for 8–10 doubles with 120 lbs of chain as a reactive method, and they all made their first 800 plus squat.

Jumping ability is developed with box squats. John Stafford, at 290 body weight, can jump onto a 35-inch box with a pair of 35 lb dumbbells. John Harper, a sophomore at Kent State University, is a discus thrower (with 189 feet) who can jump onto a 50-inch box. Maybe more extraordinary is that he is able to sit on his knees and jump onto his feet with 255 lbs on his back, which is due largely to box squatting.

Box squatting increases pulling power. It closely simulates the motion of pulling off the floor first by relaxing on the box after lowering onto it and then exploding upward. This is very close to the movement known as the modified dive. If a person suffers a knee injury, box squatting can be done while rehabilitating the injury. When sitting on a box fully and correctly, the shins are past perpendicular. This reduces the pressure on the patella tendons by placing the majority of the weight on the hamstrings, glutes and on the heels, not the toes.

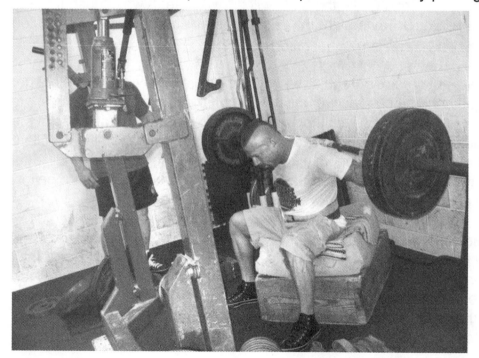

It should be noted the box itself reduces a portion of the bar weight or body weight that is being moved. After a complete patella tendon rupture, box squats helped me to go from an 821 squat in 1991 to a 920 at 235 bodyweight in 2002 after the injury, and John Bott had similar success. Also, I must not forget Jim Hoskinson, who had a horrendous injury to both knees. He had a 744 squat before the injury and had recently accomplished 1091 in the same weight class at 308.

A box squat combines two very important methods: the static dynamic method and the relaxed overcome by dynamic work. First, the static dynamic method combines two muscle activities. Static work occurs while on the box although the lifter is constantly moving backward or forward. Then, by flexing off the box, the dynamic sequence occurs.

The second method used when box squatting is the relaxed overcome by dynamic work. This occurs by sitting on the box with the hips rolling in a relaxed fashion, then switching to an explosive, or dynamic, concentric phase. Both of the above mentioned methods build explosive strength as well as absolute strength.

Why are box squats superior to conventional squats? I hope to explain it further through physics.

Lowering to the box in the eccentric phase is a form of potential energy. When sitting on the box in about 0.5 seconds, a lifter is involved in a collision. By using a box to land on, kinetic energy is produced. The amount of kinetic energy an object has depends on two things—its mass (weight) and its speed. A heavier weight means more kinetic energy., but more importantly, in a regular squat, the eccentric phase lasts about one second or about twice as long as in a box squat. By being able to relax some muscles and with the use of jump-stretch bands, the box squat is close to twice as fast. If the speed is tripled, it would represent nine times more kinetic energy during the collision.

What about the development of power? Power is defined as work done divided by the time used to do the work. Three things must be accomplished in a regular squat. The first is the eccentric phase, where the muscles lengthen. When the eccentric phase stops, a static phase begins where the muscles are not lengthening or shortening but muscle energy is decreasing. To rise concentrically, an individual must start a load while the muscles are held statically, even to a brief extent. Could this phenomenon be the reason that a person can lower 50% more than he can rise?

After all, power can be produced for only so long. In a regular squat, power must be produced during all three phases, but a box squat breaks up the eccentric and concentric phases because some of the muscles are relaxing while others are held statically by movement in the hip joints. Here is where force can be redirected very strongly. Because a heavy squat uses a large amount of energy, it makes sense to break the work into separate parts. While box squatting is not plyometrics, it builds tremendous reversal strength.

Wilson's studies (1990) have shown that the stretch reflex lasts up to two seconds. We have proven this by sitting on a box correctly the reflex lasts up to eight seconds. This is an advantage for a football lineman on a long count. Explosive strength is developed mainly by explosive efforts such as: jumps, shot put, and jerking dumbbells or a barbell. However, it is easier and safer to develop explosive strength by increasing maximal strength (Thomas Kurz's Science of Sports Training). I hope this convinces individuals to try box squatting, which many of the old champs and the new champs are doing.

Squat Training

I had a lengthy discussion with a long-time world record holder in the javelin. He told me how he trained. He threw everything but the javelin. He also said that the man who broke his record did even more specialty work and less javelin throwing than his predecessor. In turn, John Carlos was the world's fastest man in the late 1960s and was also in trouble a lot for spending most of his time in the weight room and not on the track. Valery Borsof, the Olympic champion in the 100 meter, also concentrated his efforts in the gym, building his sprinting muscles with glute ham raises and raising his GPP. A football player plays football only about 20% of the time. The other 80% is composed of special drills. I personally made a top ten squat in 1972 and placed third in 2001. The 920 I did this year ranks sixth on the 242 all-time list. At Westside Barbell, we have many all-time top ten squats. Not only do we not squat four times a week, we don't do any regular squats at all, just box squats.

Our training methods are developed after the original Culver City Westside Barbell methods of training, and we modified them to some extent to keep up with the times. In 1984, I then added the old, proven Soviet methods. If there is one thing I have learned, no one can exclusively squat to excel at squatting, and no one can squat four times a week and survive it. However, a lifter can train the squat four times a week by special means.

In 1972, the Dynamo Club in Russia came up with a method of training called the conjugate method. This club consisted of more than 70 top lifters. First, 2–40 special exercises were used. At the end of the test period, only one lifter said that was enough, but the rest wanted to choose from even more of a variety of exercises. Here at Westside, we use hundreds of combinations to increase the squat.

Our training is totally intended to raise the squat. One day, we work on special strength and at the same time build the critical squatting muscles and perfect form. Three days later, we do an exercise that builds absolute strength like deep box squatting, good mornings, or some type of pull.

That's two days a week. Thinking logically, a chain is only as strong as its weakest link, and so is the squat. There are individuals who hurt their lower back, but instead of paying more attention to it, they go back and squat again. Obviously, their lower back muscles are weak and need extra work. This extra work prevents a weak link. The rest of the squat muscles may be able to squat 75 or 100 more lbs but not as long as the lower back continues to get injured. The same holds true for hamstrings or even the upper back or abs. Again, do one dynamic squat workout a week, using multiple sets with 50–60%, and add a max effort day, working up to a max in a box squat, pull, or good morning. At certain times of the year, a lifter may not be able to break his all-time PR, but he must do all he can much like the Bulgarian method.

Two more workouts should be administered during the week for the squat. As a bonus, these also increase the deadlift. The hamstrings and glutes are the primary movers for squatting. Each workout should last 15–30 minutes. A 30-minute workout is a long, special workout. It should be almost nonstop. Always include abs in the extra workouts. First, if it is difficult to sit back in the squat, this signals the glutes and hamstrings are weak. Initiate glute ham raises because this exercise properly works the hamstrings. The hamstrings extend from the knee to the glute, and both attachments work simultaneously as if jumping , sprinting, or of course, squatting.

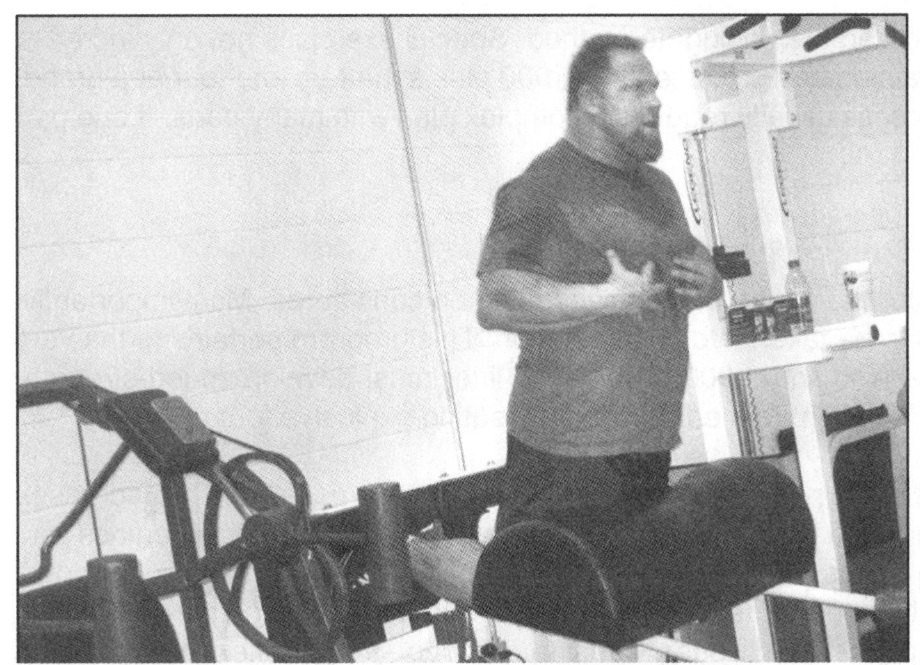

If alternating a set of abs and a set of glute ham raises, have a great extra workout designed to raise the squat. In the old USSR, 600 glute ham raises a month was just maintenance work. Westsiders like to tilt the glute ham bench as high as 30 inches, making the exercise harder.

Pull-throughs work the glutes and hamstrings very well, too. Pick an ab exercise and do supersets. When a lifter fails a squat, many times it is caused by his back bending, therefore, good mornings are in order. Try using jump-stretch bands on the bar. We prefer high reps, but I never count the reps. To change the intensity, use stronger bands. For one workout do them with a bent over style and for the next with an arched back. We also do a lot of regular weighted good mornings of all types. For squatting without placing a bar on the back, perform belt squats. One method is belt squats with weights, and a second method is to hook a jump- stretch band through an individual's power belt and stand in both ends; then, do box squats. This builds lower body flexion. An individual can also pull a weighted sled. Early in the week the heaviest weight should be used, reducing the amount as the week goes on. Reverse hypers could be substituted for a squat workout.

A number of extra workouts can be used for squatting. I suggest that all be done on a box, such as: the front squat, Zercher squat, MantaRay squat, belt squat, safety bar squat, and cambered bar squat. Immediately after squatting, go to the special exercises that fit individual needs.

If an athlete knows how to squat, there is no need to do extra actual squatting. In fact, if his squat form is not correct, more squatting will reinforce the same bad form. To become biomechanically sound, proper muscle control must be possessed. Very few people have great form. If the back is weak, bending over will occur, causing bad form. If the glutes and hamstrings are weak, it is hard to sit back properly. If the abs are weak, weakness will occur in the bottom, causing one to fold over. An extra workout can also be a flexibility workout. Whatever workout is executed, include abdominal work. Don't train longer than 30 minutes for these extra workouts. If a person is out of shape, these workouts should be done almost nonstop. The better condition an individual is in, the less stressful heavy or high volume training will be.

Matt Smith has made great progress by doing special exercises such as glute ham raises and safety squat bar squats. His squat has gone from 733 to 930 and his deadlift from 633 to 800 in, believe it or not, two years. Mike Ruggiera's squat was raised from 780 to 1000 in two and a half years. Reverse hypers and pull-throughs helped Mike.

What I have been describing is called the conjugate method. Special exercises not only increase strength but perfect form. This training has produced nine, 900 plus squatters and four at a grand, all from the same small gym. Success usually requires a complex plan with many parts. If one part is missing, failure will occur.

Periodization in Squat Training

When designing a yearly model for the squat, many things must be considered. Most importantly, the level of preparedness needs to be taken into consideration. This program pertains to the very highly trained squatter (i.e. those who squat 900 or more). A lifter must develop speed-strength, which is the ability to accelerate with light to medium loads, creating explosive force.

Strength-speed is a learned process to push maximum weights as fast as possible. This increases the powerful stretch reflex system and can be accomplished only by accelerating eccentrics and progressive concentrics. Strong bands must be used here. The bands drive an individual down at a much faster rate than gravity alone, thus creating a great amount of kinetic energy which is transferred into the muscle and connective tissues, causing a strong stretch reflex and providing an equally fast concentric phase.

Several bars can be used on squat day. I use the safety squat bar on speed day quite often and so do Dave Tate and many others at Westside. Paul Childress, a 1085 squatter, uses our 14-inch camber bar for long periods of training to give his shoulders a rest. The Buffalo bar, MantaRay and Dave Draper's device can also be used as well as belt squats. The bands solve the problem of accommodating resistance. A load may be heavy at the bottom but light at the top; therefore, half the exercise may be wasted. Fred Hatfield talked about compensatory acceleration. He was on the right track. By pushing as fast as possible against a light or heavy load, more force would be developed. However, if the weights are too light, the bar moves too fast and force is not developed.

- Dr. Squat used a very fast eccentric phase that contributed to his very quick recovery in the squat. We have added two important elements.

- Bands greatly increase the stretch reflex through accelerated eccentrics. The bands also create a greater load at the top of the lift, accommodating resistance.

Time under tension is lengthened. This time is necessary for the development of maximum force. Max force is reached in 0.3–0.4 seconds. However, it usually takes longer to complete a lift. Can the time to fully reach max force be increased with just the barbell? No, but with the addition of bands of adequate strength, the deceleration phase of the bar is greatly reduced on the ascent. The lifter must push as hard as possible for a greater length of time.

Max force is, of course, highest at the start of the ascent, with starting strength being employed. By using a large load consisting mostly of band tension and a small amount of barbell weight, I believe, the duration of maximum force and muscle tension can be lengthened, thus producing strength-speed, or the ability to push heavy resistance at a fast rate.

A four-week program of strength-speed work is made possible by combining a high percentage of band tension and a low percentage of bar weight. This cycle consists of four workouts, raising the load each week. Five sets of two reps are done each week. This is a supra- maximal method, developing maximal strength and strength speed.

	Band tension top/bottom	Bar weight	Weight at top	Weight at bottom
Week 1	635/465	135	770	600
Week 2	635/465	185	820	650
Week 3	635/465	225	860	690
Week 4	635/465	275	910	740

This is followed the next week by two reps at 325 (bar weight, same band tension), a single at 375, and a single at 415. This translates to a lift of 1050 at the top and 860 at the bottom. Lower the bar quickly but under control to a just below parallel box. (See previous articles on box squatting.) This causes a great stretch reflex and maximal acceleration. The usual special work is then performed, including glute ham raises, the reverse hyper machine, abdominal work, or similar exercises.

This cycle is very taxing and requires some short restoration work on the off days, averaging 30 minutes and including sled work, glute ham raises, the reverse hyper machine, and abdominals. The next four weeks are planned for speed and quickness. The bar weight ranges from 425–485 plus band tension of 260 at the top and 200 at the bottom. Do six sets of two reps, adding 20 lbs of plates each week.

	Band tension top/bottom	Bar weight	Weight at top	Weight at bottom
Week 1	260/200	425	685	625
Week 2	260/200	445	705	645
Week 3	260/200	465	725	665
Week 4	260/200	485	745	685

This may sound heavy, but because of the added advantage created by the bands on the eccentric phase, an individual becomes very explosive. This phase is also accompanied by special work for the abs and the posterior chain. Now, the final phase. We used three bar weights: 430, 460, and 480. The band tension is 440 at the top and 300 on the box.

	Band tension top/bottom	Bar weight	Weight at top	Weight at bottom
Week 1	430/300	430	860	730
Week 2	430/300	460	890	760
Week 3	430/300	480	910	780
Week 4	430/300	430	860	730

This four-week phase is a circa-maximal, or near maximal method. It is designed to build speed and explosive strength. It is a short meso-cycle with a mid-pendulum wave. Finally, a two-week deloading phase is done, a microcycle, to bring maximal results to the contest.

The squat day on boxes is Friday, and maximal effort day is Monday. Monday is devoted to exercises for the squat as well as the deadlift. A core lift such as a good morning or a safety squat bar squat is done followed by 2–3 special exercises for the trunk, glutes, hamstrings, or hips. These different methods, or cycles, easily blend together, creating a constant rise in performance by perfecting all special strengths while raising work capacity and mastering weaknesses through the conjugate method. This is necessary for all highly qualified lifters.

Intensity Loading for the Squat

For squatting, we use a pendulum wave of three weeks. A squat cycle of a box is 50–60% of contest max, always accommodating resistance. The simplest method is to use chains. Three of our lifters squatted 840 by using:

- Week 1: 12x2 with 405 and 80 lbs of chain
- Week 2: 12x2 with 450 and 80 lbs of chain
- Week 3: 10x2 with 480 and 80 lbs of chain

This is 50–60% of 800 lbs. A total of 24 lifts was done in weeks one and two and 20 lifts in week three. The equipment we use is groove briefs or a squat suit with the straps down. When comparing training sets to a max squat, it is:

- 58% in week 1
- 64% in week 2
- 68% in week 3

These are calculated from a box squat record. The three-week pendulum wave is continuous. If it is translated to a four-week or monthly plan it equals 92 lifts per month. For slow work or strength–speed, which is weight at 90% or above, using jump-stretch bands. Many times the total weight is over 100% of the contest max. At the bottom or box level, the weight is also extreme due to the over-speed eccentric phase.

Weekly load is five sets of two reps. For pure strength-speed, the cycle lasts two weeks. Here, a monthly total can be calculated to 20 lifts. These are done with band tension representing 65% of total load and bar weight of 35%.

The next two weeks are speed-strength and explosive power work with 40% bar weight of 1RM and 25% of band tension for a total of 65%. Twelve sets for two reps for two weeks equal 48 lifts, bringing the total lift count to 68 lifts in a mixed monthly load.

A monthly cycle like this must sometimes be used to regulate the training for an upcoming meet. When the contest is 5–7 weeks away, the last phase of training begins. It is the circa- maximal phase, which lasts four weeks. Again, always use the pendulum wave system.

- Week 1, 47%
- Week 2, 50%
- Week 3, 52%

The rest is band tension, about 40%. We know circa-max weight is 90–97% of a 1RM, but bands add kinetic energy with over-speed eccentrics. That causes additional muscle soreness and accommodates resistance maximally throughout the entire range of motion. The monthly plan, or macrocycle is ten lifts per week, five sets of two reps. At this intensity, rest periods of 60 seconds are used.

The circa-maximal as well as strength-speed work is extremely difficult. At Westside, 12 lifts per month on max effort day is constant during the year. With the ten lifts on dynamic day, 52 lifts per month are done. This can cause an individual to over train in the highest intensity range, 90–100%. For the first few circa-max phases, it is advisable to pass on the core exercises every other week. However, when becoming accustomed to intense loading, resume the max effort work as before. Instead of doing max effort work, replace it with repetition work on glute ham raises, the reverse hyper machine, lat work, and so on. During the download week, the week before the meet, drop back to the first week's weight of the pendulum wave. Check form and monitor physical state while pushing the special work.

In summary, dynamic work equates 92 lifts per month. When implementing jumping exercises, Prilepin's table should be referenced to regulate the number of jumps by intensity. When weighted jumps are employed, use the same formula to calculate the number of jumps.

Sample Squat Workouts

Though I'm repeatedly asked to make personal workout programs for lifters, this is impossible to do without seeing these people in the gym and observing their form. Their form may be terrible or they may have a blatant muscle weakness that is causing bad form. For all those people, here is a sample workout when preparing for a meet.

Shawn Nutter used the following workout for his first meet. His lifts at 242 were an 840 squat, a 575 bench, and a 650 deadlift. At his first meet, he totaled 2065. We based his attempts on a max band squat of 565 bar weight plus 375 lbs of band tension. The bands were attached to the base of our monolift, which had a 2 x 4 taped to each side. Although we don't truly cycle yearly for a meet, the circa-max, or near maximal, phase lasts three weeks plus there are two deload phase weeks. To begin, Shawn used a three-week wave with a safety squat bar. Throughout the year, we use the safety squat bar and our 14-inch cambered bar to save the shoulders and arms.

Here is Shawn's training for the IPA Nationals.

First wave with the safety squat bar:

- Week 1: 8 sets of 2 reps with 325 plus light bands
- Week 2: 8 sets of 2 reps with 375 plus light bands
- Week 3: 6 sets of 2 reps with 415 plus light bands
- Week 4: 8 sets of 2 reps with 325 plus medium bands
- Week 5: 8 sets of 2 reps with 375 plus medium bands
- Week 6: 6 sets of 2 reps with 415 plus medium bands

Switch to a 14-inch cambered bar:

- Week 7: 8 sets of 2 reps with 405 plus strong bands
- Week 8: 8 sets of 2 reps with 465 plus strong bands
- Week 9: 6 sets of 2 reps with 505 plus strong bands

Circa-max phase:

- Week 10: 5 sets of 2 reps with 435 plus medium and strong bands
- Week 11: 4 sets of 2 reps with 465 plus medium and strong bands
- Week 12: work up to 565 with medium and strong bands, about 350 lbs of band tension at the top

Deload phase:

- Week 13: work up to 565 with one strong band for 1 rep
- Week 14: work up to 405 plus 120 lbs of chain for 3 sets of 2 reps
- Week 15 (meet): 2005 IPA Nationals

I knew the training should have rendered an 860 squat at the meet, and he blew up 840 like a toy. We like to leave some on the platform and make substantial progress at the next meet. Let's look at Shawn's special exercises after the squat workout.

After Friday's squat workout:

- Speed pulls: 335 plus 100 lbs of band tension at the start and 220 at lockout, 5–8 singles
- Forty-five-degree hypers: 3–5 sets with 45–135, 2–6 reps
- Calf/ham glute raises with a 45-lb plate, 4–6 sets of 3–6 reps
- Abs of some kind
- Roller reverse hyper machine, 280 for 3x10
- Strap reverse hyper machine, 380 for 3x10

After some light stretching, he's done. Monday is max effort for the squat and deadlift. Here is Shawn's 15-week cycle, but it can vary depending up each individual.

Week 1: Raise GPP with sled pulls, 180 lbs for six trips of 200 feet as a warm up; ten-inch low box squat with the safety squat bar for max singles; good mornings on the Back Attack machine; 45-degree hypers, four sets of six reps with 90 lb; chest supported rows; five sets on the reverse hyper machine; abs

Week 2: Rack pulls with plates six inches off the floor; chest supported rows; reverse hyper, three sets; roller reverse hyper, three sets; strap reverse hyper; abs

Week 3: Sled pulls, 360 lbs, four trips of 200 feet for a warm up; cambered bar good mornings to a max triple; straight leg deadlifts, work up to 455 for five reps; barbell rows; lat pull-downs with V-bar; strap reverse hyper; abs

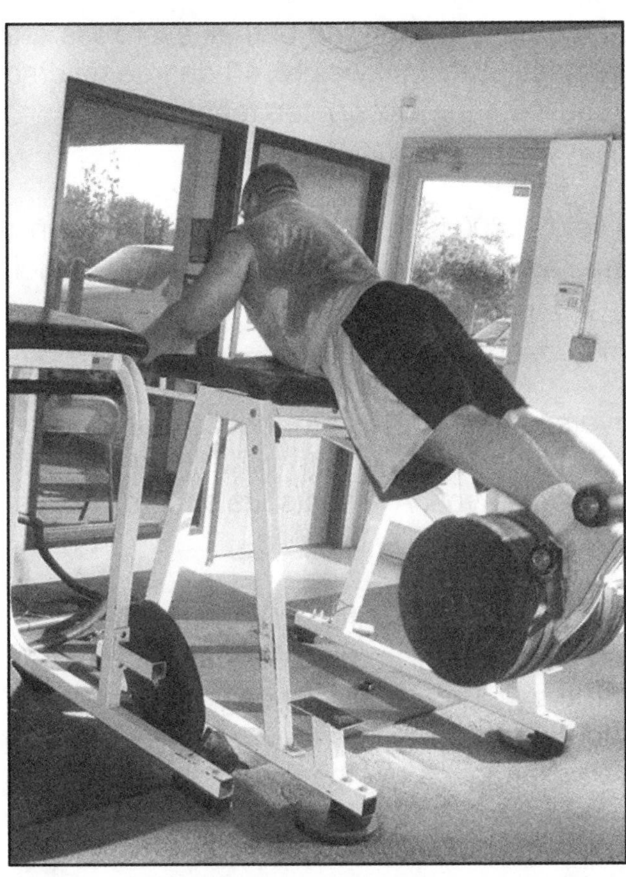

Week 4: Reverse band box squats with monster mini-bands (reduces weight on the box by 120 lbs; made 775); good mornings on the Back Attack machine; dumbbellrows; kettlebell swings; calf/ham glute raises holding a 45-lb plate; abs

Week 5: Sled pulls, 135 for eight trips of 200 feet; concentric safety squat bar squats done to a max single; 45-degree reverse hyper, 180 for three sets of two reps; chest supported rows; roller reverse hyper, three light sets; strap reverse hyper, three light sets; abs

Week 6: Close stance sumo standing on a two-inch box for a max single; front squats on a ten-inch box for 6–8 reps with moderate weight; calf/ham glute raises for sets of six reps; barbell rows; strap reverse hyper, four sets; abs

Week 7: Sled pulls, eight trips of 100 feet; lat pull-downs, wide bar and V-handle; band leg curls; band good mornings; reverse hyper; abs

Week 8: Band deadlifts, 370 lbs of tension at the top, max single (he made 405 on the bar with 370 lbs of band tension); chest supported rows; calf/ham glute raises, three sets of four reps, 90 lbs; strap reverse hper, three sets; abs

Week 9: Light sled pulls, 135 for eight sets of two reps; light lat pull-downs; roller reverse hyper, three light sets; abs

This workout is very easy because the following Friday the circa-max phase starts. Also, during the next three weeks, our max effort is changed from maxing out on a barbell lift to pushing the special exercises to high limits. Don't push the low back, lats plus abs together. Rather, we train one muscle group extensively and the others moderately hard.

Week 10: Light good mornings, work up to 70% for three reps, one set; moderate chest supported rows; three sets of three reps of calf/ham glute raises as heavy as possible; heavy reverse hypers, three sets of ten reps; roller reverse hypers with 360 lbs, three sets of ten reps; strap reverse hypers with 480 lbs; abs

Week 11: Sled pulls, 225 lbs for six trips of 200 feet; barbell rows, 135 for four sets of six reps; heavy reverse hyper, both styles, weight the same as week 10; abs

Week 12: Because we take a max on Friday with lots of band tension, no barbell exercises are done; chest supported rows; calf/ham glute raises, three sets with light weight; 45-degree reverse hyper, 200 lbs, three sets of two reps; light roller RH, 180 lbs, three sets of ten reps; abs

Week 13: This is a deload week; sled pulls, 90 lbs, six sets of 200 feet; light lat rows or pull-downs; moderate reverse hyper, two sets on roller model with 270 lbs, ten reps, two sets on strap model, 360 lbs for ten reps; abs

Week 14: This is the Monday of the meet. Do light reverse hyper. Note: After both squat day and max effort day workouts, always stretch lightly and do some joint mobility work. Most lifters at Westside never wear the straps up or knee wraps. This is up to you. All squats are done on boxes. You must taper down before meet days.

GPP is very important if a lifter wants to reach the top. If an indivual is unfit and can't do the proper exercises or do sled pulling, treadmill work, or kettlebell work, he will undoubtedly fail. I have seen men who have had to quit due to poor health because they didn't believe in being physically fit. These men are classified as "ronins," or samurais without a master. When they quit, they have no one to answer to when they could have passed on their experience to others so they won't make the same mistakes.

At the meet, an individual should open up light, something around 90% of his contest best. Don't let ego win. If there is a need, practice with gear. A lifter should know his attempts and have good help with him. Don't ask strangers to help; if they aren't training partners, they don't know an individual's needs. A total should be built from meet to meet.

At Westside, we help each other. If one of our lifters asks someone outside our gym for help, we feel betrayed. You are either with us or against us. It may take a while to master the gear because there is a lot of good gear to choose from. Don't mix and match systems. This won't work. Powerlifting is a great sport, so respect it.

DEADLIFT TRAINING

There are close to a hundred 700 lb benchers and over 50, 1000 lb squatters, but when looking at the deadlift, there are only eight, 900 plus deadlifters. The incredibly strong, Eddie Coan, made 901 at 220 in 1991, and he is by far the lightest of the group. My old friend, Danny Wohleber, of Cleveland, Ohio, was the youngest at 21-years-old in 1982 and at a bodyweight of 268. This brief bit of history illustrates how difficult the deadlift truly is.

We also got lazy in the deadlift. After all, Ted Arcidi made the first official 700 (705) bench in 1985. Now, at least 65 others have done that much. My old friend, Dave Waddington, made the first 1000 (1003) squat in 1981. Now, we have over 50, and the number is growing. I believe there are several reasons for this. One is the lack of supportive gear in the deadlift. Put down a few Benjamins for a better bench shirt and squat suit; then, the bench and squat should go up.

Although there are deadlift suits, they don't have the same impact as other power gear. Except for Eddie Coan, most men have found it necessary to gain a large amount of weight, which helped the squat but destroyed the leverage needed to pull such weight. Only three out of the eight made at least three times body weight.

I know the greatest deadlifters are built to deadlift. At Westside, we have never had the luxury of such a specimen. We had to develop the deadlift, just like Matt's increase from 633 to 825 in 30 months. September 2002 in New Orleans, I was lucky to witness not one but two, 900 plus deadlifts by Gary Frank and Andy Bolton. After trading the record back and forth, Andy reclaimed it in Columbus, Ohio, in March 2003 with 934. With Steve Goggins pulling 881 and Ano Turtiainen having made 892, it is apparent that we must work on deadlifting to keep up. Some lifters are born to deadlift (i.e. short back, long arms, and large hands). In fact, most big deadlifters lack a big bench, except for Gary. So, how can a big deadlift be obtained? Hard work and more hard work.

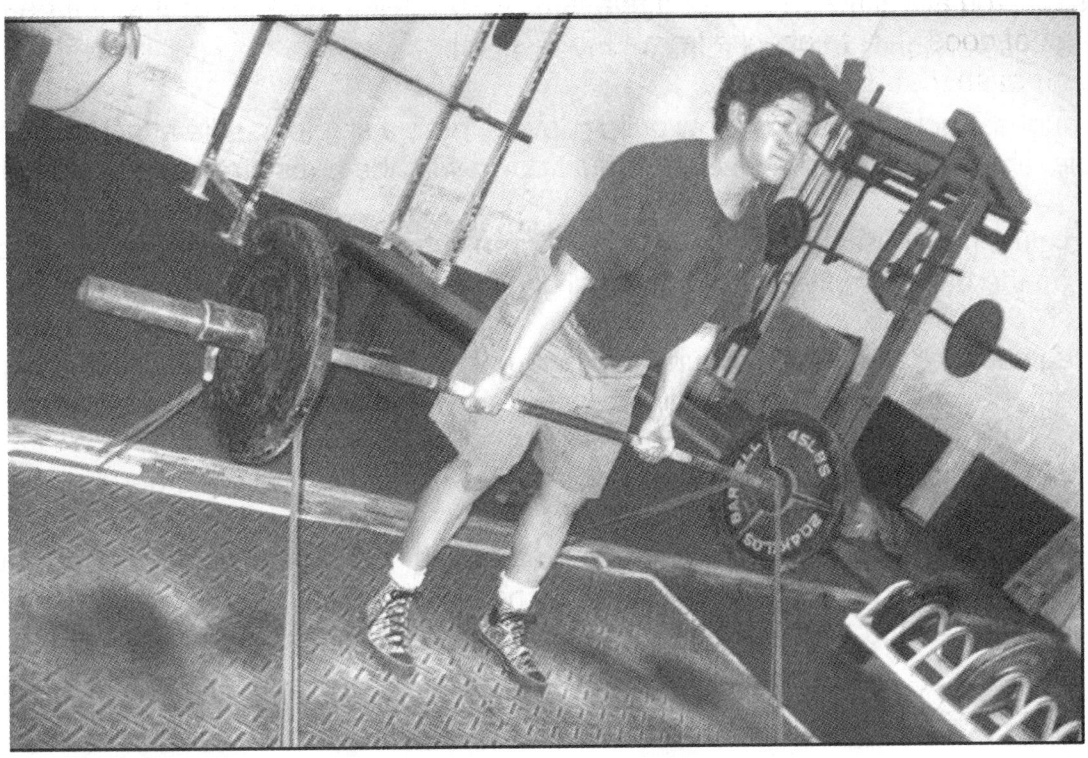

Exercises for the Deadlift

1. Jump-stretch band pulls: Our platform is designed to provide 100 lbs of tension at the start and 220 lbs at lockout. The bar weight is about 60–605% of a lifter's meet deadlift. We also will add more band tension at the lockout only, leaving the original start tension the same. A second method is to drape chains over the bar. For a 700 plus pull, use 3–4 sets of 5/8-inch chains that are five feet long. A variation of the chain method is to attach the chain to the platform on one end. As the bar is pulled upward, the chain falls on the bar at any height desired.

2.Ultra-wide deadlifts, sumo style: This develops extremely strong hip muscles. Tim Harold went from a hard 700 pull to an easy 775 pull in three months.

3. Rack pulls: Choose pins that allow only about 10% over your best regular deadlift.

4.Dave Draper's squat device: This rapidly changes the body position. This is precisely why squatting with special bars work. They artificially change the length of the spine.

5.Belt squats: These build tremendous leg strength without taxing the back. Use a belt squat machine or stand on boxes using a belt from which weight can be suspended. These not only build the entire lower body but also correct pelvic tilt.

6. Opposite style: If pulling conventional, try a sumo record. One style helps the other.
Special exercises must be used to increase the deadlift. Very few lifters can excel by only deadlifting. I've already talked about good mornings and special squats, but there are exercises that isolate certain muscle groups. The deadlift is done for singles, squats 1–3 reps, and good mornings 1–5 reps. The special exercises below are to be done in the 6–12 rep range or higher.

7. Glute ham raises: These are to be done to 2–10 reps per set, depending on the amount of weight used. Increase the difficulty of this exercise by raising the rear of the glute ham bench. Sometimes this version is referred to as an inverse curl.

8. Pull-throughs: Face away from a low pulley device, grab a single handle attachment connected to the cable, and walk forward a few feet. Squat down with the arms straight and stand back up.

9. Modified glute ham raises: Do these on a 45-degree hyper bench. While performing a back raise with a bar on the back, simply perform a partial glute ham raise simultaneously.

10. Band leg curls: Attach a band around the lower support of a power rack. Place a bench about four feet from the rack. Hook the heels in the band, sit on the bench, and do leg curls.

11. Band good mornings: Place a band around the neck and stand on the other end.

Always rotate a core exercise each week. A good morning, a low box squat, or a rack pull can be rotated. Switch the special exercises as often as necessary. One exercise may make the difference between failure and success, so pick wisely. Don't pick the ones you like but the ones that work.

Technique

For conventional deadlifts and poor lockout, the feet should be pointed straight ahead. This allows the hips to rotate forward farther and stronger. If the feet are turned out, less hip rotation is achieved. For sumo style, always push the feet apart while pulling. This brings the hips forward as fast as possible, increasing leverage. The strongest style is feet straight forward. How straight the feet will be is dependent on flexibility, which also determines the width of a person's stance.Push the feet apart and pull backward toward the body. This keeps the shoulders above or hopefully behind the bar.

Though I learned to deadlift from many, Mike Bridges was most instrumental in my practice and teaching technique. My old friend, Vince Anello, taught me that it takes many exercises besides the deadlift to excel at it. When asked what make his deadlift so great (821 at 198), Vince replied, "Anything makes my deadlift go up." He was right.For grip, Ed Coan told me to train the fingers to hold on to the bar. Training the forearms makes them bigger and the hands thicker, making one's grip worse. I hope some of these tips get you a new record in the deadlift.

The back has much potential, which is seldom reached. For such a simple lift, the deadlift can be complicated to train. If a lifter only deadlifts, progress stalls or injuries are certain. No one is totally built to deadlift. The lower back can be over trained if one bends over too much, or it can be undertrained if the legs are used too much. If sumo deadlifts are done constantly, the back becomes weak while the hips are overused. My friend, Sakari, from Finland, has surveyed the top 15 deadlifters in Finland and discovered that more than 60% of the deadlift training for sumo pullers is special exercises. The same has been found at Westside.

Using the Conjugate Method in the Deadlift

There are many styles of good mornings to choose from. Matt Smith does mostly concentric good mornings. He fixes a set of chains, hanging from the power rack with the loop of the chain three feet off the floor. He suspends the bar in the chains. As he ducks under the bar, he muscles up the weight. Once a particular style is developed, continue to use that style, and as the weight goes up, so does the squat and deadlift. Matt's best is 860 lbs. A final note: Don't swing the weight. If you do, you may start the load with the bar behind the knees. This is a squat, not a good morning. Remember, the bar must be in front of the knees to be a good morning. The concentric good morning builds little muscle mass.

The most common good morning at Westside is the bent-over style with a 14-inch cambered bar. First, stand up with the bar. Sink the chest to round the back slightly. Fill the abs with air, and bend over with the glutes pushed out to the rear as far as possible. When going from the eccentric phase to the concentric phase, try to arch the back as the lift is completed. Don't go too low.

On EMG testing, the spinal erectors will shut off and the low lumbars will be activated. This is dangerous. The next type of good morning is the arched back style. This is my favorite. I like the safety squat bar for this exercise because I don't wear gear or a belt. Push the glutes to the rear as far as possible. Very little leg bend is used. Overarch the back. In the bottom, pause for a split second, pushing the head into the pad by picking up the chin, and come up. When I break my arched back good morning record, I break my squat record. The camber of the safety squat bar places the center line of the bar well in front of the knees.

Chuck Vogelpohl and many others do a combination squat/good morning. They bend over into a good morning, and drop into a parallel squat and return to the starting position. This can be done with or without a box. Try keeping the reps to lower than three and no more than six. Whether an individual wears a belt and/or suit with the straps down is up to him and his ability. We use many special bars for squats as well as good mornings. We also sometimes raise the heels by two inches. This puts extra work on the lower back. Raising the toes 1–2 inches places pressure on the hamstrings. The legendary Paul Anderson was doing all the varieties of the good mornings I have talked about. A training partner of Paul Childress let me in on a little secret to building some very strong erectors. Place one foot on a 2 x 6 board, and do 3–5 reps in either the bent over or arched back good morning. This really isolates the spinal erectors and hamstrings. If it sounds like Westsiders do a lot of good mornings, we do.

For other sports teams, try doing walking bent over lunges with a safety squat bar. I've had NFL football players, top soccer players as well as professional rugby coaches from the United Kingdom, and MMA fighters do this, and it kicked their asses in a good way. Very low box squats are also used to build a deadlift by building a strong lower back and hips by isolating these crucial muscle groups. Some men who are very flexible will squat off a six-inch box; however, most use a ten-inch box. Reps of 1–5 works best. A strong squatter will do 60–70% of his contest squat. Use groove briefs or a suit with the straps down. Don't forget to use as many different bars as possible to break records.

After doing a max effort workout with a special squat or good morning or even a box, rack, or regular deadlift, there are very specialized exercises that must be done. The following describes some of them. In the 45-degree back raise, work up to a hard set of 3–5 reps. A decent goal would be 200 lbs for five reps. Lock the low back statically and squeeze the glutes as hard as possible. We use our own C/H/G design with a three-foot wide pad. After all, a wider base is best. If a lifter's base is narrower than the top, it is unstable and so is any coach who preaches this style.

Pull-throughs are very productive. They can be done with a jump-stretch band or a low pulley machine. Do high reps of about 10–15. When doing heavy weight on a low pulley, it is hard to stay balanced because the weight on the cable may exceed the individual's bodyweight. Another way to do pull-throughs, the original way, is with a kettlebell. Use a shoulder width stance. Place both hands on the kettlebell, and swing it through the legs until the hamstrings and glutes stop the bell. This sets the stretch reflex into action. Very quickly, swing to the front to waist height or higher and repeat for 6–12 reps depending on the weight. Do 3–4 sets. These can be done with one arm, two arms, or alternating hands.

Try some one-arm deadlifts. Sumo style works best. Use straps or a hook grip. They work muscles you didn't know you had. Reps of 3–5 work best. Herman Gonner has done 727 lbs. Zercher lifts will build every squat and deadlift muscle in your body with the exception of your hands. Westside does a lot of grip work with various devices such as: the Rolling Thunder from Ironmind, the G-Rex Grip from Sorinex, the Telegraph Key, and by holding the bell end of a hex dumbbell.

Pay attention to stretching and joint mobility work. Ab work is also essential. I prefer the stand up style. Kettlebell swings work the abs as well. Some Westsiders do weighted sit-ups, flat or decline. We also use a device from Pat Roberts that has helped a lot. It's a wheel with metal foot straps with which an individual walks on his hands or does push-ups. We also do a lot of static holds with the wheel. It not only builds the abs, but it works the upper and lower back. An added plus for me is that it works my groin and legs.

The Reverse Hyper Extension Machine

The reverse hyper machine is crucial; it not only builds the hamstrings, glutes, and spinal erectors but also traction the low back by rotating the sacrum and rehydrating the disks. The reverse hyper machine has two U.S. patents, a third patent pending, and a U.S. trademark. This machine is used at least four times a week. On a strap Pro model, Chuck's normal weight is 480–520 for three sets of ten reps. The same day, Chuck also does three sets on a roller Pro model. The usual weight is 360 for ten reps. This workout is completed on Monday and Friday. On bench days, he performs two sets of 15 reps on just one machine with about 70% of the weight of the heavy day. Also, a lot of leg curls are executed with the roller Pro model.

Westside Favorite Types of Deadlifts

1.Jump-stretch band pulls: Our platform is designed to provide 100 lbs of tension at the start and 220 lbs at lockout. The bar weight is about 60–65% of one's meet deadlift. We also add more tension at the lockout, leaving the original start tension the same. A second method is to drape chains over the bar. For a 700 plus pull, use 3–4 sets of 5/8-inch chains that are five feet long. A variation of the chain method is to attach the chain to the platform on one end. As the bar is pulled upward, the chain falls on the bar at any height desired.

2. Ultra-wide deadlifts, sumo style: This develops extremely strong hip muscles. Tim Harold went from a hard 700 pull to an easy 775 pull in three months.

3. Box deadlifts: This is a productive method done by standing on a platform, ranging in height from 1–4 inches. A conventional or sumo deadlifter can use four levels up to four inches. Keep track of each box record for a single. To increase grip strength, do a triple, pausing each rep on the floor. Pulling off a platform builds the start or finish of the deadlift regardless which portion of the deadlift which is lagging. This is done by increasing the range of motion by 1–4 inches, depending on box height. A bonus is developing the grip by having to hold on to the bar longer than a regular deadlift. My old friend, Jerry Bell (the first 165 to pull 700 officially) from Toledo, Ohio, would stand on a four-inch platform to train his deadlift with obvious results. Rick Crain made a 716 deadlift at 165, a world record at the time in 1982. He did both wide and close stance deadlift training off a coke crate to build his phenomenal pulling power. Don Blue, a 148 king, did the same. Unfortunately, Don was in an altercation and was stabbed in the eye and lung, yet he recovered enough in eight weeks to again break the deadlift record.

4. Rack pulls: These are also effective. Most lifters do rack pulls incorrectly; the bar is too high off the floor, allowing one to lift a weight would never be attempted in a meet. This can cause a total breakdown of the central nervous system. An Olympic lifting guideline contends that the optimal weight percent for pulls be restricted to 10% above the best clean or snatch. This was discovered by Ermakov and Atanasov (1975) by accumulating the results of 780 highly skilled weight lifters. Lifts at 85% were primarily used at 22.9%. Ninety percent of the lifts were done 16.7% of the time, and lifts of 80% were done 14% of the time. Compare this with weights of 100%, which were done only 2.5% of the time. In 1982, I made a 722 deadlift at 220. My best rack pulls were 705 at two inches off the floor, 730 at four inches off the floor, and 760 at six inches off the floor. I later made 855 eight inches off the floor and 805 six inches off the floor with straps. However, it was not until I recently made a 715 PR with no straps two inches off the floor did I make progress again. I realized that I will never make an 855 or even 805 deadlift; I was wearing myself out for nothing.

The law of accentuation states that strength should be trained only in the range or sport movement where the need for high force production is maximal (V. Zatsiorsky). It would seem that to lift weights not remotely possible is a waste of time and energy. Rather, it is beneficial to do several singles, ranging from about 80–90% of a maximum deadlift. I recommend the guidelines set forth by Prilepin (1974). Because the deadlift is very taxing on the central nervous system, I recommend the minimal number of lifts to be ten at 80%, reducing to four lifts at 90% of a particular pin record.

Periodization for the Deadlift

What can be done for the deadlift? Try training! A lifter must train the deadlift in a multi- year plan. An 8–12 week cycle won't work. For example, it may take six months to raise an individual's hamstrings up to acceptable levels. Deadlift records have made little progress in recent years. I believe, it is easy to add pounds to a squat or bench press due to more progressive equipment. The supportive gear, in Westside's opinion, pushes a lifter to gain bodyweight to increase the squat and bench press. However, anyone, including myself, can tell a person if he is too heavy, his pull is destroyed.

With all that said, how does someone train the deadlift for a meet? He doesn't. The deadlift must be trained in a multi-year plan. An 8- or 12-week cycle won't work. For example, it may take six months to raise the hamstrings up to acceptable levels. If not, an individual will never reach his potential. Consider Matt Smith's progress in a 30-month period. Matt had a 633 deadlift meet PR. Two and a half years later, it is 825. This deadlift completed a nine for nine day, which gave Matt a 2445 total at SHW.

Matt used the conjugate method, which links special exercises that increase awareness and coordination. Its purpose is to raise the classical lifts. First used for the Olympic lifting team at the Dynamo Club in the old USSR, this method was tested on 70 top lifters. It consisted of 25–40 special exercises.

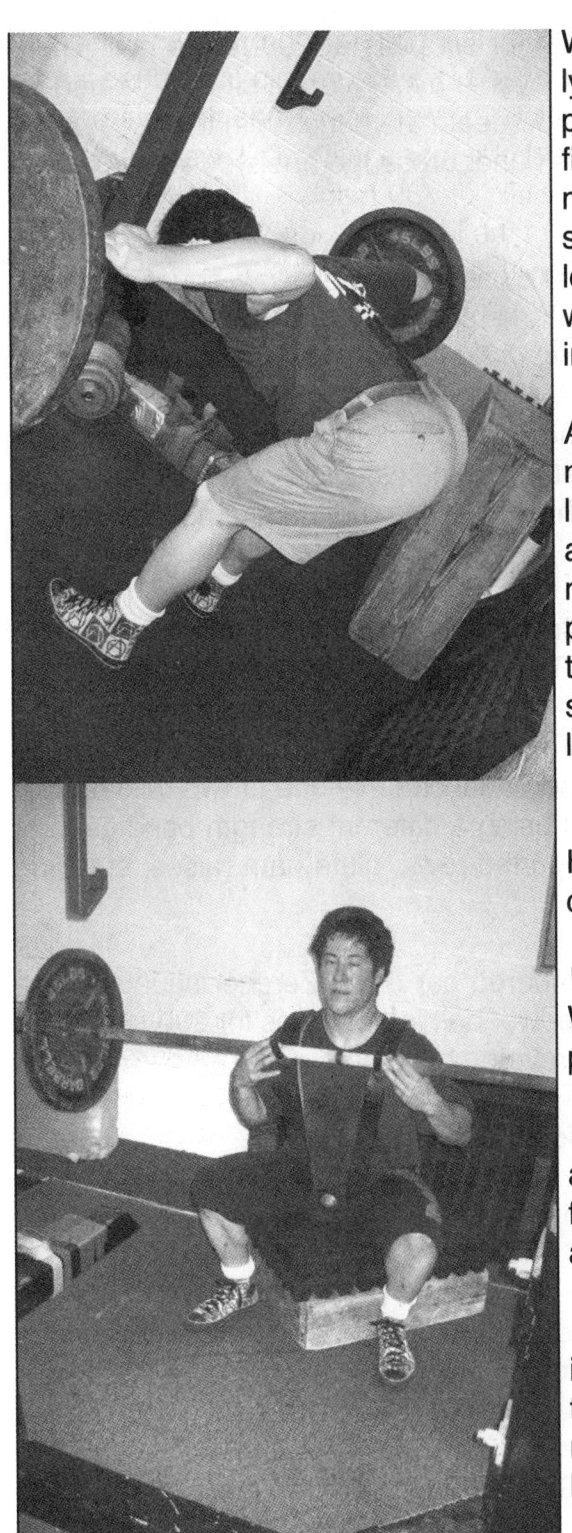

Westside Barbell also began using this system in the early 1970s. If I put one million dollars under a rock in the parking lot and told someone to find it, chances are the first rock picked up would have nothing under it. I bet that million the same person would keep searching until he strikes it rich. It's the same with exercises. If an individual looks long enough, he'll find methods and exercises that work best for him while realizing that many are worthless in comparison.

A constantly revolving system of exercises is used on max effort day, always trying for a PR. For the advanced lifter, complete three lifts, all singles—one at roughly 90% and then a PR, and if it is truly a max, stop. If not, try one more. It is much better to break new ground as often as possible. Lifting weights of 90% or more for more than three weeks will stop progress, but by rotating the core special exercises each week, one can max out all year long. This system is the super-maximal method.

Here are several workouts for the deadlift that can be coupled in a variety of ways.

Workout 1: Safety squat bar squats on a 12-inch box. Work up to max. Next, glute ham raises, the reverse hyper, and abs.

Workout 2: Bent-over good mornings to a max single or a three rep max. Then, sled pulling for eight trips of 200 feet with moderate weight, the reverse hyper, lat rows on a chest supported machine, and abs.

Workout 3: Deadlift using the lightened method by placing the jump-stretch bands at 5 feet 6 inches off the floor to lighten the load by 65, 110, or 150 lbs, working up to a max. Next, do pull-throughs, dumbbell rows, the reverse hyper machine, and leg raises.

Workout 4: Front squat on a parallel box. Try a new max, a single or a three rep max. Next, do glute ham raises, sled pulling with ankle straps, the reverse hyper machine, and standing ab work.

Workout 5: Rack pulls with the plates two inches off the floor for a max single, pull-throughs, incline sit ups, barbell rows, and the reverse hyper.

Workout 6: Heavy sled pulls with a belt around the waist for six pulls at 200 feet a pull. Then, glute ham raises, dumbbell rows, Janda sit-ups, and the reverse hyper. Janda sit-ups, named for Professor Vladimir Janda, are done by hooking a band underneath the bench with the feet not anchored to eliminate hip flexor involvement. Hold on to the band, press the heels downward, push out on the abs, and pull up on the band.

Workout 7: Cambered bar good mornings. First, bend over close to parallel. Now, squat as low as comfortable, and then, raise up. Work up to a single or a three rep max. Follow with pull-throughs, snatch grip rows, standing abs, side rows for obliques, and the reverse hyper.

Workout 8: Arched back good mornings. Remember, when doing a good morning, the bar must be in front of the knees. If not, it is a quarter squat. Work up to a max single or a triple. Pull a sled backward for six trips of 200 feet each. Barbell rows with a close grip, Janda sit-ups, and the reverse hyper machine.

Workout 9: Concentric safety squat bar good mornings. Crawl under a bar that is suspended three feet off the floor and do good mornings for a max single. Then, glute ham raises, chest supported rows, standing abs, and the reverse hyper.

Workout 10–14: Band deadlifts on a platform. Here, an individual can use one or two mini-bands, or purple, green, or blue bands. This is workout 10–14 if using a different strength band each of these weeks. Work up to a max single. Then, chest supported rows, glute ham raises, standing abs, and the reverse hyper machine.

Workout 15–17: Suspend the Buffalo bar or 14-inch cambered bar or do Zercher squats with a suspended bar. This is workout 15–17. Pull a sled with a power belt for four trips for 200 feet backward. Follow with dumbbell rows, Janda sit-ups, and the reverse hyper.

Workout 18: Box deadlifts off a four-inch box for conventional dead-lifts.

Workout 19: Sumo deadlifts off a two-inch box. Do hanging leg raises, pull-throughs, and the reverse hyper machine.

Workout 20–22: Belt squats off a low box. Workout 21 is off a parallel box, and workout 22 is off a high box. Use a very wide stance for each of these workouts. If using the same boxes but with a very close stance, this would be workouts 23–25.

Workout 26: One-legged squats with a straddle stance. Support the back foot on a box while the front foot is far out in front. This builds the entire leg while increasing flexibility in the hip and groin. Then, do Janda sit-ups, backward sled pulling for six trips of 200 feet each, side bends, and the reverse hyper machine.

Here is a total of 26 workouts, which is not even close to the amount we do. There are many methods combined in our workouts (concentric, eccentric, accommodating resistance, flexibility, awareness, and coordination). Do a new task each week, and max out continuously with exercises that build strength-speed.

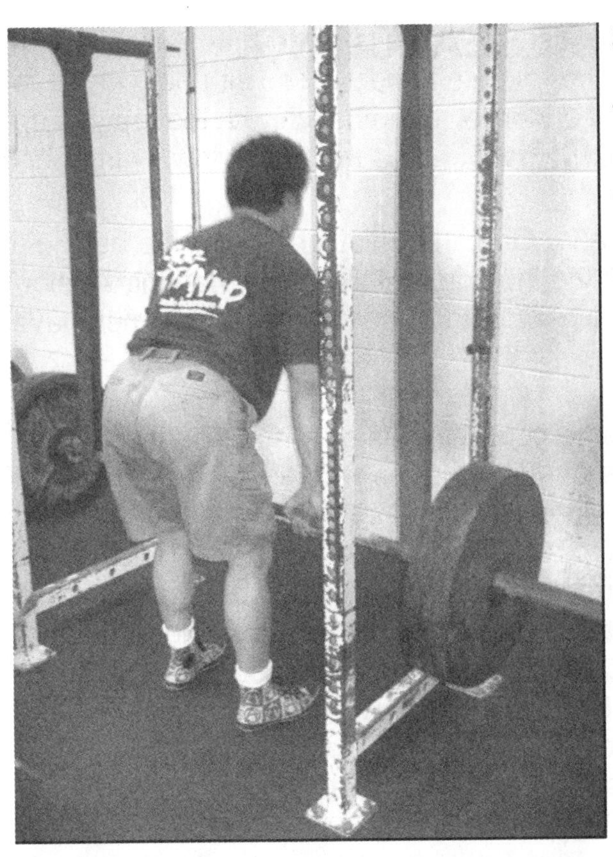

Speed Training for the Deadlifts

These can be done on either dynamic squat day or max effort day. When using 60–70%, do between 6–10 singles. The rest intervals are important, 30–45 seconds between singles. Do not do reps on speed deadlifts. The reason for this is that no eccentric work is being done during a deadlift. The CNS is stressed more when deadlifting than when squatting or benching, so do only the optimal number of reps according to Prilepin's table, not the maximal number. All the speed pulls should be very fast.

If a Tendo unit is available, results between 0.9 m/s and 1.2 m/s are optimal.

Bands: The most common method is to place mini-bands over the bar. Depending on how explosive an individual is, train with a bar weight between 50–55% of your max. Use about 80–100 lbs of band tension on the bottom and 180–220 on the top.

Light band tension: Again, use bands over the bar but use a band tension that is light at the start and about 100 lbs on lockout. Use 70% bar weight.

Lightened method: Attach blue bands over the power rack pins at 5–6 inches off the floor. This causes the bar weight to be close to zero at the start. At the lockout, a true bar weight is released. Use 70% of a 1RM.

Chain pulls: Attach 5/8-inch chains to only the front of the platform and drape a five-foot length of chain over the bar, causing a moveable static overcome by dynamic effect. Set the chains evenly over the bar, and adjust them to fall off the bar at one's mini-max.

BANDS AND CHAINS – RESEARCHING RESISTANCE

There are many things about strength I don't understand. One, in particular, is how the heck did the father in "The Courtship of Eddie's Father" turn into the Incredible Hulk? Even Vladimir Zatsiorsky, Lazar Baroga, and Alexei Medvedyev could not help me with this. However, these men have taught me many things, most of all to think.

Using chains, bands, or weight releases is known as the contrast method where the weight varies at different points of the lift. Remember, all angles of a lift must be worked. Good equipment is important. Learn how to use a shirt, suits, and the training equipment available today. In the immortal words of the Road Warriors, "If you are going to a knife fight take your guns." That is precisely what we do. Don't let resistance stop you in your tracks. Use it to your advantage. Because the human body is stronger at some positions than at others, we are limited as to the amount of weight we can use in a certain movement. For instance, a lifter may be able to do a quarter squat with 600 lbs, but he may be able to only full squat 400 lbs. We all know through practical experience that while doing a simple curl, the start of the movement is very hard; whereas, the finish is somewhat easier because of changing leverage. This problem was first addressed around 1900 by Max Herz. His solution was the oblong cam, which he patented. Years later, the Nautilus line of exercise equipment tried to solve this age old problem, in my opinion, unsuccessfully. One lifter's strength is certainly different from another lifter's at the same joint angle.

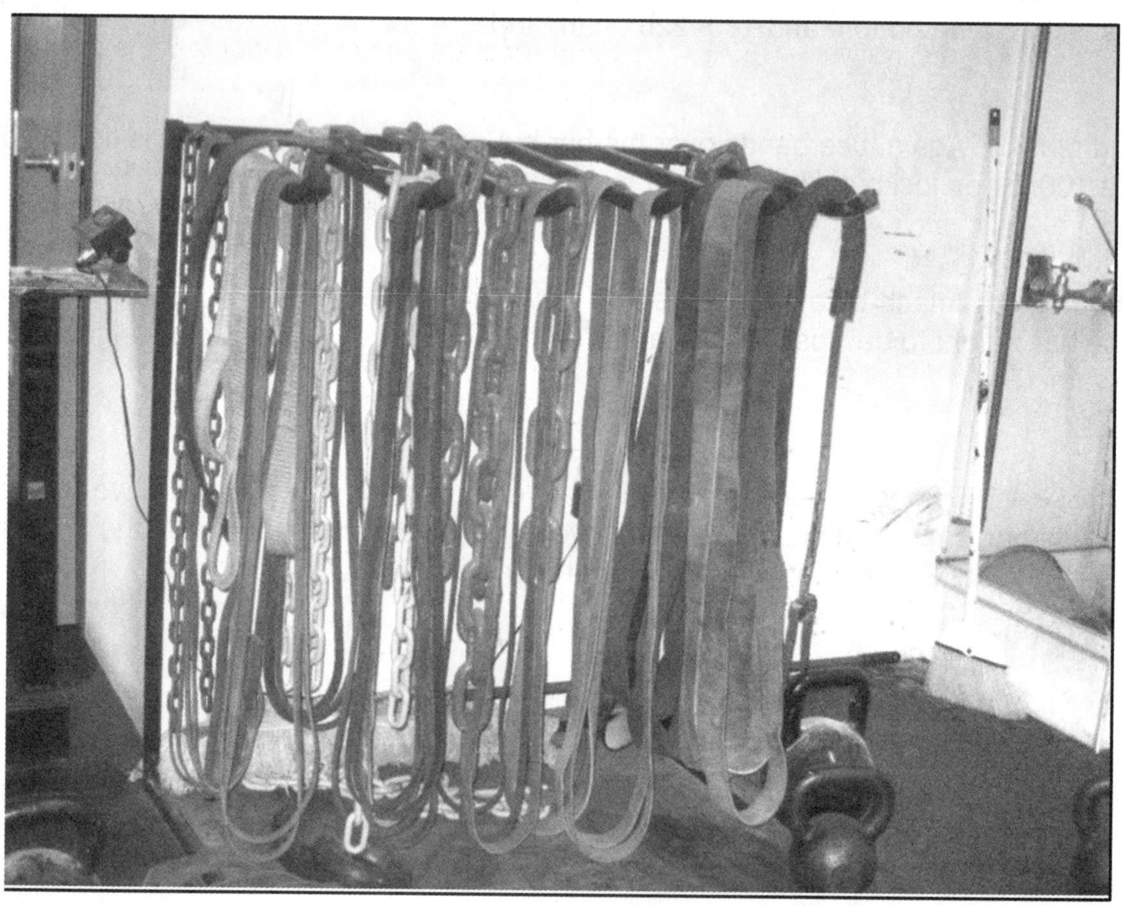

Let's go back to the 1960s and power rack training. A power rack will in one way address this problem. For example, a lifter deadlifts 600 lbs off the floor. Utilizing a power rack with the weight two inches off the floor, he can pull, 625, and four inches off the floor, 650. By setting the weight as high as eight inches off the floor, he may be able to pull 750. In this manner, we have solved, at least partly, the problem of overloading or providing adequate resistance as joint angles change. However, it's difficult for some to display this new found strength from pin height to pin height. This can be explained by the fact that it is very seldom that one's body positions the same while pulling off the floor as pulling off the rack. Isokinetics may be a partial solution.

As with most machines, a person must follow the path of the machine, which is different from the path of a free weight. The path of a barbell is somewhat unpredictable at times. Another drawback is that prior to the start as well as the finish, there is no load bearing on the lifter with this type of apparatus. Is there an answer to the problem of how to overload or adequately load the body to match the body's increase in leverage? Yes, there is.

Accommodating Resistance

Everyone should know what accommodation is. Accommodation causes performance to stagnate or decrease. Zatsiorsky stated that the response of a biological object to a given constant stimulus decreases over time.

Let's take a look to the past…on March 7, 1997, at the Arnold Classic, George Halbert benched a world record 657 (298 kg), weighing 220. George dropped to 220 on October 18, 1997, and he made a 600-lb bench. In five months, he achieved 657 by doing special work with bands and chains. On speed day, which is Sunday for us, George does his benches with 335 for eight sets of three reps, which is slightly over 50%. The three reps are completed within the same timeframe that his max single requires, and they are very explosive.
For example, a football team practices for hours and hours, but when game time arrives, there are off-sides, holding, missed tackles, and fumbles. Why? Could it be they practice the game too much and not the parts of the game, which cause the difficulties on game day? How can a high school basketball player like LeBron James be the number one pick in the NBA? Is it because he has forgotten the fundamentals of basketball and merely play the game as a whole? Now, a junior high school player from Indianapolis is projected to be the top NBA pick after graduation next year. How? Are they concerned only with the entertainment value of the game and nothing else? Perhaps. Is that why we can't win Olympic gold with superstar millionaires?

The U.S. Olympic lifters have a technique day. Why? The last world record by a male U.S. Lifter, Joe Dube, was in 1969. Olympic lifters, like ballplayers, repeat the same activities over and over, only to stagnate after a short time. I had to mention Olympic lifters, so I can receive my fair share of hate email. I always have the door open at Westside for them, but only Glen Pendlay has made the trip.

Of course, all of us can experience becoming stale. How can we train the squat without experiencing accommodation? At Westside, we box squat, but we change the box height occasionally or use a soft box (hassock) instead. Most of us manipulate the width of our stance during the same workout or point the feet at different angles, but everyone carries the bar at the same place on the back. We instinctively do this to take advantage of our best leverage.

This is in itself good. However, what about the muscles avoided training by doing this? How can they be trained? Using different bars can train neglected areas. We use a three-week pendulum wave, going from 50–60% in three weeks and returning to 50%. A safety squat bar may be used for three weeks, and a second loading may be done with a cambered bar for the next three weeks. Then, perhaps a straight bar or even a MantaRay can be implemented for a wave. To reduce accommodation to a greater extent, one must include methods to accommodate resistance. This is done by including chains, bands, or weight releasers to the amount of bands and chains added to the barbell weight.

Another proven method of changing the amount of work being done is to control the length of the rest time between sets. This is reflected by the intensity zone being used. Speed-strength rest intervals can vary from 30–90 seconds between sets. For circa-max weights, the rest can be 60 seconds to two minutes and 30 seconds. This max depends on an individual's GPP. For bench pressing, the same procedure is executed. For dynamic benching, a person can use chains, bands, weight releasers, or a combination of the three. Instead of the regular bench press for speed work, he can floor press, breaking up the eccentric/concentric chain. A different method is to do speed work by lowering the bar to power rack pins. Relax the muscles on the pins and then press up. The type of bar used can also disrupt the process of accommodation. A fat bar, a Buffalo bar, or a MacDonald bar can be used with a five-inch to one-inch camber. Every time you change something and master its performance, you become a better lifter or athlete.

The deadlift can be trained by doing box deadlifts off a two- or four-inch box, or by completing rack pulls, varying from having the plates two inches off the floor to having the bar set at knee height or slightly higher. It is important to do both sumo and conventional styles.

The deadlift can be done with jump-stretch bands over the bar. A doubled mini-band adds 220 lbs at the top and about 100 lbs at the floor level. A monster mini-band adds 280 lbs at the top and 125 at the start. For more top end tension, a single light band adds 100 lbs mostly at lockout. The lightened method is also used frequently at Westside.

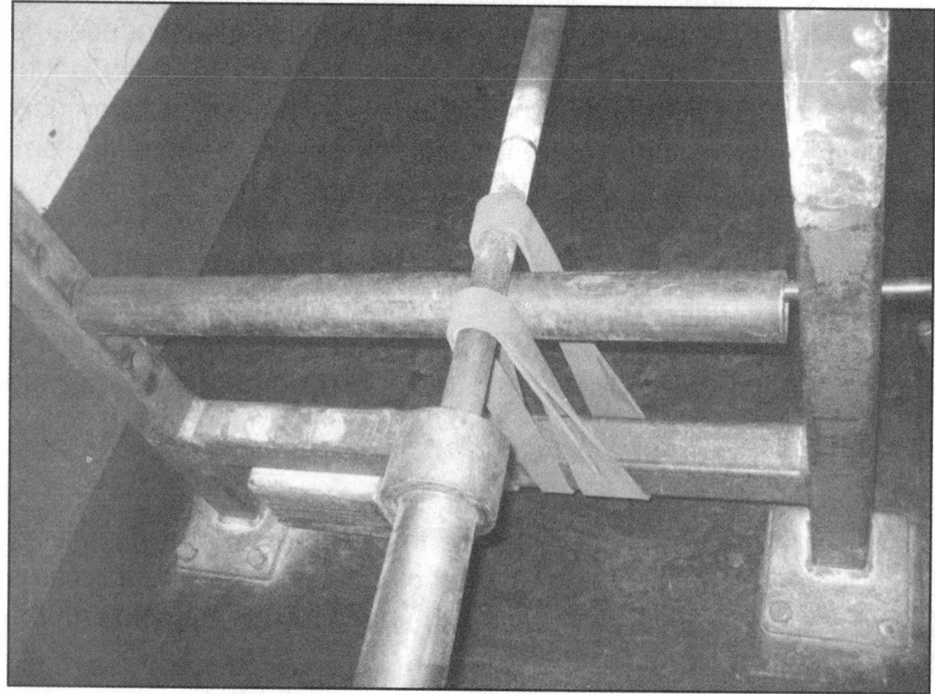

This is done by suspending the bar in strong bands five feet off the floor, reducing the bar weight by 135 lbs at the floor level. At lockout, the entire bar weight originates from the bands. This creates a different type of speed of resistance. Don't forget good mornings of different types.

Finally, let's look at the Olympic lifts. We know because of accommodation that it is not advised to use standard exercises for a long cycle. The loading system must change as well. We have found that a three-week wave works best.

A note to college coaches: A full clean and jerk is two lifts: a front squat and the jerk. If an athlete simply tries to increase the clean and jerk, it is only a matter of time before failure strikes. A lifter may be quick to jump under the bar but may not be able to recover from the squat. The front squat must be pushed up, not by front squatting but by doing special exercises for the front squat. For example, back squat off a low box with a full two second relaxed pause or front squat off a box with a long relaxed pause. Employ a variety of bars (e.g. Buffalo bar, 14-inch cambered bar, safety squat bar) in addition to the reverse hyper machine, pull-throughs, 45-degree hypers, heavy glute ham raises, inverse curls, belt squats, weighted sled pulls, and pistol squats. Use bands and chains plus weight releasers. For pulling, use at least two grips for cleans and snatches. Stand on a two-inch platform for power cleans and power snatches, and complete straight leg power cleans and power snatches. Use kettlebells with one or both hands. Do functional isometric pulls adjusted with bands. This is just a small list.

Proper form should be taught early in the training of novices. Then, more exercises for strength can be added to the training. This is the conjugate method where special exercises correct technical flaws. Most of the exercises I have talked about are close in form to the classical lifts. Chains or bands are used to accommodate resistance (40–60 lbs of chains, 100–160 lbs of resistance with bands). If an athlete does the power or Olympic lifts with only a barbell, his potential to create additional speed or force is limited by the one- dimensional weight on the bar. If he is to do speed work, no more than 50% for the 8–10 sets of three reps should be used. This is based on a no-bench shirt record and is for explosiveness, strength, and acceleration. This is exactly why bands or chains must be employed to accommodate resistance. Without them, the bar moves too fast at the top. George knew his mini-max, or sticking point, was about 2–3 inches from the top, so after speed work, he hit the triceps first, then the delts and lats. George also did a small amount of lat and triceps work on Monday and Friday.

On Wednesday, max effort day, George's favorite exercise is to use a bar with a five-inch camber. He places two, 2 x 6s on his chest. By doing this, the bar descends only one and a half-inches below his chest, not the full five inches, which would be too stressful for our lifters. He implements flex bands, adding 160 lbs of tension to the bar, and he either works up to a max single or does three sets of three reps. His best was 475 for three triples. With the flex bands, it is 635 at the top.

The flex bands provide added eccentric overload, which not only builds muscle size but also increases reversal or starting strength. Because of the added tension, George uses the bands for only three weeks because of the additional muscle soreness.

George also likes to do floor press with chains. Because the bar rack is so close to the floor, the chains are dropped over the sleeve of the bar. He warms up with the bar and then adds chains until he has 200 lbs of chain. Then, weight is added, and he works up to a max single. His best is 445 plus 200 lbs of chain. George always goes for a new max, and many times he misses. As the chains come off the floor and the weight accumulates at the top, he sometimes falls at his mini-max, or sticking point. He pushes as hard and as long as possible at this point, about three inches from lockout. By doing this, he is working at his weak point, devoting valuable time to it.

At the Arnold Classic, when the 298 kg hit George's sticking point, he blew past it to lockout. How? He developed a tremendous start and increased the bar speed on speed day. On max effort day, the chains develop and teach acceleration merely through trying to outrun the chains. Also, when George misses at his mini-max, he is performing functional isometrics in the best possible way. As the chains add to the weight of the bar, we can determine the precise point where George fails. We know where his weak point is with a particular weight. Conventional isometrics (that joint jarring pressing against immovable pins) is unnecessary. The bands work in the same way but with added eccentric work from the bands pulling a lifter down. This additional eccentric work also builds muscle mass.

After each workout, George tries to increase his tricep work in volume and weight. The triceps are worked first after the main exercise followed by the delts, lats, and upper back. Remember, this is done after dynamic day work on Sunday and after max effort day work on Wednesday.

An individual must bring up his weaknesses through special work and develop special strength such as starting, accelerating, eccentric, and concentric strength. We do primarily slow work on the stability ball. Always try to cover everything. At 50-years-old, I benched 600 on February 15,

1998. I like to do three sets of heavy (155s or 125s) dumbbells to failure on a stability ball. This is commonly known as the repetition method. We throw in weight releases on speed day or max effort day, get a good response for a few weeks, and then switch to something else.

Using Chains in Training

There are many keys to success, but two invaluable ones are accelerating strength training and accommodating resistance by adding chains or bands or sometimes both. Chains and bands are used in all of our training, be it the dynamic method for speed-strength and acceleration or the maximum effort day to develop absolute strength. In the bench press, bands and chains have helped 17 of our lifters achieve 550 or more and seven lifters have done 600 or more. When I talk about bench training, I am referring to my lifters with a 550 bench or better. That's whom we experiment with. On speed day for the bench, while doing the 8–10 sets of three reps, the chains are attached in the following manner. Loop a 1/4-inch link chain with a hook around the bar sleeve, regulating the height of the 5/8-inch link chain (five feet long). Run the 5/8 chain through the metal loop and adjust it so that half of the 5/8 chain is lying on the floor while the bars in the rack. Use 60% of a no-shirt max on the bar. For example, if a lifter's max is 500, put 300 lbs on the bar. When the bar is on the chest, only the weight of the bar should be on the chest. That is, all the 5/8 chain should be on the floor.

If a lifter's best bench is 250 lbs or less, use one pair of 1/2-inch link chains. These weigh 23 lbs a set, so he is locking out an extra 11.5 lbs. A 350 or more bencher should use one pair of 5/8-inch link chain. By doing this, he'll be locking out an extra 20 lbs. (They weigh 20 lbs each but half is on the floor at lockout.) A 500 lb bencher can use both the 5/8- and ½-inch chains for a combined added weight of 31 lbs. A 600 bencher uses two, 5/8 chains and sometimes adds a 1/2-inch chain

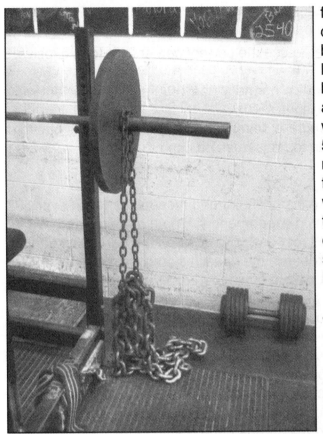

for 40–51 added lbs at lockout. You can experiment on your own, but remember this process is to build bar speed and acceleration. It also teaches how to launch the bar off the chest. A special note: Lower the bar quickly and try to catch and reverse the weight as fast as possible. Never pause. On max effort day, warm up to 315, and then, do a single. Next, add a 5/8-inch chain on each side and do a single. On the next set, use two sets of chain, then three sets, and so forth. This is similar to how a bench shirt works. The weight is less at the bottom and much greater at the top. The chains build not only acceleration but also a quick start and a strong lockout. For floor pressing, simply drape the 5/8-inch chain over the sleeve of the bar and you're ready.

JM Blakley and George Halbert do a lot of floor presses like this. George uses 200 lbs of chain (five sets of chain) and works up to a single. His best at a bodyweight of 220 is 440 plus 200 lbs of chain, which is 640 at the top. JM uses a different combination of weight and chains. His best was 400 lbs on the bar with seven sets of chains for a combined weight of 680 at lockout. Try any weight-to-chain ratio; feel free to experiment. A cambered bar can be used as well. These are a few methods to add to max effort day.

While many people call me for advice, others give me information that I pass along. A gentleman, whose name I don't remember, related to me some training he had done with chains. This was a few years ago, but we finally got around to using chains in an experiment with Amy Weisberger (a world champion whose best total in 12 weeks went from 975 to 1025 at 123), Vanessa Schwenker (a national champion whose total went from 1030 to 1100 in 12 weeks), Traci Tate (a novice lifter who increased her bench from 180 to 210), and Dave Tate. (Dave Tate, Traci's husband, is a 308 with a previous total of 2028. He went from 782 to 830 in the squat, 540 to 585 in the bench, and 705 to 720 in the deadlift for a total of 2135. After being stuck at 710 on a low box squat for two years, he made 765 after six workouts.) Now with these examples in mind, here's how we use chains in our training.

The chains are five feet long with a 5/8-inch link size and weighing 20 lbs each. They can be found at most industrial tool supply companies. For bench pressing, we attach the chains to the bar, so when the arms are fully extended, half the chain is resting on the floor. After lowering the bar to the chest, all the chain is on the floor. By doing this, the original bar weight is maintained. Let's go over this again. If 300 lbs is on the bar plus 80 lbs of chains attached (two sets of chains) with half the chain already on the floor, that adds up to 340 at the lockout position. When the bar is lowered, all the chain is on the floor, and the total weight on the bar is reduced to the original 300 at chest level. As a lifter presses, the weight gradually increases to 340.

Training with chains in this manner accomplishes three things:

1. We have maintained our original weight in order to use the correct percentage for explosive training.
2. We have overloaded the top portion of the lift, which normally does not receive sufficient work because of increased body leverage at this position.
3. A neurological response to build explosive strength is developed. This training trains one to drive to the top because he can't slack off at the top phase as he used to.

Those who bench press 400 lbs or less should use 40 lbs of chain, and those who bench over 500 should use 80 lbs of chain. Individuals in between should experiment with both amounts and aim for adequate bar speed. Remember, half the chain should rest on the floor when the bar is racked. Lifters who have a sticking point at or slightly above the knees in the deadlift also find great benefit from using chains. Attach the chains to the bar with a light weight chain to adjust where the heavy chain leaves the floor and contributes to the weight on the bar. Tom Waddle uses 405–455 of regular bar weight on the deadlift bar. To that, he adds up to 200 lbs of chain. As he lifts the 405, it gradually turns into 605 as the chains leave the floor.

The chains compensate for added leverage near the lockout. If a lifter is weak at the top, this will solve his problem. Also, it will develop starting strength. Because the chains make it more difficult to press as the bar ascends, the lifter will instinctively try to accelerate the bar from start to finish. The effects of special training normally occur in 2–4 weeks, but to my surprise, the training effect with chains is immediate.

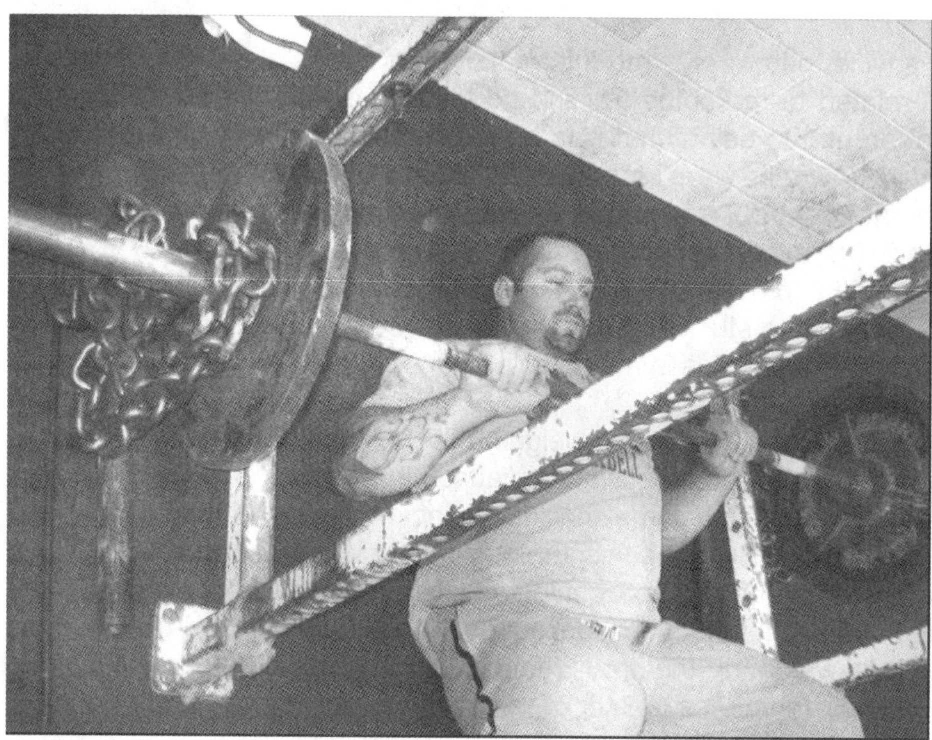

As an experiment, we loaded the squat bar to 415 and did two reps. Next, a set of chains was added. They were attached so that all the chain weight was on the bar at the top of 455 and half was unloaded at the bottom or 435. Four additional sets were executed for a total of five with 415 or more. On set six, two sets of chains were placed on the bar.

The top weight was 495, and the bottom weight was 455. On set seven, three sets of chains were used. The top weight was 535, and the bottom weight was 475.

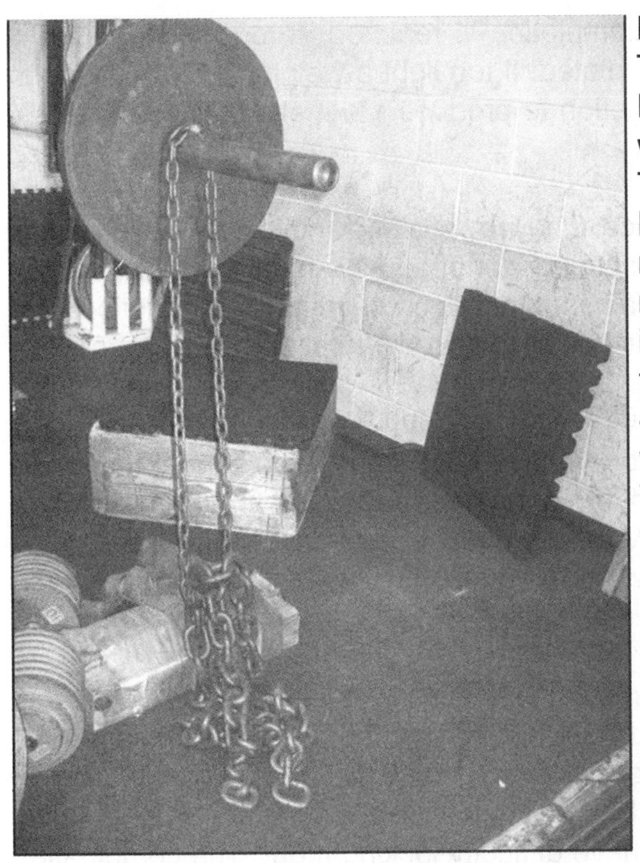

For set eight, four sets of chains were employed. The top weight was 575, and the bottom weight 495. For set nine, five sets of chains were used. The top weight was 615, and the bottom weight was 515. These sets were done with 50 second rest periods. Next, we removed all the chains, so that the bar was reduced to the original 415. The box, which was already an inch below parallel, was lowered another inch. Four more sets were done. To our surprise, they were more explosive than our first sets with 415. After 13 sets with 50-second rest periods, we were actually more explosive because of the chains. This immediate benefit is unheard of with conventional training.

At Westside, we all use chains and bands even to squat. Here's how. First use a set of 1/4-inch link chains that attach to the bar sleeves. We suspend a metal ring from the 1/4-inch chains, regulating the height of the 5/8 chain from the floor. Loop the 5/8-inch chain through the metal ring so about three chain links are lying on the floor when standing. When sitting on the box slightly below parallel, half of the chain will be unloaded onto the floor.

How much chain should be used? If an individual squats 350 or less, he should use one set of 5/8-inch chains, equaling 40 lbs at the top. If a person squats about 600 lbs, he should use about 60–70 lbs of chain at the top. If someone squats 800 lbs, he should use 80–120 lbs of chain at the top. About 10% of one's squat weight should be added with chain. If a lifter is doing sets with 400 on the bar, she should be standing up with 520. An 800 squatter whose top training weight is 480, or 60%, will add 80–120 lbs of chain to the bar, equaling 600 at the top.

I don't sell chains, but I hope you buy this idea. It is one of the most effective ways to train that I have encountered. The chains build starting strength and overload the body at the top of all three lifts, where due to added leverage, the muscles receive little work compared to the bottom portion of the lift. At the bottom, the chains work as a lightening device, enabling one to handle the most weight at any one position of the lift. I am passing this on in the hopes of helping you reach your goals no matter what they are.

The Force—Velocity Curve, Science Behind Bands

Looking at the relationship between force and velocity, we know that while using light loads an increase in speed has little effect. An example is throwing a whiffle ball. The load is so light that even throwing it twice as fast will propel it no farther. In contrast, strength becomes much more important when the load or external resistance is increased. When doing a barbell lift, the bar speed at the beginning is zero, and of course, at its completion, it is reduced to zero again.

After accelerating to top speed, it decelerates as completion is reached. If too much weight is used, the start may be too hard for the lift to be completed. If too light a weight is used, although the start will be quick, it will be too light at its completion to produce a beneficial effect. In either case, an unsatisfactory result will occur.

This brings us to a solution: accommodating resistance. One way of achieving this is with isokinetic devices with variable speeds. They can be set for fast speed for speed-strength or slow speed for strength-speed. There are drawbacks to these machines. Most don't have eccentric motion, and because they are machines, they do not increase stability. However, by using rubber bands with barbell weight, many things can be accomplished.

When training with bar weight alone, the weight is too heavy at the start or too light at the top. If only bands are used, the weight is too light in the bottom and too heavy at the top. With a combination of bands and bar weight, an athlete can truly accommodate resistance. Whether training for speed-strength or strength-speed, the ratio between band tension and weight can be altered to accomplish a set goal.

When implementing the theory of accommodating resistance, one must look at the relationship between force and posture. At different joint angle positions, the amount of weight lifted varies because of one's mini-max, or sticking point. At some joint angles, great force can be generated. For example, the deadlift is a fairly simple task. Yet one lifter will experience a hard start and an easy finish and another will blast the bar off the floor but have difficulty locking it out. The combination of band tension and bar weight allows maximal tension throughout the entire range of motion, not just at the weakest point. This is the peak contraction principle at its best.

The bands may not out-accelerate gravity, but they will significantly increase the eccentric phase as illustrated by our experiments with one of our 1008 squatters, Matt Smith. With 550 lbs of only weight on the bar, the eccentric portion took 0.9 seconds and the concentric 1.35 seconds. With a combination of weight and bands (375 + 175, 550 at the top and 375 at the bottom), the eccentric phase was 0.55 seconds and the concentric 0.76 seconds. When only bands were used (750 at the top and 550 at the bottom), the eccentric phase was 0.53 seconds and the concentric 0.57. Bands work like muscle and connective tissue, lengthening and contracting in addition to absorbing kinetic energy.

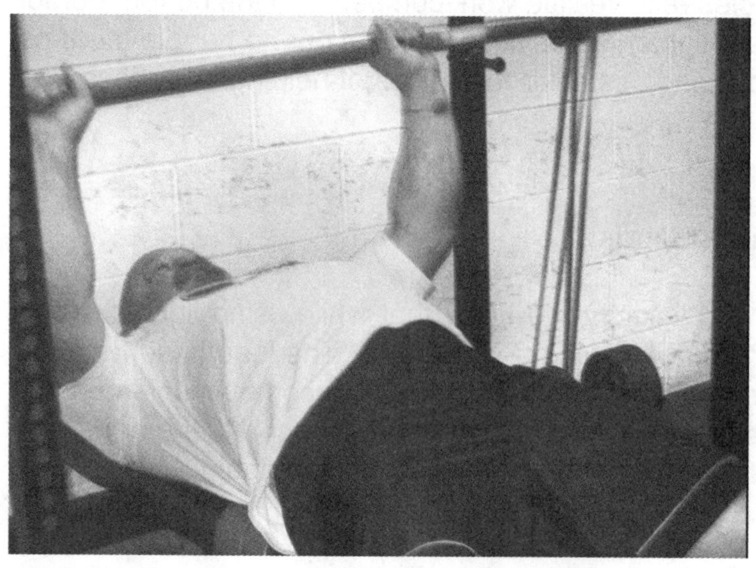

The Effect of Bands—Virtual Force

To test the effects of bands on speed-strength, Ano Turtiainen, Chuck Vogelpohl, Mike Ruggiera, Tony Hutson, Paul Childress, and Keiran Kidder use 40% bar weight and 25% band tension at the top and 10% band tension at the bottom. This equals 65% at the top and 50% at the bottom: 405 lbs of bar weight, 250 lbs of band tension at the top, and 100 at the bottom. The above mentioned lifters all squat 1000 or more officially.

For strength-speed, or slow strength, the band tension is 44% or 440 at the top and 20%, or 200 at the bottom. The bar weight ranges from 450–500 lbs. The top would equate to 940 total and the bottom 700 for the top weights used for five sets of two reps. This phase is known as the circa-max, or near maximal phase.

The relationship between force and posture can't be matched correctly with barbell weight alone. Weights are much too heavy at the bottom and too light at the top. Bands alone are too light at the bottom and too heavy at the top. With a combination of bands and weight, the relationship between force and posture can be matched more precisely.

Compensatory acceleration can't be accomplished effectively with light or moderate weight because these weights are too light at near completion. At this point, the lifter is much stronger than the load and a deceleration occurs. The answer is to employ bands or chains. If a person has ever lifted in a power rack, he has noticed that as he raises the pin levels, he can lift more. Each time he raises the pins two inches, he can lift 50 more lbs. It makes sense to attach bands to add that 50 lbs every two inches. If he places his lowest pin record on the highest pin, it would be much too light. Conversely, if someone places his highest pin record on the lowest pin, he can't budge it. By merely attaching bands to the bar, an individual can maximally lift the most weight at each level (i.e. accommodating resistance). This is also a contrast method where the weight is much heavier at the top than the bottom. Unlike using weight releasers where the additional weight is released at the bottom, it is regained during the concentric phase.

Zatsiorsky states, "The magnitude of weight that an athlete can lift in a given motion is limited by the strength attainable at the weakest point of the full range of joint motion" (Practice and Science of Strength Training, 1995). In other words, muscles are activated maximally only at the weakest point of motion (peak contraction principle). There are four methods to approach this concept: (1) accommodating resistance, (2) the peak contraction principle, (3) accentuation of muscular efforts, and (4) ignorance of the issue, the approach followed by most. At Westside, we use the three methods that work all the time.

When using chains, the proper method is to have them unload at the bottom, or starting position, known as the concentric phase. Using a large load of chain at the bottom teaches a lifter to explode at the start, enabling him to overcome the additional load as it reloads onto the bar becoming heavier toward completion.

Bands have an added value of kinetic energy. A larger, moving mass results in more kinetic energy. In reversible movement exercises such as squatting to a box, an increase in mass leads to a decrease in rebound velocity, but a moderate increase in velocity when approaching a box leads to an increase in rebound velocity. This is why box squatting is essential to the stretch reflex action. The stretch reflex lasts up to two seconds and longer in trained athletes (Wilson, Supertraining).

Unlike a conventional squat where an athlete lower himself to a certain position and reaches zero velocity at that point before overcoming the load, in a box squat he is moving when contact is made. This is kinetic energy. This helps increase the velocity of the eccentric phase, causing added kinetic energy (over speed eccentrics). I have named this process virtual loading.

To observe an example of virtual loading, jump on a bathroom scale and see what it registers for a split second. The readout is much heavier than one's actual body weight. This is virtual force from virtual loading. Joe Dell-Aquila, who has a doctorate in physics, helped to name this phenomenon.

A test was performed with a 970 lb squatter, Matt Smith (who also has a 2470 total at 345 lbs). First, Matt squatted 550 of barbell weight only. The eccentric phase was 15 inches to the box. The duration of this phase was 0.9 seconds. The duration of the concentric phase was 1.35 seconds.

Dr. Akita, who has a doctorate in calculus, measured the time in this study. Then the bands were attached to the bar, producing a weight of 750 lbs at the top and 550 at the bottom on the same height box. The duration of the eccentric phase with bands was 0.53 seconds. This was due to the over-speed eccentrics caused by the bands pulling Matt down, causing added kinetic energy as stated by Zatsiorsky in Science and Practice of Strength Training. The duration of the concentric phase, returning the bar to the top, was 0.57 seconds. That's right, 0.57 seconds with an extra 250 lbs of resistance at the top.

To develop speed in the eccentric phase, six males who squat 1004–1080 with bodyweights ranging from 220–365 used four phases of special strength work.

Phase I: Lactic acid tolerance training
Squat sets were performed, 15–20 sets of two reps with about 45-seconds rest between sets. One quarter of the weight was contributed by bands.

Phase II: Strength-speed
This phase is nearly impossible and dangerous for the untrained college student. Band tension is 60% of the total bar weight. To lift limit weights, one must be under max or near max tension for the length of time it takes to complete a max squat, which may be up to three seconds.

Phase III: Speed-strength
Squats were done with a bar weight of 40% for 10–12 sets of two reps. The band tension at the top was 200 lbs and 100 lbs at the bottom.

Phase IV: Circa-max phase
This phase employs a three-week pendulum wave. The bar weight is 45–50%, and the bands contribute 40%. This is slightly under the recommended 90–97%, but the bands cause a total reduction in momentum. Also, eccentric work creates the most muscular soreness. The over-speed is very stressful on the lifter. Five sets of two reps are done.

When done correctly, the bands exert a force on the body over a distance (in Matt's case, 15 inches), resulting in potential energy. That energy is transferred into the muscles and soft tissues of the body. This is a form of the shock method, or plyometrics. Plyometrics should be used only by those capable of squatting two times their bodyweight. The box makes it possible for not only the feet but also the hamstrings and glutes to absorb energy. The amount of kinetic energy an object has also depends on the object's mass as well as its speed. That's why fully sitting on a box is essential. Remember also that the stretch reflex lasts a full two seconds, so there is no need to touch and go off the box.

When using chains, the chain must be almost totally deloaded onto the floor. A large chain cannot merely be connected to the sleeve on the bar. Rather, a special attachment should be used on the bar to hook the working chains securely. When most of the resistance is made up by bands, the slower the bar travels. Thus, strength-speed is being developed. As the bar weight and band resistance is lowered, bar speed is increased for the development of speed-strength and even explosive strength.

Training with the Bands – An Overview

Bands are a little tough for some on speed day because of the added eccentric properties they create. Weight resistance is also much more radical at different positions. It's much less at the bottom but much greater at the top. The bands are literally pulling down on the lifter.

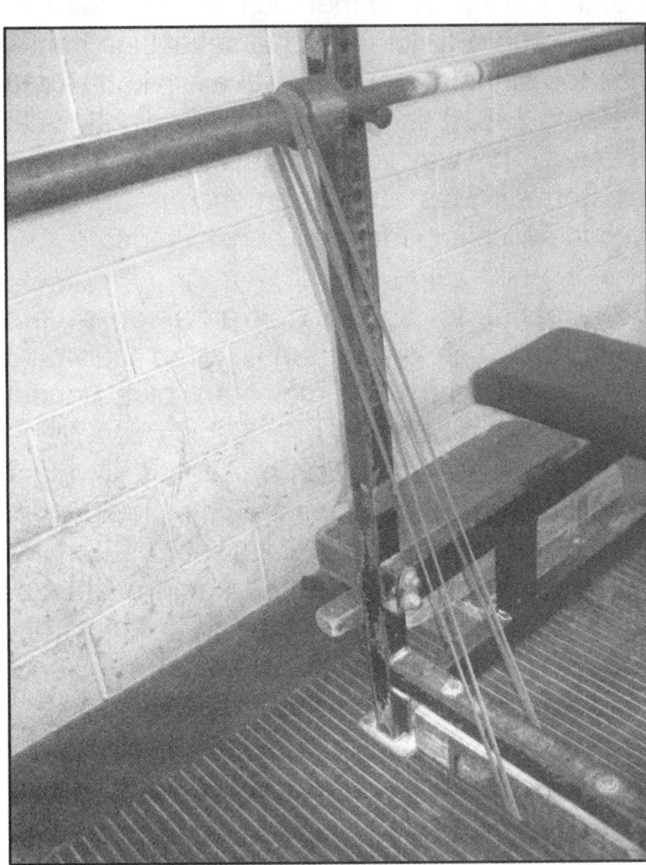

Bands have many benefits:

- accommodating resistance
- added kinetic energy in the eccentric phase by out-acceleration
- gravity
- similarity to muscle and connective tissue
- tremendous stability

When using bands, be careful not to over do it. The bands produce a large amount of eccentric overloading and can cause excessive soreness, but they are more than worth it. They build the lockout as well as the start. A lifter has to outrun the bands, so he develops a quick start, enabling him to lockout a heavy weight.

The most popular methods implementing the bands are as follows. On max effort day, do board presses with four, 2 x 6s. Loop the bands through the bottom supports of the bench and then around

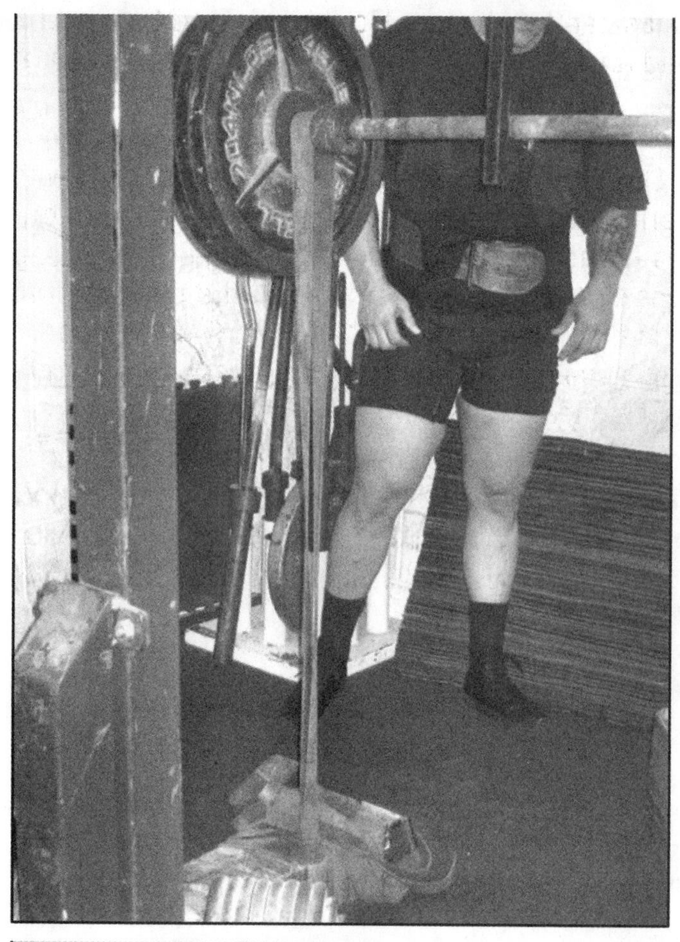

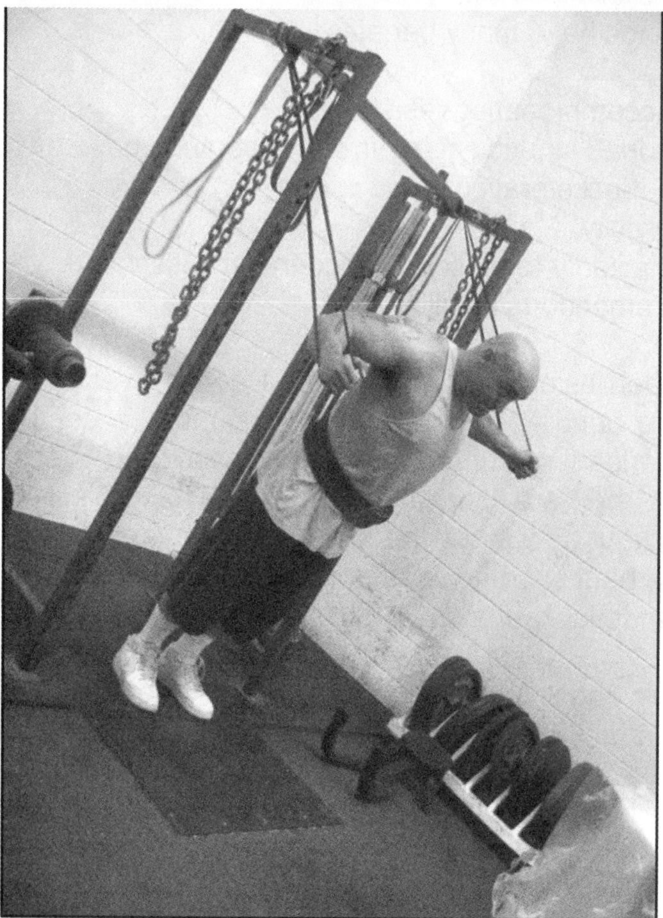

the sleeve of the bar. When using 4-boards, the tension is never released. Because of this, a quick start is impossible and locking out a heavy weight is really tough. To make it even more difficult, use a cambered bar. JM presses with bands are very popular at Westside. Use several bands to increase the challenge. Lower the bar straight down, aiming between the nipples and chin and stop 4–5 inches off the chest; then, press back up. Use a close grip.

Bands and chains are often employed for triceps extensions. This radically changes the strength curve of the movement by accommodating resistance (lifts are usually easier at the top). Thanks to Doug Ebert for the following band exercise. Attach a blue band to the bar and start with 95–135 lbs. Take a pink or green band, depending on individual strength, twist it once, and place it around the upper back, so the tension is pulling back the hands. Now, lie down on the bench, stretching the band to grab the bar, and start benching. This "double" tension is unreal. Also, try the lightened method recommended by Carl of Jump- Stretch. Attach a set of blue bands to the top of the power rack with a slip knot. Load the bar to 135. It should be almost weightless at the chest. This way you can bench 135 lbs more than normal. This builds tremendous power at lockout, which is perfect for bench shirts.

To use bands for squatting, if a person squats 650 or less, use green bands. If an individual squats more than 650, implement blue bands. Here are two examples of 900 plus squatters. Billy Masters and Dave Barno used a top weight of 500 lbs and 150 lbs of tension with blue bands. Billy did 909, and Dave did a perfect 925. Neither train at Westside, but they use our methods. When squatting, wave the training weights from 50–60% in 3–4-week cycles. Do mostly 6–8 sets of two reps with 45-seconds rest between sets.

For max effort work, a bar weight of say 400–500 lbs can be chosen. Do a single and then add a set of chains. Keep doing singles and add a second and third set of chains until a PR is broken or a miss occurs.

The same can be accomplished with flex bands. Good mornings are a great exercise to do with chains and bands. High pulls with the pink or green bands are also great. I have seen one of our lifters with a 600 deadlift go to 670 in six months by adding bands on the deadlift. Bob Young used 275–315 on the bar with about 200 lbs of tension from the bands. We use the platform that Jump-Stretch sells with their bands to do this exercise. To excel at powerlifting or any sport, speed-strength must be developed, along with increasing acceleration, and gaining absolute strength. Bands and chains can be instrumental in developing these aspects of strength. I highly recommend that trying them as soon as possible.

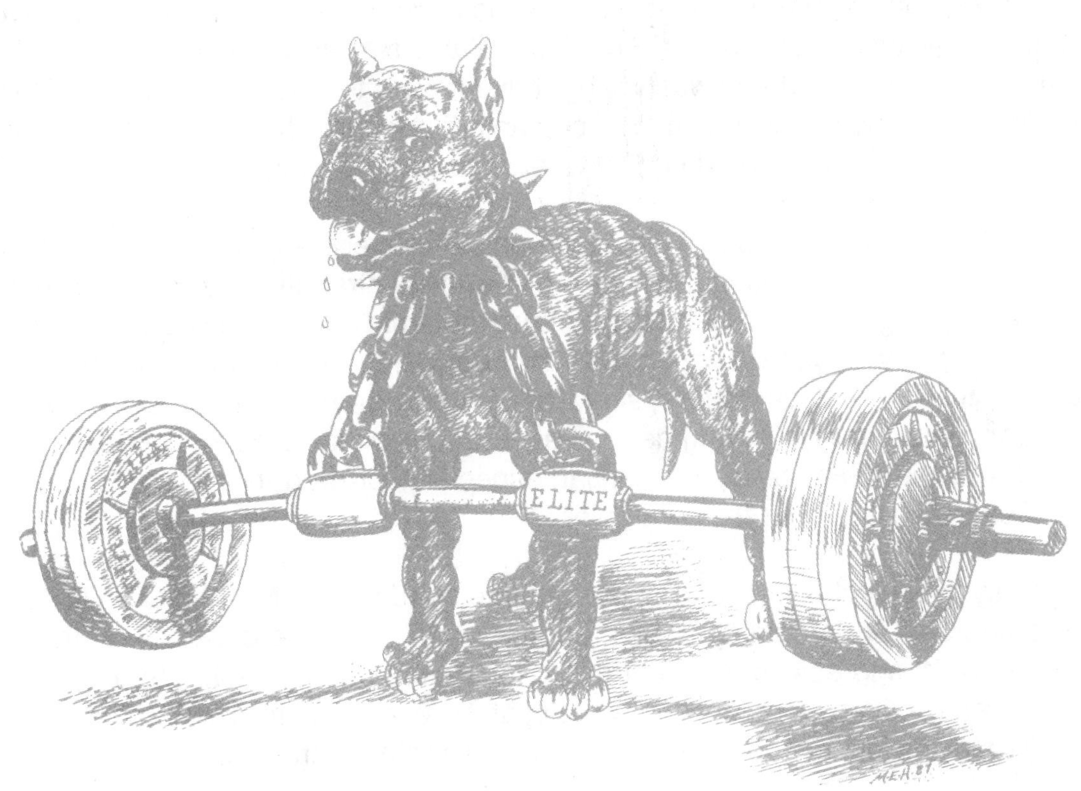

WESTSIDE BARBELL™

OVERCOMING PLATEAUS

There are basically four reasons for failing or succeeding:

1. physiological
2. psychological
3. technical
4. exercise selection

As for psychological, don't have deadbeats hanging around. Stay in a positive mental state. If your training partner can't hang, no matter what their age, give them the hook. You must be competitive even while training. You also must want your training partner to succeed, so you can be pushed even more.

On maximum effort day, go until only the top man is left. On dynamic day, try to hurt your training partner with short rest periods. To win, you have to put yourself through hell. Have training partners that want to kick your ass all the time (during the workout). Trash talk is always present at Westside. A new lifter at the gym wanted to load my plates for me during one of his first workouts. I asked him if he respected me. He said he did. I said, "If you respect me while we train, Ill boot you out of here." He got the idea. When I was young, I didn't want to lose to an old man. Now that I'm an old man, I don't like to lose to young men. I cop an attitude, and that attitude kept only five men on the top 100 list kicking my ass (and I know where they live).

What about the physiological aspects? This encompasses several aspects of training such as: the development of starting, accelerating, absolute, and special strength. These are primarily developed with barbell training. The correct loading on the dynamic day as well as the maximum effort day is essential. The physiological aspects also include the development of muscle hypertrophy. This can be accomplished with dumbbells, sled work, and the proper use of special exercises such as: chins, rows, triceps extensions, and delt raises. Exercises that raise work capacity or general physical preparedness (GPP) are also essential, especially for drug-free lifters. Men such as Bill Gillespie and Sean Culnan are perfect examples.

To sum up the psychological aspect of training with the words of Dr. Mel Siff and Dr. Yuri Verkhoshansky, the authors of Supertraining, a high degree of performance depends on the motivation to reach certain goals, aggression, concentration, focus, the ability to tolerate pain while coping with anxiety or stress, the development of a winning attitude, and the ability to manage distractions and relax. While striving to develop the best method of resistance training, we are led down many paths.

The three most common approaches:

1. accentuation
2. peak contraction
3. accommodating resistance

Accentuation: Accentuation occurs when exercises are used at precise angular positions in which maximal efforts are developed during a specific, sport movement. The greater the force contributes to greater the velocity.

Peak contraction: With the peak contraction principle, maximal force is developed at the weakest body position such as at the start of a pec deck.

Accomodating resistance: Accommodating resistance refers to maximizing muscular tension throughout the entire range of motion. This is done with bands or chains added to the bar, which is called the reactive method. The weight is different at one position of the lift than another, causing one to react to a contrasting effect. Reactive methods build power and explosive strength by imposing great demands on the central nervous system. The most common reactive method is plyometrics, but because this system is well documented and thought out, the term powermetrics applies. What we are looking at is resistance training with a second or third type of resistance other than barbell weight such as bands and chains.

The Mini-max Point

Using only bar weight causes the optimal training weight to be too heavy at the bottom and too light at the top of the lift. Bands on a bar with no weight make the resistance too heavy at the top and too light at the bottom. However, a combination of both bands and weight creates a near perfect situation.

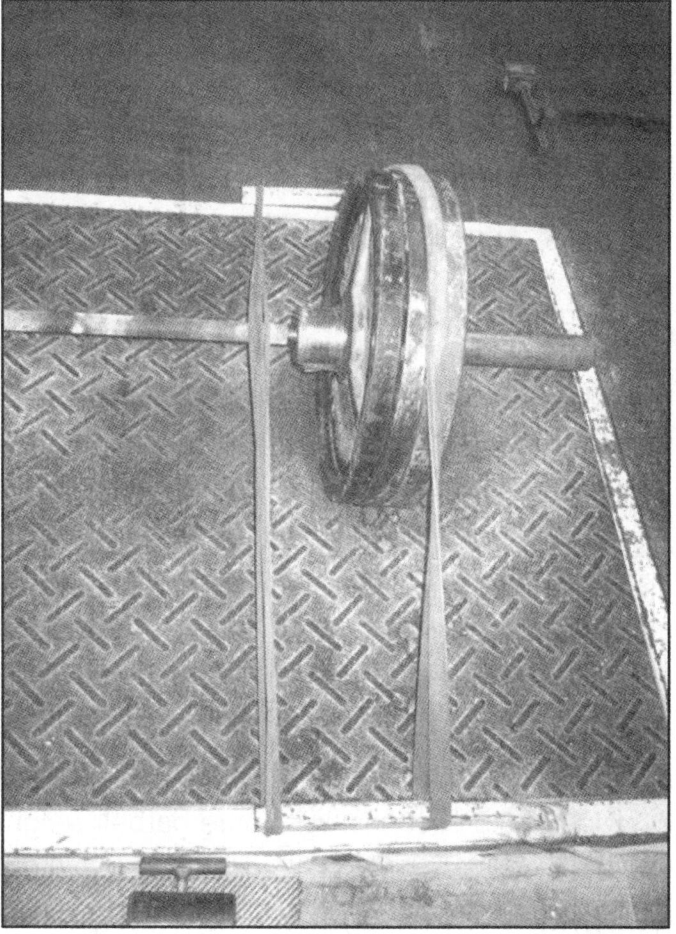

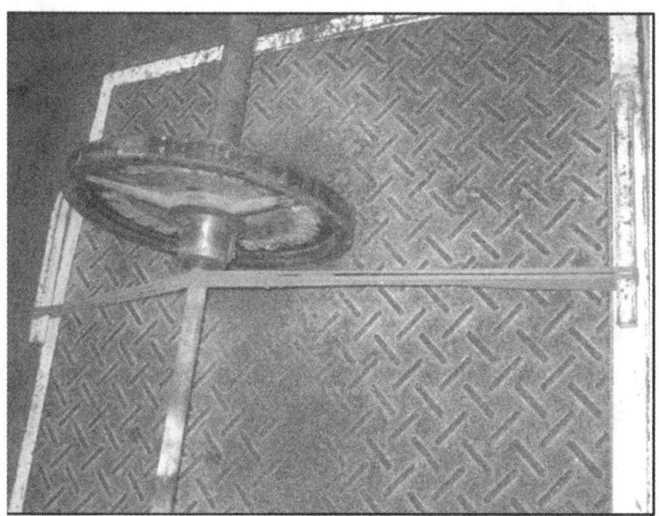

But is it? Because of the mini-max position, when hip extension strength is greatest, the knee extension is poorest. The opposite is true in other force-posture situations. The maximum strength value of hip extension is 150 degrees. For knee extension, it is 120 degrees. For the layman, what does this mean? It simply explains why some are strong at the bottom of a squat or deadlift and bench press while others are stronger at the top.

The low back can be a factor in how strong a lifter is at the halfway point. The same is true in the bench press. Bands added to the bar can accomplish many things. They can help reduce bar deceleration on the concentric phase, accommodate resistance, eliminate momentum, and increase the stretch reflex function, causing over-speed eccentrics, producing a virtual force effect, which is a loading that is there but not recognized. How can people with different mini- maxes benefit from the same band training?

The staggered system is a method of combining chains and bands of different amounts.

Method 1: Bands are available of variable tension. Tension can be by placing more than one band on the bar (up to three) but not just on the bar. Westside lifters may place one band over the bar and then a band over 25 lb plates on the bar or over 45 lb plates. Where the strongest band for loading or deloading is placed depends on an individual's mini-max.

Method 2: Chains are used when looking for an abrupt loading effect. For the strongest squatters (800 plus), a combination of bands is used for a constant loading/deloading effect and 120–160 lbs of chains that can be totally unloaded at the bottom, partially deloaded, or completely reloaded at the top.

Method 3: Ano Turtiainen, the super 1080 squatter from Finland, implements bands over the bar and then adds weight releasers, overloading the eccentric phase. When the releasers unload, a contrast effect results, causing a lighter concentric phase.

Method 4: Ano also attaches a strong band to the top of the Monolift, creating a lightened effect. He will set the bands to reduce the load by 130 lbs at the bottom. When the load is lifted, the 130 lbs is again applied to the bar.

Method 5: To ultimately overload the eccentric phase, weight releasers and the lightened method are used concurrently.

Method 6: Use chains only, not bands with the weight releasers. Chain weight does not cause over-speed eccentrics. To achieve the highest results, switch the combination of resistance often, usually every three weeks. This places maximal demands on the body regardless of one's mini-max.

Never do sets with a large amount of band tension and then remove the bands and try a heavy weight. Timing on the eccentric phase will be off. This was confirmed by Professor Akita. Using a large percentage of bands above 40% causes a super over-speed eccentric phase lasting an average of 0.5 seconds. With pure barbell weight, it is 1.5 seconds. The reversal muscle action is confused. This occurs in squatting or benching.

Staggered Loading Effect

For more staggered deadlift loading, try using mini-bands doubled over the bar. Here at Westside, the added band tension looks like this:

- Mini doubled adds 220 lbs
- Jumbo mini doubled adds 280 lbs
- Light single adds 100 lbs
- Medium single adds 150 lbs
- Strong single adds 220 lbs

To achieve a staggered effect, place a doubled mini-band over the bar. To add tension starting at the knee, add light, medium, or strong bands over the bar. To increase tension below knee level, place the bands over a 25-lb plate on the bar. To intensify tension close to the platform, place bands over 45-lb plates. To achieve a triple staggered load, place mini-bands doubled over the bar, green or blue bands over 25-lb plates, and finally a light (purple) band over the 45s. It is recommended to do this extreme loading for only –2 weeks and then return to speed-strength work.

Remember, if you don't apply bands, chains, or weight releasers correctly, you won't get the desired results. Review Westside's reactive method video for the correct use. Most of what you see is for the advanced lifter or athlete. Pay close attention to proper loading (i.e. the number of lifts at certain percentages). This is essential.

The Squat

Your squat is going nowhere. No matter what you do, it won't increase. What can you do? First, let's talk about form; box squatting is a must. Use a box that is slightly below parallel. Sit fully on the box, keeping all muscles tight, most importantly the abs and the obliques. By releasing only the hip muscles, you are going from a relaxed state to a dynamic phase. This is one of the best methods of developing absolute strength as well as explosive strength. Lowering the bar produces a great amount of kinetic energy, which is stored in the body resulting in reversal strength.

For box squatting, the form is the same as regular squatting. Before descending, the glutes must be pushed out to the rear. Because you are going to squat to the rear and not down, this sets up the body for a stretch reflex. Next, push the knees out to the sides. This accomplishes two things. It places much of the stress, or work, on the hips, and it will greatly increase your leverage in the bottom of the squat. By pushing the knees out, you are at least attempting to keep the knee joint in line with the hip joint. In theory, if you can stand up with 1000 lbs while your shoulder, hip, knee, and ankle joints are in line, you could squat to parallel with the same weight if the above joints are kept in line. That is why it is so important to super arch the back, keeping the chest up while in the bottom of a squat.

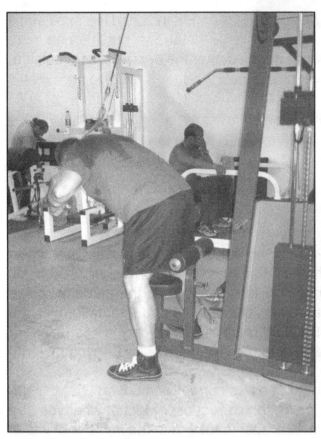

If you correctly push the glutes out first on the descent, the head will move last. On the ascending phase, the reverse is true. The head must come up first by pushing the head into the traps. It is then natural for the hips and glutes to follow. Also, never push down with the feet when squatting. Instead, push out to the sides on the eccentric and concentric phases. That's why we recommend Chuck Taylor shoes. The feet can be pushed out to the sides without them rolling over. When sitting on the box, it is possible, and desirable, for the shins to be past perpendicular. This places all the work on the vital squat muscles, which is impossible with regular squatting.

Train on a box with 50–60% of your best contest squat. A 500 lb squatter would start at 250 and jump 10 lbs a week for six weeks. Now, the weight is 300 lbs. On week seven, drop back to 250 (50%) and a new wave. This is done for ten sets of two reps for four weeks.

Then, drop to eight sets. This keeps the bar volume relatively the same. The volume changes dramatically when starting the wave again. Add 3–4 special exercises that have not been used for a period of time.

The combination of varying special exercises and using short rest periods (about 40 seconds between sets) has proven to be most effective for producing growth hormone. The short rest causes lactic acid to build up.

When fighting through this discomfort, the most growth hormone is produced. Also, when using maximal weights in the same exercise for more than three weeks, growth hormone production stops! Wusef Omar, a colleague of the renowned Tudor Bompa, with the help of top exercise physiologists validated this at York University in Toronto.

After box squatting on the dynamic day, select 2–4 special exercises to improve. Because all the muscles that squat are located in the back of the body with the exception of the abs, select exercises for the spinal erectors, glutes, and hamstrings such as back raises, reverse hyperextensions, pull-throughs, sled dragging, and calf/ham glute raises.

The abs are essential for squatting, and abdominal training is very serious. When squatting or deadlifting, a person is standing up; therefore, we do the majority of our abdominal work standing. This is done on the lat machine. Face away from the machine and pull a triceps rope down to the base of the neck. Hold the ends of the rope against the chest. Now, bend over by forcing the abs to flex downward into the hips, which is exactly how the abs are designed to work. The obliques are the most important ab muscles. When flexing a weight off the floor or starting out of a heavy squat, it is the lower obliques that initiate the entire upward motion.

What I have been discussing is correct exercise selection. Note I have not included leg extensions and leg press. Leg extensions are a waste; it's true that they isolate the quads, but the amount of weight is insignificant. Leg press machines are very dangerous in general. They place a tremendous amount of strain on the lower back. A leg curl machine is designed for bodybuilding. While it does build the hamstrings between the knee and hip, bodybuilders use it because it does not build size at the knee or the glute tie in. It starts with knee extension and ends with hip extension but in a biomechanically unsound fashion. A glute ham machine works both the knee and hip extenders simultaneously. As in running and jumping, the quads do very little in squatting. Don't waste too much time on quads. When accommodating resistance, use chains or bands. Weight releasers are useful for building reversal strength.

I have discussed Friday's speed day for squats. In the development of absolute strength, we have a max effort day three days later. On this day, we never do regular squats. About seven weeks out of ten, we do some kind of good mornings for a 3RM, using special bars including the safety squat bar, Buffalo bar, bent bars, and a special cambered bar that has a 14-inch camber, which takes the upper back out and makes the mid to lower back work overtime. Two out of ten workouts are some type of squatting on a variety of boxes from 8–17-inches high and with a variety of bars or with the MantaRay or front squat harness. Do a 1–3 rep max in these special squats. Switch the core exercises every two weeks again to maintain production of growth hormone. One out of ten workouts should be some kind of pull for a 1RM.

After the core lift, use 2–4 special exercises (glute ham raise, reverse hyperextensions, or pull-throughs). Raise special work for 3–4 weeks. This is the correct method to raise volume with special work, not the classical exercises. Note: Close to a meet, work on speed and raise special exercises for the abs, low back, hamstrings, glutes, and hips.

The Bench Press

Everyone likes to bench press, but no one likes to get stuck. Not making progress is no fun and sometimes grounds for retirement. Only the strong at heart will continue. Should anyone ever stall out? The answer is no. The problem is if a lifter does the same training, he will get the same results.

To address the technical aspects of benching, it must be determined what is proper bench press form. It has always been thought that an individual should push the bar back over the face. However, it makes little sense to do so. When a bar moves toward the face, bad things occur. The delts are placed under great stress, especially the rotators, and no one wants that. Also, the lats are no longer involved in the lift when the bar moves toward the face. The bar should be lowered with the lats, not the arms. Without strong lat involvement, there is little chance that the bar can be placed on the chest correctly. It may land too high or too low. If it is too low, the delts are involved too much, and if the bar lands too high, the triceps are involved too much. Strong lats ensure the bar is placed in the correct position, that is, with the forearms vertical. In this position, an equal amount of delt, pec, and triceps are used in pressing. If the bar is not placed in the correct position, delt and pec injuries are more likely to occur.

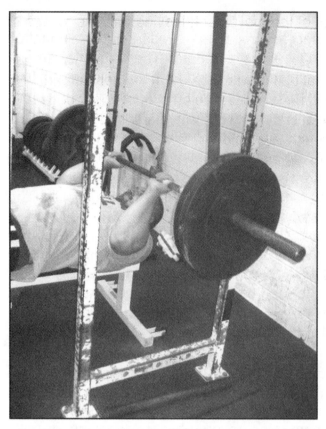

The path of the bar in the concentric phase (raising) should be a straight line, which requires the correct use of the muscles. When the Clemson University coaching staff wanted to know which are the most important muscle groups for benching, George Halbert told them triceps are first, lats second, upper back third, and delts last. George holds the world record in the 220s at 657, a world record of 688 in the 242s, and a 683 at 227, the heaviest triple bodyweight bench of all time (457 lbs over body weight!).

The delts are almost always overworked, and the triceps are underworked. A lot of delt and pec injuries occur but not a lot of triceps injuries. This tells me that most lifters don't train their triceps to the max. When the triceps, upper back, and lats are the strongest muscle groups, the bar travels in a straight line, making the distance to lockout much shorter. Also, it does not require the arms to rotate outward, which causes injuries to the pecs and rotators.

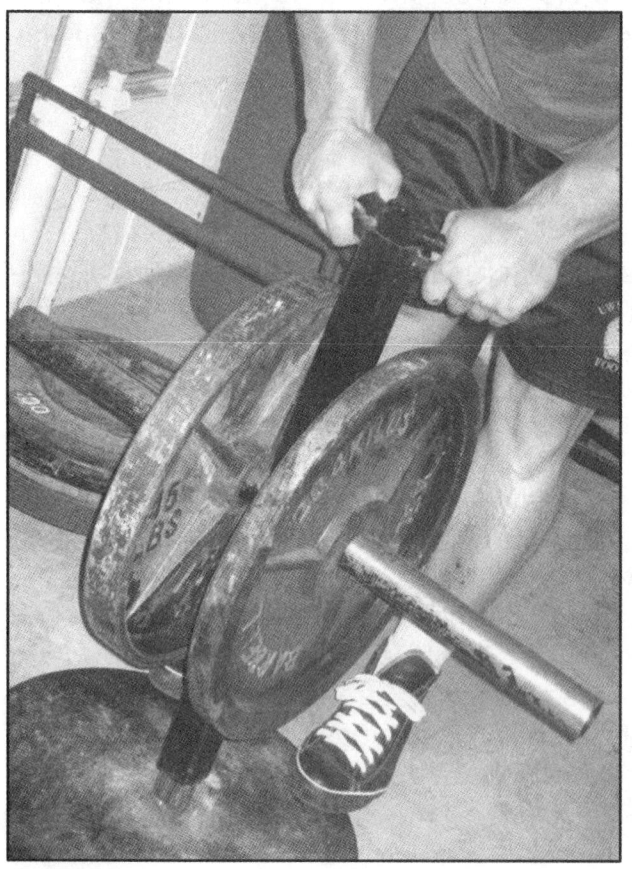

Exercise selection is crucial. On dynamic day, after doing 8–10 sets of three reps at 60% of a shirtless max, train the triceps first. It is quite common for our guys to do 14–18 sets of triceps extensions, which are done mostly with a straight bar. One frequently used exercise is JM presses for 3–5 reps, working up to as heavy as possible. Always try for a new PR. The same applies to straight bar extensions to the chin, forehead, or throat. Heavy dumbbell extensions are also implemented for 6–10 reps for 6–10 sets. Take short rests between sets, usually 30 seconds or less. For the bar work, 90 seconds is advised.

For advanced lifters, such as Phil Guarino, superset light push-downs or light dumbbells in between bar extensions or JM presses.This greatly increases GPP and thus the bench press. Phil used this method for one year and pushed up his bench from 525 to 633 at 242 and recently made a 661 at 253 body weight. Also, for the triceps, try adding flex bands while benching off five 2 x 6s.

This takes the delts and chest almost completely out of the movement, leaving only the triceps to do the work.

Lats are next. Rows of all kinds are done as well as lat pull-downs with a wide variety of bars. We don't do many chins, but they are a good way to work the lats also. We do a lot of upper body sled work, which is my personal favorite. We also do a lot of static lat work with the flex bands by hooking one band around one of the uprights of the power rack and holding the ends of the band, so the lats are contracted for a long period of time (about 2–4 minutes). When a lifter becomes fatigued at one position, he should change the position by slightly bending or straightening the arms and continue to hold the tension. Remember, when bench pressing, the lats are held statically. The delts rotate and the arms bend, but the lats stay contracted.

The sled and bands work perfectly for the upper back as well. Inverted flyes, dumbbell power cleans, and lat pulls to the face can also be done. Choke a set of flex bands to the top of the power rack, one on each side. Place a bar in the loops. Lie down as if to bench, and pull the bar to the chest or belly using various grips. This simulates the action of the lats while benching. Tuck the elbows in tight.

Strong forearms are imperative. I have never seen a strong bencher who doesn't have large, powerful forearms. The tighter the grip, the easier it is to activate the triceps. To use the biceps fully when benching, imagine stretching the bar apart. The first muscle to flex while pushing a bar concentrically is the biceps. This technique of pushing the bar apart is very important and requires external rotator work, which can be done with rubber bands. Older lifters may remember the chest expanders that Bob Hoffman sold. When these were popular, there seemed to be fewer shoulder injuries. Could it be that all of that external rotating prevented rotator injuries, which we see so many of today?

If one's bench press is not progressing, it could be poor form, which could be a result of a lagging muscle group or not knowing how to bench correctly. Don't merely take someone else's advice on how to bench, but think for a minute and review what was discussed here. On speed day, speed is what we are after—starting and accelerating as well as reversal strength. Train with 45–50 % of a no-shirt max. This utilizes power production maximally. Do 8–10 sets of three reps.

On the maximum effort day, max out on one core exercise and don't be afraid to miss. Do a final warm up with 90%; then, try a PR. This workout should occur three days after speed day. On both days, push up the special exercises such as: triceps extensions, delt raises, lat work, and forearm work. After the core lift, pick 3–4 exercises and never work out longer than 60 minutes. Do triceps first and forearms last. If possible, do a second workout later in the day. This workout should be 20–30 minutes long and should consist of extensions, raises, lat work, and curls. No bar pressing should be done.

Does this work? Check out the records and clubs of our lifters. Bill Gillespie, strength coach for the Washington Huskies, has gone from 480 to 782 in about seven years and has passed every drug test he was given. This should be proof that this system works for anyone, not just those at Westside.

The Deadlift

Squat and bench press records are continually being set in recent years. It's easy to see why. Most federations have a 24-hour weigh-in rule, which is a positive thing for the health of the lifter. It is easy to rehydrate in 24 hours, which results in fewer cramps, muscle pulls and tears. In the old days, it was common for lifters to pass out while squatting or to drop the squat bar because they were dizzy. Of course, the more a lifter weighs, the more he can squat or bench. In addition, the introduction of power suits, groove briefs, and bench shirts has enabled the lifter to make bigger and bigger lifts.

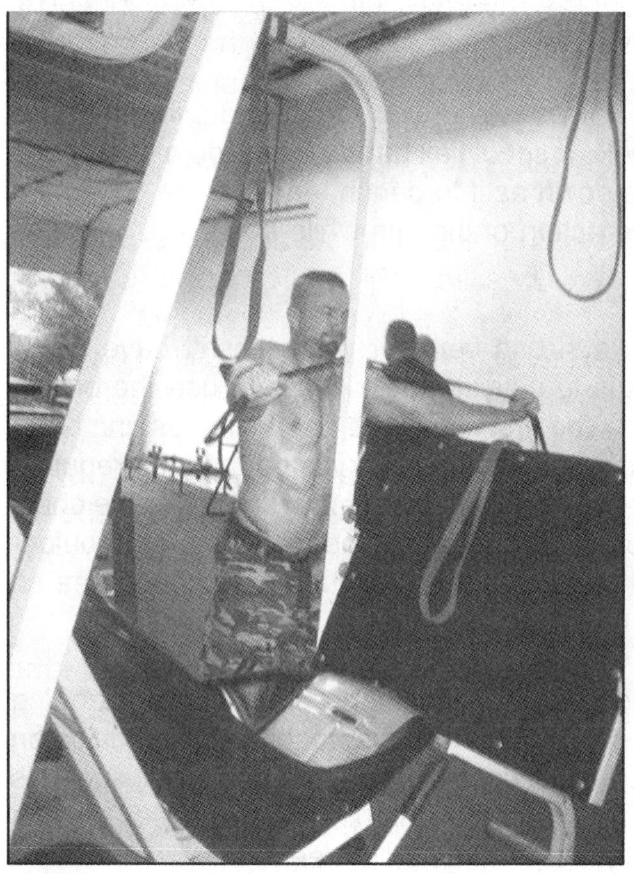

What about the deadlift? Does equipment help in this lift? Shawn Coleman said that using a larger deadlift suit helped him get into a better starting position to pull a PR 835 deadlift. While supportive gear can help the squat and bench and prolong one's lifting career, more times than not it can be a hindrance for deadlifting. If equipment is of little benefit, what's the answer when it comes to the deadlift? Training.

Most lifters deadlift too often and too heavy. This has an ill effect on the central nervous system. A better method is to use a variety of exercises that mimic the deadlift or special exercises that develop the individual muscles that are used while deadlifting (the conjugate method). One must build the muscles that start and finish the lift. There must be methods used to develop speed and acceleration. The quicker the bar is locked out, the less chance for the grip to give out.

Vince Anello, an 821 deadlifter at 198, once told me that anything he did would make his deadlift go up. Bill Starr said that if you want to deadlift more, don't deadlift. Bill was an excellent Olympic lifter who pulled a 666 national record in 1970, having concentrated on powerlifting for only a short time. Whether they knew it or not, both men were utilizing the conjugate method, which was devised to develop the muscles and special strengths (starting, accelerating, and absolute).

The good morning is a valuable exercise in the conjugate method; for deadlifting, the bent over version is the best. Bend at the upper back first and round over while lowering the bar. The legs can be slightly bent to prevent hyperextension of the knee. While doing good mornings, always think about duplicating the motion of a deadlift. Only the person doing the good morning can gauge its effectiveness by the stress on the spinal erectors, hamstrings or glutes, and hips, and of course by whether or not the deadlift goes up.

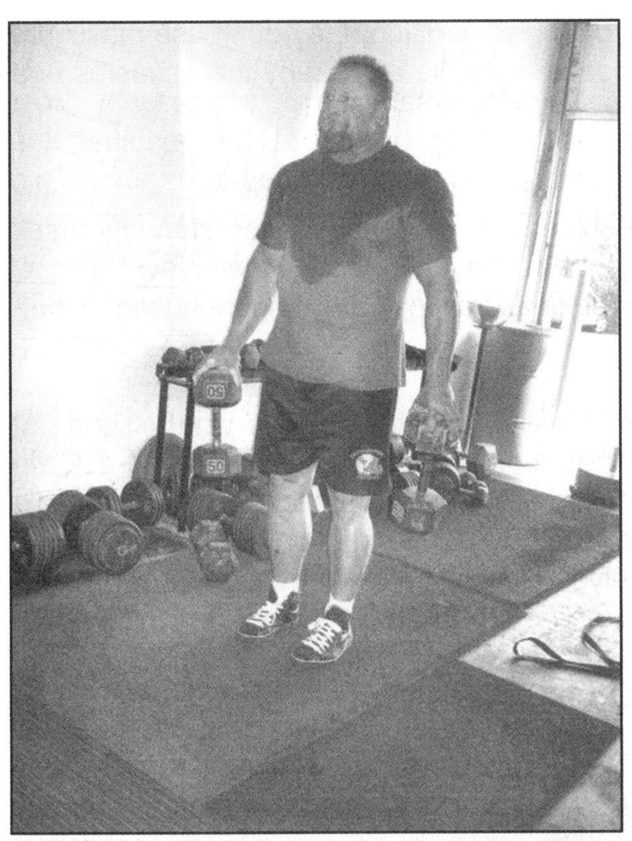

Shawn Coleman did 600 for five reps in the good morning prior to his 835 deadlift. If a lifter is doing 600 for five reps and his deadlift is 700 lbs, he is just kidding himself, and he must change his training. Employ a variety of bars in the good morning: straight, cambered, and the safety power squat bar. Use a high bar placement and a low bar placement, a close stance and a wide stance, and sometimes do them seated. Bands and chains as well as weight releasers can be added. One to six reps works best. Stockier men should do at least three reps to increase muscle tension. Because a max deadlift can take several seconds to complete, the duration of a set of reps in this lift must also be several seconds.

Various types of squatting should also be done to increase the deadlift. Michael Brugger of Germany related to me that the Olympic style squat was his favorite exercise to increase his deadlift of 887. Eddie Coppin of Belgium made an 826 deadlift at a body weight of 186. The front squat was a major part of his training. In the early 1970s, George Clark pulled 700 at 181 and just missed 735, the world record held by Vince Anello. George's main exercise was the hack squat deadlift with the bar held behind his back. These are three examples of great lifters using a form of the squat to raise their deadlift.

Squatting with a bar held in various ways places the stress on the erectors, hips, and glutes—the primary muscles that deadlift.

We advise using a group of specialty bars including the Buffalo bar, safety power squat bar, and MantaRay. This teaches how to maintain a more upright position, which is conducive to a good deadlift.

If an individual does all deadlifting, it is a matter of time before his deadlift will stall, or even worse, injury will stop all progress. Why? No one's body can equally distribute the work evenly between the lower, mid, and upper back. If the lower back takes the major role in deadlifting, which is most often the case, eventually an injury will occur. By doing a variety of special exercises for the upper back, the muscles of the entire back are more likely to receive equal work. These exercises include shrugs, lat work, spinal erector work, good mornings, back raises, reverse hyperextensions, glute ham raises, sled work, and pull-throughs.

What about starting and accelerating strength? The best way to develop these strengths is by using flex bands. By attaching the bands over the bar, the resistance is applied to the bar evenly. The higher the bar is raised, the more resistance applied to the bar. If an athlete is weak at the top, with the bands he learns learn to pull faster at the start so momentum and then acceleration can help carry the bar to lockout. It he is weak at the start, the bands teach him to start off the floor faster because without the fast start, he will not be able to lockout a heavy deadlift. For those who have said this will not build acceleration, they don't use maximum weight with the bands but rather 60%. More resistance is added to the bar by the bands as one lifts the bar, which is called accommodating resistance.

Concerning contradictory information on this subject, research in the United States is invariably done in a college environment. It is conducted with students as subjects. These students many times are not avid weight lifters, nor are they of high standard such as Elite lifters. Nevertheless, conclusions from these studies are put forth as a model for all training, including that used at football and weight lifting facilities.

The most usable results are obtained by testing high skilled athletes. This is what is done at Westside, where only Elite lifters are tested. Someone must have a qualified trainer to ask the right questions and highly qualified lifters to test to help answer those questions. Poor testing also occurs when two different training methods are tested together. This example also points out the misuse of plyometrics. A lifter had tried a program of plyometrics in between deadlift sets. Not only did the plyometrics dampen the central nervous system for the following sets of deadlifts, but in fact, the deadlifts also negatively affected the plyometrics. He raised his pull 2.5 kg, an insignificant amount to register a valid training effect. Plyometrics and the maximal effort method cannot be trained at the same time.

Plyometrics help the separation phase only when the bar separates from the floor. This particular lifter had difficulty above the knee level and locking out. He was also doing rack work above the knee at the same time and sled pulling. These two exercises build the top part of the deadlift where he would fail. The plyometrics build the start, not where he needed help. In the United States, plyometrics are misused more times than not. They are so draining on the central nervous system that heavy pulls and squats must be decreased or done during the non-competing months of the year. In summary, please be careful what you read. Not all conclusions are valid.

The abdominal muscles are extremely important in deadlifting. The abs must flex first before the lower back starts to do its work. Lifters with weak abs and a strong back invariably hurt their backs. When the back flexes first without the abs working as stabilizers, the back is put under great stress. Learning to increase intra-abdominal pressure while lifting is essential. This reduces the risk of a hernia and greatly reduces pressure on the disks.

The internal and external obliques play a great role in stabilizing the hips, and they initiate straightening the legs in the deadlift. Years ago, when powerlifters could deadlift more than they squatted, the obliques were often much more developed than they are today. Lifters did side presses and one-armed deadlifts to develop the obliques.

All types of ab work must be completed. In addition to standing ab work, which is done by Westsiders, leg raises and straight leg sit-ups are beneficial. Don't be confused by the way bodybuilders look. Every time I watch one of those fitness shows, some big time bodybuilder is telling everyone to keep his or her knees bent to take pressure off the lower back. I guess sucking in those abs is a bunch of crap, huh. Because if their abs were half as strong as they look, they wouldn't be worrying about their lower back.

Although a smaller waist makes it easier to deadlift, it must be very strong. One could see John Kuc's abs through his super suit from 100 feet away when he made 870 at 242. Bob Peoples taught me the best method of using the abs in the deadlift. He said it was better to breath into the stomach only, not the chest. This stabilizes and supports the lower back, and it does not elongate the spine. The shorter the spine makes a better deadlifter. If a lifter has long legs, a short torso, and long arms, he has the perfect build for deadlifting. More important than the right build is attitude. The deadlift is a tough lift, especially at the conclusion of a long meet.

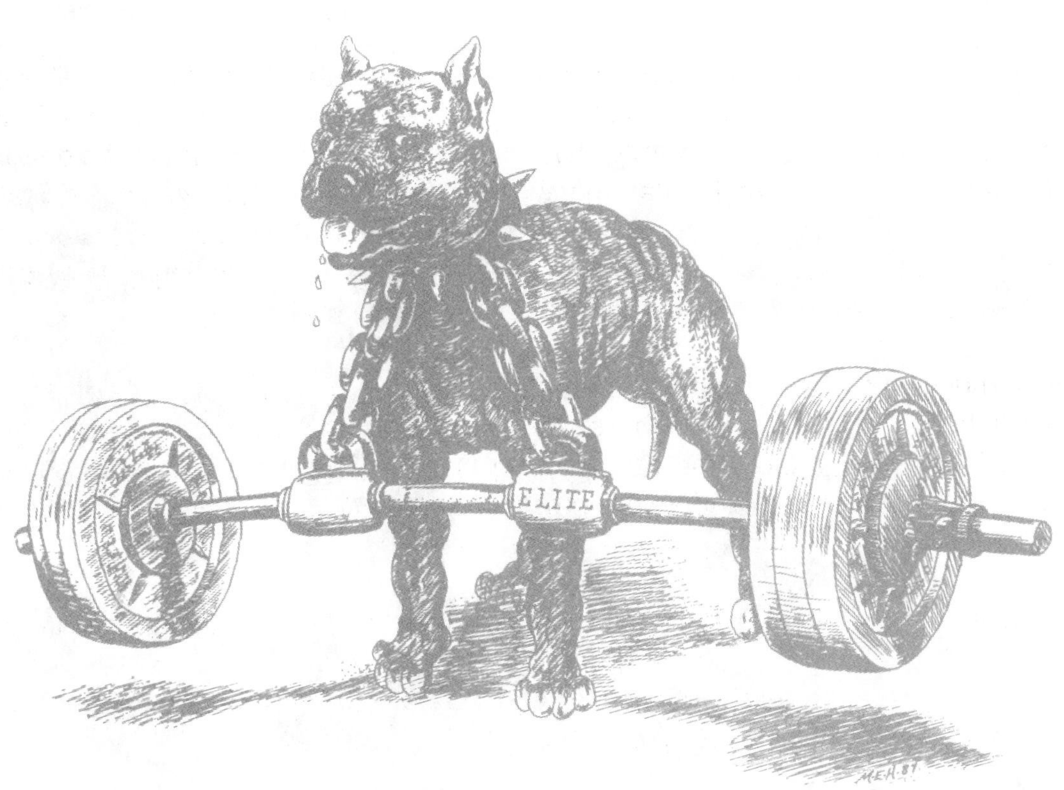

PREPARING FOR A CONTEST

Training for an upcoming contest must be thought out precisely. Muscle mass, speed, strength, and coordination must be added. The simplest method of progression (10s, 8s, 6s—progressive gradual overload) works in the beginning, but what doesn't? As a lifter becomes more advanced, he needs a more sophisticated method. If he chooses to go from 10s, 8s, and 6s down to 2s and singles, many bad things happen. One is that the volume and intensity are impossible to control. There is an optimal number of lifts at certain percentages. For example, weights at or above 90% of a 1RM are to be done for 2–4 lifts, but many do 3–5 lifts on a regular basis. An Olympic lifter can do 4–10 lifts per workout with 90% while a powerlifter should do 2–4 singles per workout with 90% and above. With the old progressive overload method, 10 reps with 70% is common. What a waste. Through extensive tests of high-skilled lifters, 4–6 reps with 70% was shown to be optimal. For all athletes, the better one is with reps, the worse he is with a single.

Think about this. Throw a basketball as high as possible. The ball reaches its highest point before it lands and bounces. The first bounce is the highest bounce. Each successive bounce is lower as the ball's energy dissipates. Similarly, when doing reps, a lifter has a limited amount of energy. With each rep, he is a little less effective in force production. Unlike the ball, he has a brain and spinal cord, and he must learn to conserve energy to perform more reps. This is a mistake because the lifter becomes slower and unable to push effectively with heavier weights. Remember, we are striving for speed, explosiveness, and absolute strength.

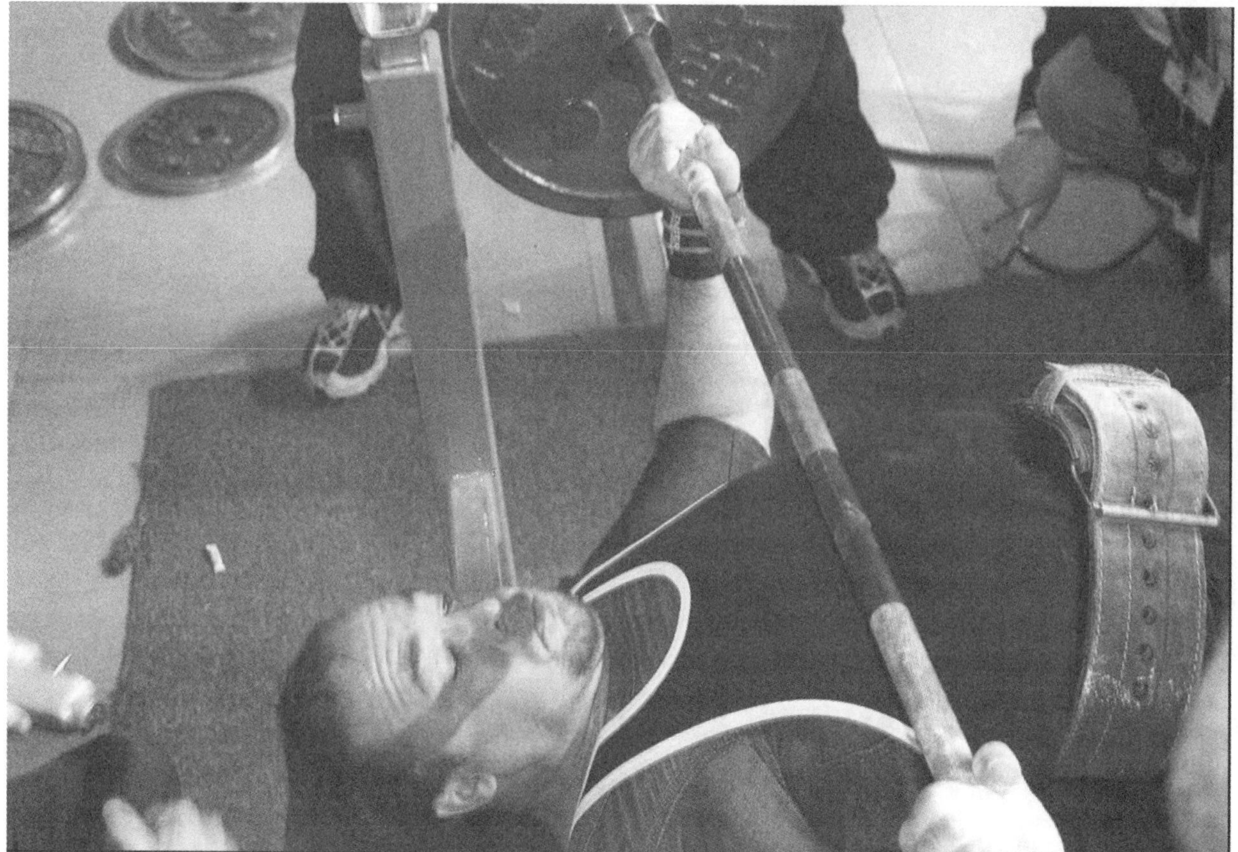

Competition picture

Like everyone else, I watch TV. One of my favorite shows is Kiana's Flex Appeal on ESPN. Well, you've probably guessed the main reason I watch, but I also watch the high rep bodybuilding boys do their best imitation of plyometric training. They are slower than my grandmother. Why? This is the result of slow, high rep training (similar to HIT).

The old progressive method is based on a hypothetical max. No one can project hypothetical max. This throws off the entire training cycle. One thinks he's at 80% when he's really at 90% of his true max. Again, remember what training at 90% does to CNS. After three weeks, progress ceases. Another reason for the failure of the progressive overload method is that close to the meet, most lifters will drop assistance exercises. Why do them at all if they are going to be dropped? The effectiveness of these exercises is almost completely lost in two weeks. Also, because of the stress of doing max singles in all three competition lifts, a lifter is mentally and emotionally worn out before the meet. It's stupid to spar with Mike Tyson if the fight is with are Cecily Tyson.

With the progressive overload system, every type of training is used in one workout. However, body doesn't know what to do with so many different demands placed on it. For example, speed and endurance must be trained separately.

Overall Program Guidelines

So, what's right? Personally, I look at weight training for what it is—mathematics, biomechanics, and physics. This is what we do at Westside (and the results speak for themselves). The work must be divided into special days: a dynamic method day for the bench and one dynamic day for the squat and deadlift, a maximal effort day for benching, occuring three days after the dynamic day, and a maximal effort day for the squat and deadlift. The week should look like this: dynamic squat on Friday, dynamic bench on Sunday, max effort squat/deadlift on Monday, and max effort bench on Wednesday. This sequence works best for weekend meets.

Always box squat just below parallel. Without bands or chains, the bar weight is 50–60% of a 1RM. During the cycle, do 12 sets of two reps with 50, 52.5, and 55% and ten sets of two reps with 57.5 and 60%, using only one percentage per week. When a lifter reaches 60%, he starts over with 50% the next week. This is a pendulum wave much like that used by Alexiev. It is easy to improve form and build speed and starting strength by training with weights at these percentages.

When using bands or chains, 6–8 sets of two reps are used even during the circa-maximal phase. It is easy to monitor volume and intensity with this system. After box squats on Friday, special work for glutes and hamstrings, abs, hips, and spinal erectors are completed. Every other week, we do six speed deadlifts with 60–70% with short rest periods of 45 seconds.

With progressive gradual overload training, which is used more often than any other method of training, in the beginning the intensity is low and the volume is high. Later in the cycle, the structure is reversed close to a contest. The injury rate is higher with this type of loading, and the volume is impossible to control because several intensity zones are used in one workout.

This is very ineffective. As the weight gets heavy closer to the contest, the special exercises for individual muscles is neglected. This is when the injuries occur because of a lack of GPP. Let's forget progressive gradual overload; it's a dead-end street, which I found out 17 years ago. By the way, this system was invented and abandoned in the old Soviet Union over 40 years ago. One should learn about other periodization models such as those of Verkhoshansky, Vorobyev, and Medvedev. I personally thank these men as well as Dr. Siff and Dr. Zatsiorskl for making it possible for me to lift more at age 52 than I have ever dreamed possible.

Designing Your Training Outline

When is the most stressful two weeks of your life? Two weeks before graduation and flunking out? Two weeks before your wedding and you know your whole life will be ruined forever? Or how about the last two weeks before a power meet? This is the most important time in training. It is "make or break" for many of us. How much or how little should you do? When is the last workout? What about taking openers? Should you use meet equipment?

As you know, we use a wave mini-cycle for the squat. We also train with a box at or below parallel. I will use Rob Fusner as an example. His best squat was 875 at 275 at the time.

- Week 1 425 x 8 sets of 2 reps
- Week 2 455 x 8 sets of 2 reps
- Week 3 475 x 8 sets of 2 reps
- Week 4 495 x 6 sets of 2 reps
- Week 5 425 x 8 sets of 2 reps
- Week 6 455 x 8 sets of 2 reps
- Week 7 475 x 8 sets of 2 reps
- Week 8 425 x 8 sets of 2 reps

In addition to the normal bar weight, we use chains (about 120 lbs) or bands (about 150 lbs of tension). These sets are done on Friday's dynamic method day, combined with the contrast method through the use of bands or chains.

The objective is to move the weights:

- Week 5 faster than in week 1
- Week 7 faster than in week 3

This shows the development of force. The purpose of the dynamic method is to build acceleration and reversal strength. Short rests between sets are important for increasing intensity. Forty-five seconds is recommended.

We have found that 40-60% weights work best for the squat. It is very important to push up and rotate the special exercises such as: the reverse hyper, abs, sled work, and belt squats. Use only 3-4 exercises after squatting. The goal is to become faster with the same weights on each new wave.

This can be accomplished by the use of flex bands or chains or by increasing the special exercises that build strength in the glutes, hips, hamstrings, and abs. This also builds form by increasing the strength in the vital squat muscles. Do not do regular squats after a box squat workout. The squats completely wear the vital squat muscles and make a regular squat seem very hard and sluggish. We do a contest style squat only at the contest, never in the gym. Also, if a max box squat is achieved, don't do it the week before the meet. Two weeks out is okay, but four weeks out is best. Don't get psyched up. Get motivated but don't burn adrenaline. We never use knee wraps or pull up the straps on the suit. Don't do an opener. Needing to do this is just a lack of confidence. Think about it. If a lifter is worried about his opener, he's in trouble. Rather, think PR.

Here are two examples of a comparison of box squat maxes to a contest best. Amy Weisberger's best parallel box squat is 82%, and her best contest squat 445 at 123. Todd Brock had a parallel box squat of 710 (86%) and a contest squat of 820 at 270. This shows a 15–20% carryover to a contest squat from a squat PR. Most can use this reference. We seldom do any regular deadlifting at Westside. Jerry Obradovic does rack pulls with the plates 2–4 inches off the floor. This is done only one time per month. The result is the highest deadlift/bench combine in the 275 class of all time: an 804 deadlift and a 644 bench. It is a rare combination to be such a good bench presser and deadlifter. It requires two different body structures.

Monday's max effort work is comprised of squatting and deadlifting. About six out of ten workouts are good mornings because they work most major muscle groups used in the squat and deadlift: the glutes, hamstrings, spinal erectors, and hips. About three of ten workouts are special squats, using a variety of bars. Sometimes, especially during a heavy mini-period like circa max, we don't do any max effort work but rather train the muscles using the repetition method.

Each time the bar is changed, there is a variance the length between the sacrum and the center of the bar. This is possible by using a MantaRay. It raises the bar approximately 1–2 inches above the top of the delts. A safety squat bar, with its cambered design, also changes this length. On max effort day, you must push the muscles to their fullest extent. Try records in all types of good mornings, squats, and pulls. On both the dynamic effort and max effort days, push not only the major core exercises but also the special work such as: reverse hyperextensions, pull- throughs, back raises, glute ham raises, and lat and abdominal work.

An individual does not have to squat or deadlift to become a good squatter or deadlifter. If it takes three seconds to do a max squat or deadlift and the lifter places the right muscles into play with a good morning or special squat, he has accomplished the same thing. The more exercises he becomes accomplished in, the easier it is to master any exercise including squatting and deadlifting. Even football players play football only 20% of the training time; the other 80% is for special drills and to raise GPP. Individuals should pick the exercises that work best for him and use them closest to a meet. Rotate every two weeks and always max out. Do singles in squatting and pulling and triples in the good mornings. When performing pulls, don't do them for more than two weeks and never the last two weeks before a meet.

This is the conjugate method. Use special exercises to raise absolute strength and perfect form. This method will allow you to max out week after week, year after year. My friends, this is the only way to do so. If you choose to max out in one particular exercise for 3–4 weeks, you will stop making progress for neurological reasons. Check your training log if you don't believe me.

Delayed Transformation

The biggest obstacle for Elite lifters is displaying efforts from training at meet time. I frequently hear of lifters taking their openers before the meet. If the lifters at Westside were worried about their openers, we would not go to the meet.

What is the proper method of tapering training for the meet? Much depends on the weight class the lifter is competing. The heavy weight classes may need more time to reach full peaking. Leading up to any meet, the training should be divided into three-week waves. For squatting, the months before the meet should consist of light speed-strength work, 10–12 sets of two reps with less than 60-second rest intervals. This results in good form, raises work capacity, and above all, builds speed-strength qualities, which all are important in order to exhibit maximum force production.

We focus on maximal speed with submaximal weights. With max speed, 154 lbs can produce 264 lbs of force. Most training sets average 40–50% of our top meet squat, but remember, we squat on a box. For one wave, we may use a blue band (200 lbs of tension at the top) or a green band (120 lbs of tension at the top) with three sets of 5/8-inch chain correctly hung from the bar (120 extra lbs at the top) or a purple band (80 lbs more at the top). It is essential to constantly change the rate of bar acceleration by different means. We may also use weight releasers with about 12% of our best squat weight, or the lightened method, where bands are hung from the top of the rack to support, or lighten, the bar load at the bottom of the lift.

After heavy training, such as the circa-max phase, one can't get any stronger. This is because of the accommodation effect of the near maximal efforts over a three-week phase. The logical thing to do is to reduce the training load. This improves the lifter's strength or performance by transferring the previous training weeks into performance growth. The circa-max squat phase is very strenuous, consisting of 6–10 lifts close to max to achieve strength-speed, leading to a gain in absolute strength. The training volume must be changed, not the exercise. If not, no satisfactory result will be achieved. Two to four weeks are needed for the realization of better results at contest time. Only the top Elite powerlifter should use the circa-max method, which uses weights between 90–97% of a 1RM. It is very severe, and most at Westside use it for meets. We recommend that a four-week deloading occur (including the week of the meet) after the circa-max phase.

Here is an example using Paul Childress's final six-week training period before a meet. Leading up to the seventh week, Paul uses a high volume system of training, working on speed- strength exclusively with weights ranging from 40–55% for 8–12 sets of two reps. When Paul starts the circa-max phase, it looks like this:

- Week 1: 455 for 5 sets of 2 reps plus 500 lbs of band tension
- Week 2: 475 of 4 sets of 2 reps plus 500 lbs of band tension
- Week 3: 500 for 3 sets of 2 reps plus 500 lbs of band tension
- Week 4: 500 for 5 sets of 2 reps plus 250 lbs of band tension
- Week 5: 500 for 4 sets of 2 reps plus 125 lbs of band tension
- Week 6: 500 for 3 sets of 2 reps, no bands
- Week 7: meet result, 1052 at 308

At the 2005 Arnold Classic, Paul squatted 1085, a world record. If this extremely heavy workload had continued up to meet time, he would likely have failed to make a big squat because he would have had CNS fatigue as well as physical and emotional fatigue. This explains why a four-week cycle, or mesocycle, is needed to validate the previous training and express it at the meet. During this deloading phase, the number of workouts is reduced as well as the number of exercises per workout. The last four-week phase calls for full restoration and calmness. Fewer bar exercises are performed and more specific exercises for building hamstring, glute, low back, and abdominal strength are implemented along with stretching.

By stopping the circa-max phase so far out from the meet, Paul was able to do a max effort day three days later on Monday. On this day, he did triples in the 80% range. This pendulum training system works in direct line with the three-week pendulum wave that I have repeatedly written about. The fourth week is, of course, the meet.

The number of weeks of deloading necessary depends on a lifter's level of preparedness. Ano Turtianen uses a similar circa-max phase and then a two-week deloading phase. He recently squatted 1080 at 286. His bar weight varies from 540 (50%) to 628 (65%) plus a couple of singles at 705. The band tension is 220 at the top and 100 at the bottom. Chuck Vogelpohl was the lightest man to squat 1000 and 1025 at 220. His circa-max phase looked like this:

- Week 1: 455 for 5 sets of 2 reps with 375 lbs of band tension at top
- Week 2: 555 for 4 sets of 2 reps plus 375 lbs of band tension at top
- Week 3: 575 for 3 sets of 2 reps plus 375 lbs of band tension at top

Because of Chuck's high level of fitness, he uses two weeks to deload, lifting at the meet on the third week and realizing a total delayed transformation. Learn to balance the very intense training while preparing for a meet with the efficiency to produce a high total at meet time. At Westside, this is done with a system of yearly, monthly, and weekly (macro-, meso-, and micro-cycles, respectively) cycles for the dynamic and maximal effort days.

Of course, delayed transformation occurs in bench pressing and deadlifting as well. There is no need to take an opener the week before the meet. In summary, delayed transformation occurs by reducing the number of exercises of all types, and in turn, decreasing the total training load due to the period of non-improvement that is caused by accumulated fatigue. This deloading for three weeks leads to an increase in strength. Its purpose is to prepare the lifter for a major competition. The higher the level a lifter achieves with a greater work capacity, the longer the delayed transformation is carried out. For those with a lower work capacity and usually a lower rank, the delayed transformation phase is shorter because they don't endure the same extreme rigors as the more advanced lifter. Lower skilled lifters don't use the same amount of muscle fiber as top lifters.

Our lifters at 275 and above always require a longer time to peak or realize the training loads as a high meet result. Even when a contest is not close, the total volume must be waved up and down to achieve higher results in a yearly plan. Changing exercises continuously helps recuperation. Westside lifters never do the same exercise on max effort day two weeks in a row. This is to avoid accommodation. The more exercises completed in a yearly plan, the more fully prepared a lifter will be.

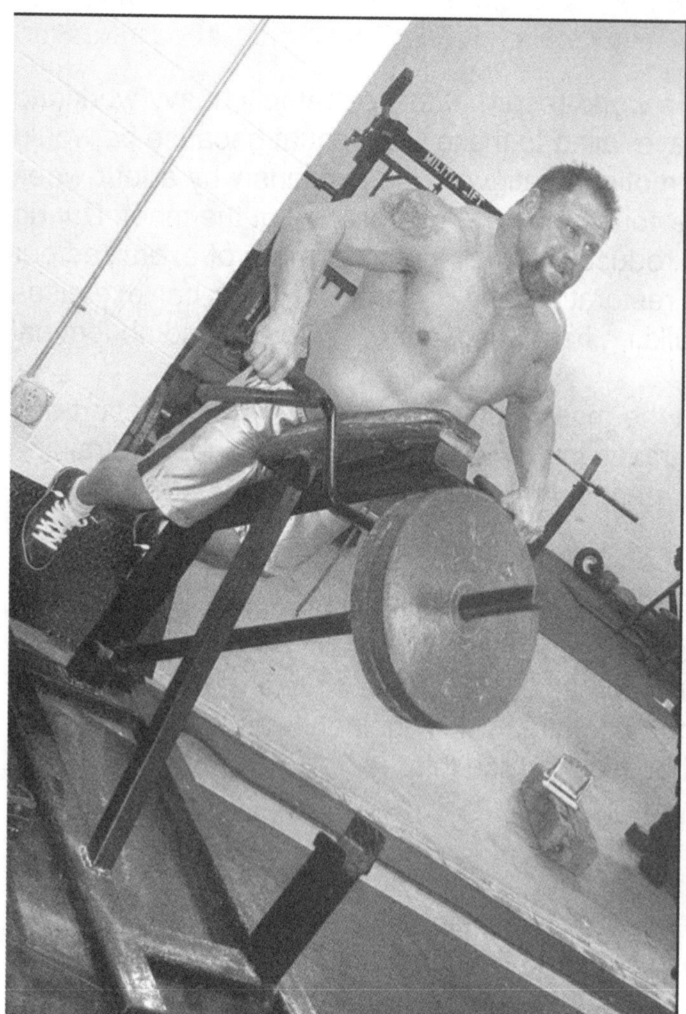

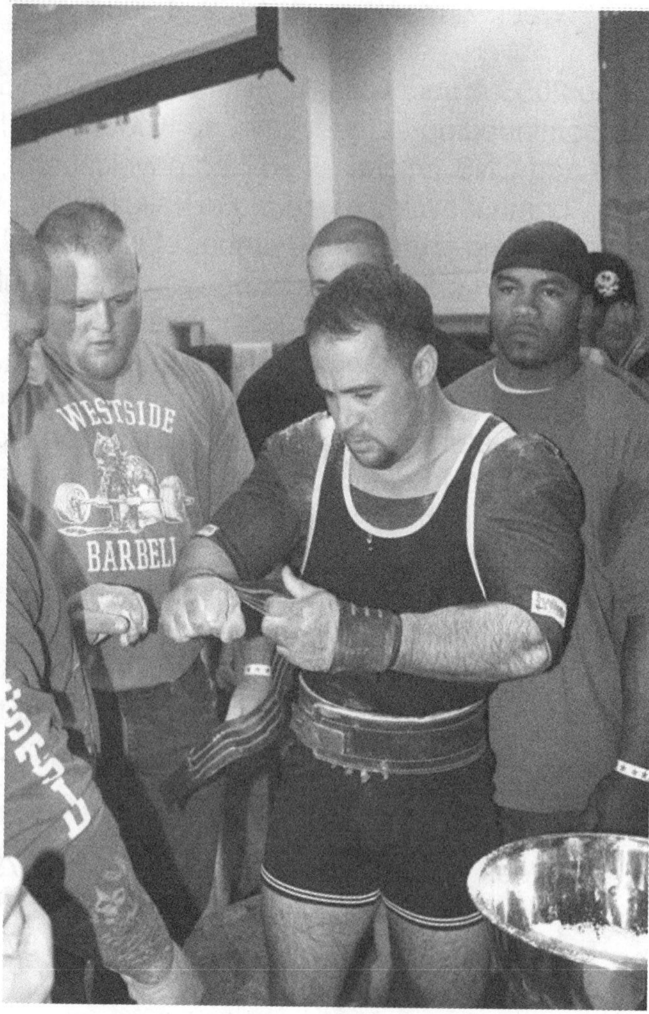

GENERAL PHYSICAL PREPARATION

Though I write to all powerlifters, I am always amazed to hear a drug-free lifter say he can't train the Westside way. Although these lifters are going nowhere fast, they choose to use the progressive gradual overload method, going heavier and heavier each week. In most cases, they stop making records and are stuck for years. Yet, they still choose not to use a more sophisticated method of training such as that used at Westside and presently used worldwide. These drug-free lifters train so heavy that they can't do the special work that is required to excel at powerlifting. They do most of their training at over 90% of their max; whereas, we do most of our training at 60%. Doesn't this make more sense? A drug-free lifter trains only three, sometimes two times a week. No wonder he gets sore. This style of training is similar to a weekend warrior playing basketball.

Many major college and NFL football teams train in the same manner as Westside, and guess what? They are drug-free. During spring training, three practices a day are common. That is 15 workouts a week. Why do you think you should train only 2–3 times a week? We are on the same side folks, so let's look at a systematic program that allows progress.

What is GPP?

General physical preparedness (GPP) is a term that refers to a degree of fitness, which is an extension of absolute strength. Many don't believe in it at all. Here, I'm referring to those who say that if you want to be good at the power lifts, just practice the power lifts. Of course, this leads others to say that powerlifters are out of shape and the above-mentioned group is in shape. Many times the ones who advocate for only the classical lifts are the very ones who complain that powerlifters are out of shape. We all squat, yet we are not built identically. Some develop large quads, some develop big glutes and hips, and others may have very powerful hamstrings. It's obvious to me that if one muscle group is developed to a greater degree than another, then the smaller muscle groups are holding back lifts.

What's the answer? Special exercises must be done for the lagging muscle groups. Before you can pursue an increase in volume by way of special exercises, you must be in excellent shape. GPP raises the ability to do more work by special means. Rest periods should be 45–60 seconds between sets for explosive and speed work, and the muscles should be in an excitable state or slightly fatigued. This causes an increase in difficulty of training. If this is impossible for you, your GPP through small workouts is low. You can raise your GPP through small workouts between days and even prior to training.

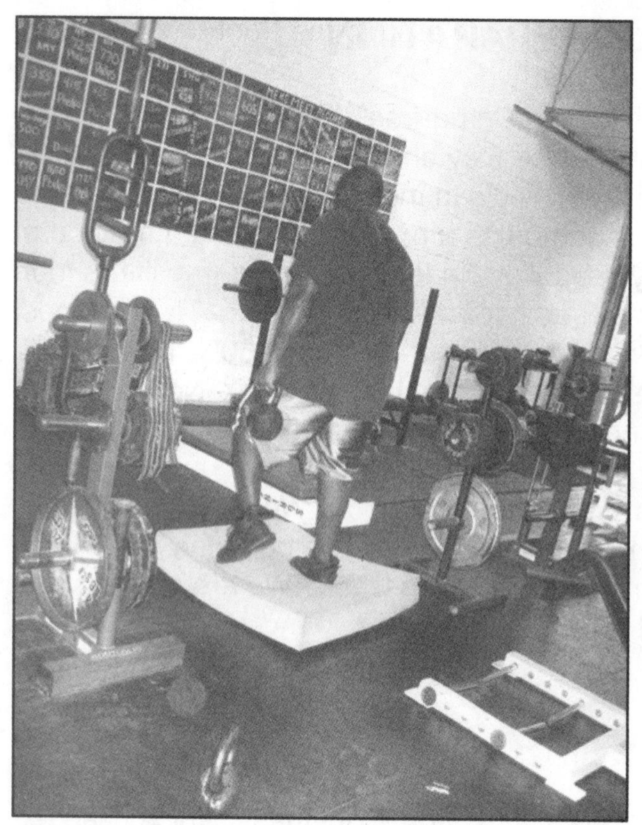

Chuck Vogelpohl and I commonly go heavy on the reverse hyper machine and do abs, lats, and sometimes reversal action workouts before a squat or max effort workout. Small workouts during the week greatly increase the chances of raising a lifter's total. Some of these workouts should be for special strength and some for restoration. This is a must for drug-free lifters. I've had many drug- free lifters here who have greatly pushed up their lifts by doing extra workouts. It's okay to be drug-free, but don't be brain-free. If you don't do more, you will not make progress. A lot of you dudes played high school football, which included two and three a day practice sessions. You were drug-free then, so what's the difference? If these workouts are done systematically, you can't over train. Remember when your squat was 400? 500? 600? 700? But now you squat 800. How did you get stronger without doing more work but without over training? You merely raised the amount of work systematically over the years. Simply stated, you raised your GPP.

Sled Work

There are several ways of raising work capacity. One method that we use at Westside is pulling the sled for the hips and glutes. We pull the sled with the strap attached to the back of our power belts. We walk with long, powerful strides, maintaining an upright body position, pulling through with the feet, which stress the hamstrings and glutes. This is common practice for throwers overseas.

I learned about pulling from Eskil Thomasson, who is Swedish. Before he moved to Columbus, Ohio, he visited Finland to see why so many Finns deadlift so well. Many of these strong deadlifters were lumberjacks. They routinely had to pull paper wood down to the main trail where the tractors could pick it up.

Another style of pulling is with a double handle held behind the back and below the knees. The torso is bent over, and the strides are long. This is great for building the hamstrings. To work the front of the hips and lower abs, attach a strap to each ankle and walk, pulling the sled by the feet. Vasily Alexiev used to walk in knee deep water for roughly 1000 steps after a workout. This is similar to what we are doing but with the advantage of being able to add or reduce weight, which varies the resistance.

For building the outside of the hips and the inside of the legs, position the straps around the ankles and walk sideways, first one way, then the other, left then right, forward and backward.

For the quads and front of the hips, walk backward with the strap around the front of the belt. To start this type of work, I recommend doing six trips of 200 feet each. Use only one style of dragging until you feel confident of your ability to include more work. We do this lower body work on squat day, Friday, and on max effort day, Monday, in addition to the days after (Saturday and Tuesday) using 60% of what was done on the previous day. This contributes greatly to restoration.

For the legs, upper back and grip building, try pushing and pulling a weighted wheelbarrow. This has had a great effect on my knee that suffered a patella tendon rupture. I thank Jesse Kellum for this exercise. He used this for knee rehab for professional football players. Pushing the wheelbarrow up a mild grade really increases the work on the lower thigh muscles. Again, start with six trips of 200 feet. Only when a lifter has adjusted to the additional work should he increase the number of trips.

Now, let's go back to the sled, but this time for the upper body. When George Halbert sees an increase in upper body mass, the process must be working, and that process is pulling a sled with the upper body. There are many methods for doing this. Duplicate the motion of a pec machine. Start with the arms behind the back, and slowly pull the arms to the front. Walk forward slowly, and let the tension in the strap pull the arms to the rear, and again pull forward.

A front raise motion can be executed with the palms facing down. For the lats, start with the arms behind the back and raise the arms, palms up like a double upper-cut by first flexing the lower lats. The farther forward the hands go, the more the upper lats are worked. By walking backwards, rear delt work can be implemented along with upright rowing, and external shoulder work.

A good reactive method for the bench press is to hold the straps out in front of the body, and while walking forward the slack is removed, so drive the sled forward in a shock fashion. This is very taxing but is great for reversal strength. Do the upper body sled work for time, not distance. Mix the different styles together. Start with five minutes of pulling, and work up to at least 20 minutes.

I do 30–40 minutes, walking slowly and not jerking the sled. Only the reactive bench press method should be jerked. Use the rule of 60%. Start heavy on day one and reduce the weight each day for three consecutive days. Go back to a heavy weight the fourth day (e.g. 90 lbs, 70 lbs, and 50 lbs with each weight representing one day). The same applies to pulling the sled for lower body power and to the wheelbarrow. This work increases the physical ability to train and doubles as restoration. This style of resistance work is for those seeking greater overall strength and power. This includes weight lifters, football players, or anyone who needs to raise work capacity to reach a higher level of excellence, which is anyone who took the time to read this book. However, are there different routes to this type of work? Yes.

As outlined above, there are several ways to drag the sled:

1. forward with strap attached to your belt
2. backward with the strap attached to your belt
3. forward with bent over style
4. forward going one side in front
5. forward doing triceps extensions
6. forward doing presses

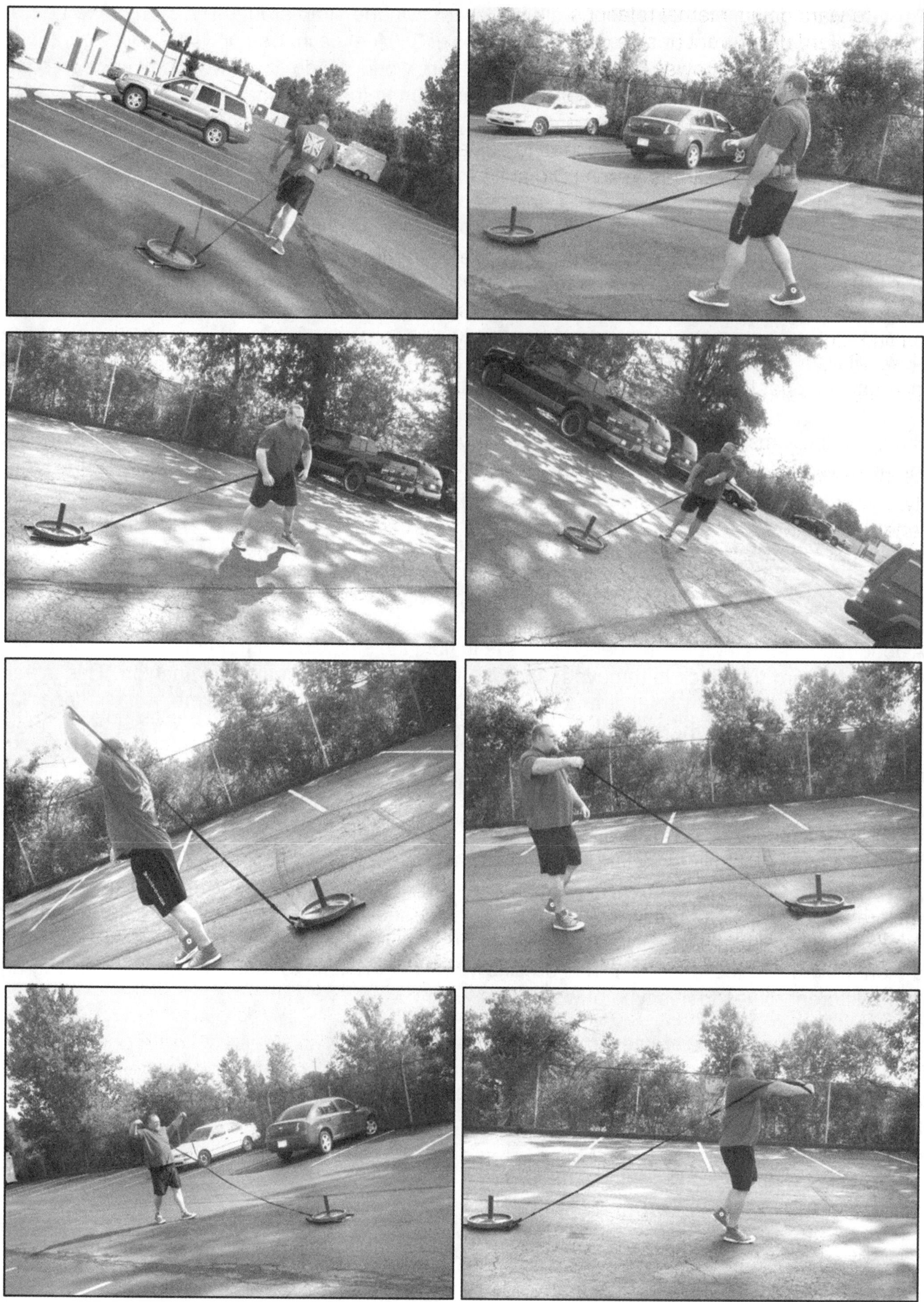

7. forward doing internal rotations
8. forward doing front or side delt raises
9. backward doing rows
10. backward doing external rotations
11. backward doing rear delt raises
12. backward with the straps attached to ankles
13. forward with the straps attached to ankles

GPP work is very common in track and field overseas, but it is still very much overlooked in the United States. An experiment was conducted at the University of Pittsburgh. Head strength coach, Buddy Morris, brought in a sprint expert, John Davies, who is very well versed in GPP work for running. John works with many professional players and has consistently lowered their 40 yard times. While his GPP work consists of weightless drills such as: jumping jacks, line hops, mountain climbers, and shuffle splits, it perfects running and jumping skills in addition to lateral speed.

As John simply puts it, "I have never met a North American athlete from the major team sports who the inclusion of this work will not cause a remarkable change in their optimum performance. Simply, without this solid base, substantial gains are limited and success is restricted to those more genetically gifted. The median improvement in 40 yard dash times over eight weeks was 0.25. This work is not for the weak of heart as the overall work volumes are enormous."

Extra Workouts

I recall reading about a great Chinese fighter named Chen Fake (Fay-kee). When he was a child, he was very small, weak and lagged behind the other students. He asked the master how he would ever be able to catch the better students when they were progressing at the same rate. The master thought for a while and said, "While the others take their afternoon nap, you train. And at night while they sleep, you train." After taking the master's advice and doing extra workouts for some years, Chen Fake surpassed the top students and eventually became Grand Master of the Chen style, Tai It Juan. This is a true story, and what I am about to describe is also true.

Like Chen Fake, if you are to become better, you must do more work. How? We know that a workout should last 45 minutes, 60 minutes at the most. Energy and testosterone levels fall off greatly after that. Commonsense tells us that longer workouts are not the answer. However, we must spend more time in the gym. This can be done by adding more workouts. At Westside, we hold three of the 12 all-time bench press records. How? We do a dynamic method workout, using 60% of a 1RM for force development. It is also intended to build starting and reversal strength, and with the help of bands, eliminate the deceleration phase of the bench press. After the bench press, triceps, lats, and delts are trained maximally for the development of absolute strength in each of the individual muscle groups, which is completed on Sunday.

On Wednesday, we do max effort exercises with a barbell. Many core exercises are done but only one per workout (e.g. floor press, steep incline, chain press). Remember, just one per workout. This is followed by pushing the triceps, lats, and delts to the max. All workouts should last no more than an hour. As of October 1999, we have eight men with a 600 or more bench. The biggest triple body weight bench (683 at 227) is a 657 world record at 220, a 701 world record at 238, and a 728 world record at 275. How do we do this? We do this by adding special workouts, which last 20–30 minutes. They are intended to raise work capacity, or GPP.

For example, George and Kenny do two special workouts per week. They are done on Monday and Friday. Each workout begins with the triceps. They use several exercises such as: barbell or dumbbell extensions, cable push-downs for high reps or heavy weight (always changing the bar attachments or the angle of the exercise), push-ups, or super high rep medicine ball throws. The same approach is used for the delts and lats; upper back exercises are rotated in the same way. These workouts are done for restoration as well as for raising work capacity. Why is this so important? The more special workouts that George and Kenny do, the harder the two main workouts can be without them experiencing ill effects. If you want to do more, your workout must be continually harder. This means higher intensity and greater volume. You must also be able to recover from the workouts.

There are three main methods of restoration:

- Anabolic: This is, of course, out of the question for the truly drug-free lifter.
- Therapeutic: This includes massage, sauna, whirlpool, ice, electric stimulation, and so forth.
- Small workouts: These should last 20–30 minutes and should be done 24 hours after major workouts.

These workouts have the advantage that work can be done on a particular muscle group, one that needs attention for either strength building or restoration. Let's say at first glance a lifter appears to have very large arms, but on closer inspection, his delts and lats look underdeveloped. Although he may have a good bench, what would occur if his delts and lats matched the development of his arms? His bench would certainly be much greater. That is what special workouts are for. If this lifter continues to neglect his lagging muscle groups, his bench will never increase. Also, he may be risking injury by not attending to his weaknesses. Even anabolics or massage can't cure a weak muscle group.

In the old Soviet system, 10–16 workouts per week were prescribed. In football, three workouts a day are quite common. That's 15 a week, but no one seems to think that's unreasonable. Here is an example of our major and extra workouts. The squat and deadlift use the same muscle groups, so we use a speed day for squatting with 50–60% of a 1RM for multiple sets and perhaps 4–8 singles in the deadlift with 50–70% (using only one percentage per workout). Both the squat and deadlift must be emphasized for speed. After the percent training, we move to special exercises for the glutes, hams, torso, and hips. We pick exercises that work at least two muscle groups concurrently such as: the glute ham raise, reverse hyper extensions, pull-throughs, and sled work. This saves time and is very productive. Remember to train the abs standing up.

On max effort day, we max out on good mornings, super low box squats with different bars, heavy sled pulling, bent over rows, and rack pulls. In addition to regular weights, add chains and bands and adjust the resistance. Do the special exercises after maxing out on the core exercises. On max effort day, use only one core lift followed by 2–4 special exercises. The extra workouts may consist of sled pulling.

Here are some typical workouts. Pull the sled for ten minutes, and do glute ham raises for five minutes and abs for five minutes (20-minute workout). Perform reverse hypers for ten minutes, lats for ten minutes, and abs for five minutes (25-minute workout). Do pull-throughs for ten minutes, abs for ten minutes, and dumbbell shrugs for five minutes (25-minute workout); any combination works.

Johnny Parker, the longtime strength coach of the Patriots, told us a story about an old Soviet coach. Johnny asked him what to do on Monday after a game on Sunday. The coach said to work the player's legs. "What about Tuesday?" Johnny asked. The coach replied, "Work their legs." Johnny asked, "What about Wednesday?" The coach said, "Work their legs." Johnny said, "Wait a minute." The coach laughed and explained to work the legs everyday as long as possible, switching exercises. That is what Westside does. We constantly change exercises, so the body won't adapt to the stimulus. One can mix and match 2–3 special exercises in a short, intense workout lasting no more than 30 minutes. The lower or upper body can be trained like this. Start with two additional workouts a week and slowly increase to 3–4. The more advanced a lifter becomes, the more special work is required. Powerlifting is like any other sport. To become better, more work must be performed.

Remember to use exercises that build the muscles. The muscles can be trained very hard and often. Large muscle groups can be trained every 72 hours and smaller muscle groups every 24 hours or less. If baseball pitching coaches understood this, perhaps they would use a three-day rotation, working half the staff every three days for a month and then the other half for a month while the resting half would go through a series of restorations. It is almost impossible to win 30 games with a five day rotation; yet, there used to be 30-game winners. It's all about GPP and special physical preparedness (SPP).

If I may go where I don't belong again, let's look at the home run race. Ken Griffey, Jr. started out like fire in the home run race doing quite well until the All-Star break. Then, a meltdown occurred. His physique showed that he did little GPP work. As a result, he faded badly near the end of the season mostly from small injuries. On the other hand, it is obvious that Sosa and Mac do extra workouts outside of baseball. Doing so enables them to hit home runs right into October.

Let's review. Extra workouts work for great fighters and baseball players, and—of course— they will work for you. They may help make that third attempt in the squat, bench, or deadlift. Remember, for benching only, add two workouts per week. They must consist of special exercises for the pressing muscles: triceps, delts, lats, upper back, and abs. Do only 2–3 per workout, which should last less than 30 minutes. Rotate the exercises as often as necessary. The extra workouts for the squat and deadlift should be no longer than 30 minutes, paying special attention to the abs, entire back, hams, and glutes. Again, only do 2–3 exercises per workout. Always work the abs in each workout plus 1–2 other exercises. The main purpose is restoration and raising the weakest muscle groups up to or surpassing the stronger ones. We must learn to train scientifically. The man whose mind won't change also has a total that won't change.

Designing Your Extra Workouts

First of all, an individual must be fast and very strong to excel at powerlifting. This requires a training program that is 50% for the development of absolute strength. The workouts must be separated by 72 hours! What can be done in between? Small workouts, 15–30 minutes per workout can be implemented.

Let's look at bench pressing.

Workout #1:
Lat pull-downs, dumbbell extensions, and side delt raises. Always do abdominal work.

Workout #2:
Perform barbell rows and four sets of dumbbell presses to failure. Use a weight where 15–20 reps can be done. Rotate from flat, incline, decline, and seated press. Also do abs.

Workout #3:
Three sets of seated dumbbell power cleans. Use a weight where 20 reps can be done but with much effort. Also do one-arm dumbbell rows, 2–4 sets, and two sets of push-ups to failure as well as abs.

Workout #4:
Two sets of benching for 25 reps. Use a different grip—wide, close, thumb or thumbless, or even reverse. Also do chin-ups, inverted flies, and abs.

Workout #5:
One of our 198s, Sonny Kerschner, had a 410 bench and was stuck. He began doing triceps push-downs with a pink flex band looped over a door at his house. Using strict form and a moderate tempo, he did 100 total reps three times a week. Six months later, his bench press was an official 470.

All of the above workouts must be brisk and almost nonstop. Not only will this build substantial muscle mass in the precise area needed, but it raises work capacity. There are countless combinations to choose from. Remember to switch often and always think, "What do I need to raise my bench press?" Then, do only that for 15–30 minutes tops. Start by adding one small workout a week and increase to a second and so forth when you feel capable. For the squat and deadlift, the same exercises work for both. It is important to do ab work in every workout; sometimes abs can be the only muscle group worked.

Workout #1:
Pull-throughs, leg raises, and dumbbell rows.

Workout #2:
Reverse hypers, stability ball, and abdominal work.

Workout #3:
Pull a sled from a belt, rows, and standing abdominals.

Workout #4:
Pull a sled from the ankles and lat pull-downs.

Workout #5:
Perform glute ham raises, weighted leg raises, and dumbbell power cleans.

Workout #6:
Implement walking lunges, side bends, and sit-ups.

Workout #7:
Do flex band good mornings and chest supported rows.

Workout #8:
Box squat with a band looped through your belt and stand through both ends. Don't remove the band between sets. Then, hook a band to the top of a rack and over your head to do standing abs.

Workout #9:
Choke a band around the base of a rack and do seated leg curls. Then, do lying leg raises with chains draped over the ankles.

Workout #10:
Perform good mornings with a band looped through the belt, standing in the loops, plus a second band over the neck and under the feet. Note: When using bands, contract the muscles forcefully and beware—band work is very taxing.

I have outlined many workouts here. Use 1–3 exercises per workout; limit the workout time to 30 minutes including abdominal work. This time can also be used for flexibility work, which is important but often overlooked.

These special workouts are intended to raise the lagging muscle groups that we all possess. While working almost nonstop, GPP is also raised, something else that is often overlooked. For sports other than powerlifting, many drills can be used. Agility, flexibility, and dexterity can also be improved.

There are many lifters who deadlift or squat over 800 and also total 2000 drug-free, so I know it is possible for anyone to make great progress if approaching training in a more scientific light. It must be realized that large muscle groups recuperate in 72 hours and small ones in 24 hours or less.

It is quite possible to train many times a week.

Powerlifting, even with the advances in equipment, still is light years behind all other sports. Tracks have been made for sprinting and better poles and pits have been made for pole vaulting. New advances in football equipment including helmets, pads, and turf have evolved. Unfortunately, powerlifters train with the IQ of a caveman. The IPF refuses to use a monolift, and lifters are actually lifting in what is called raw or no equipment meets. What gives? We are going backward, not forward. Take advantage of technology and a scientific approach to training and you just might succeed.

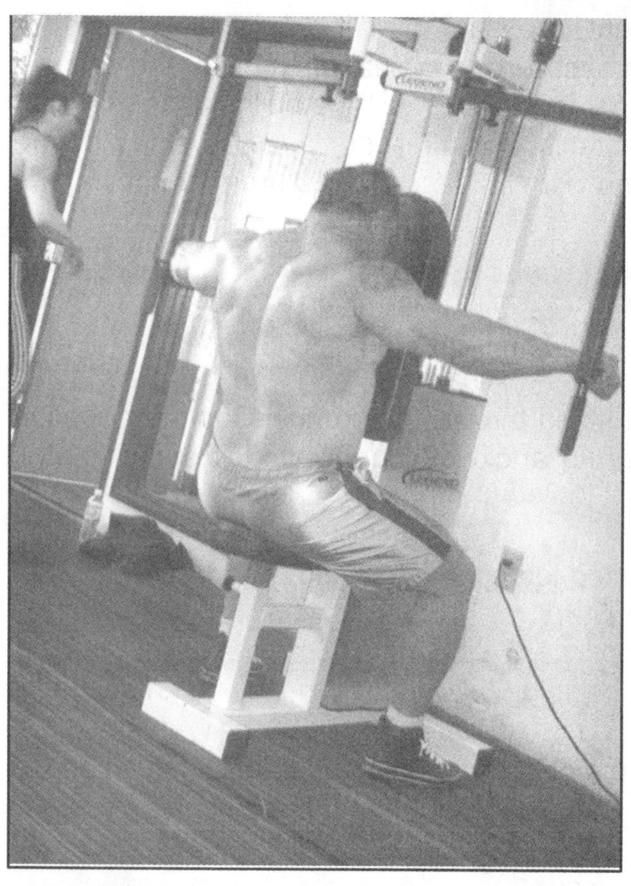

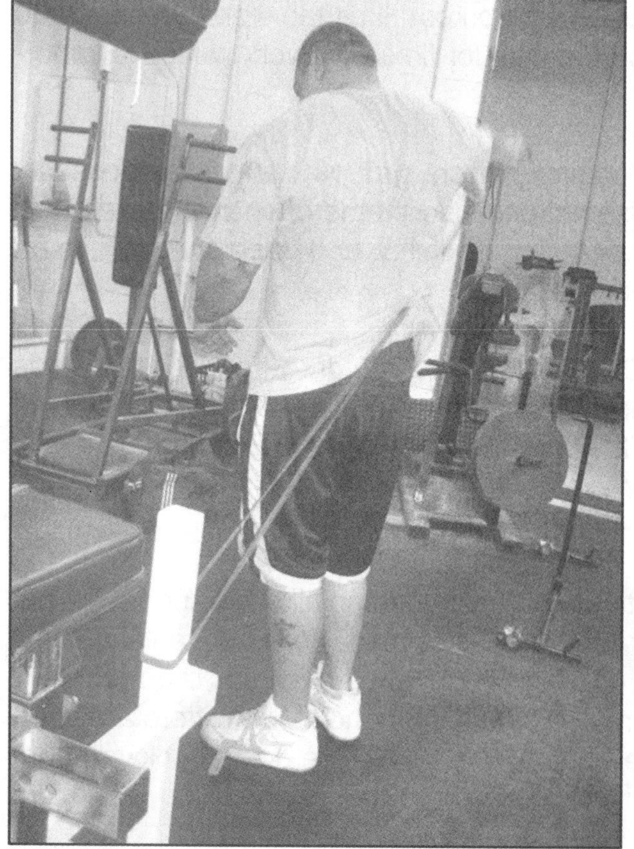

Foundational Training for the Powerlifts

When I was a little boy, I remember building a club house. I worked very hard on the foundation and was ready to start the frame when my dog started barking and poking me with his nose to get my attention. I realized he was trying to tell me I had built the foundation on my neighbor's property (he was a smart dog). Sure enough, my neighbor was looking out her window laughing at me. Needless to say, I hated that girl, but she and my dog were right. All that foundation work was wasted. Years later, after talking to hundreds of lifters, I have discovered that many of them build their foun- dation in the wrong place as well, so here I am talking about lifting.

Bench Press

These lifters read too many bodybuilding magazines and build their foundation for a big bench by doing countless chest exercises and bicep work. Just like me, they built their foundation in the wrong area. By doing so much chest work, the body automatically lets the arms turn out prematurely in the bench press, thus placing all the stress on the pecs and taking the lats, which act as stabilizers, out of the press. This causes soft tissue damage to the pec tie in. Sound familiar? I have heard so-called experts say that the lats don't aid in the bench press. It is apparent that these so-called, well-read experts are not experts at bench pressing. One only has to look at the great bench predecessors who all possess well-developed lats.

At Westside, we instruct all lifters to lower the bar with the lats. The lats work as stabilizers to keep the bar in line. Lowering the bar with the lats primarily and the arms secondarily allows for an explosive start by contracting the triceps in the concentric phase. If a lifter lowers the bar with the arms alone, the bar shakes and the elbows fly out to the sides, causing peck injuries. Perhaps worst of all, the shoulders are rotated severely, causing rotator injuries which are hard to get rid of. Many are taught to press the bar over the face.

This is incorrect. The bar should be pressed in a straight line. Why? First, it is the shortest distance between two points. Second, there is no shoulder rotation, which is much safer for the rotators and the pecs. How is this technique possible? The right foundation must be built; this requires an enormous amount of work for the triceps first, then the delts, and finally the lats. I have said before that there are many shoulder and pec injuries, but how many triceps injuries (from benching) are heard of?

There are very few because the triceps are never stressed as much as they could be. First, pick 3–5 triceps exercises: dumbbell extensions; straight bar attentions to the forehead, chin, and throat; and maybe JM presses. The bar extensions can be done with chains or flex bands. Basically, use one exercise until the triceps are exhausted. Then, finish with some push-downs to hit the parts of the triceps missed by extensions. By rotating a different type of extension when it ceases to work, the triceps can be made stronger year after year. After 3–6 weeks, switch to a different extension, and always try for heavier weights.

Delts are trained the same way. Front delt work with a bar, dumbbells, a cable, or a plate can be used. Again, push up the weight as well as the number of reps. Side delt raises with dumbbells standing or with a cable device and rear delt work while standing with a lat machine can be implemented. Just pull a lat bar to the face or chest or to the top of the head. Dumbbell power cleans and inverted flyes work great. Remember to switch to a different delt exercise for a particular delt angle—front, side, or rear—and change again when it stops working.

This is the correct base, or foundation work, that is needed for a huge bench. One final note—when the triceps become strong, try to stretch the bar apart when pressing a weight. That's what happens when a reverse grip is used. By doing this, the triceps are really put into action.

The Squat and Deadlift

Almost every time a squat article is written, it concludes with assistance work for the legs such as leg presses, leg extensions, and leg curls. With the exception of non-machine leg curls, the foundation work is all wrong. When a lifter misses a squat, it is because the lower back is giving out. This was brought to my attention by Bill Starr in an article in MILO.

If an individual overdevelops the quads, he is likely to go forward when squatting. This can cause two problems: knee pain from overstretching the patella tendon and difficulty breaking parallel. If he goes forward, hypothetically his knees would touch the floor and the hip joint would still be above parallel.

Leg curls are adequate but not nearly as effective as glute ham raises. A leg curl activates the lower insertion that ties in behind the knee and then the knee and the attachment that ties into the glute. Because squatting is a multi-joint activity, the hamstring contracts and stretches while ascending and descending at both the hip and knee, respectively. That is why the glute ham raise was developed; it is beneficial for both squatting and pulling. Kenny Patterson recently pulled a 650 deadlift, a 65-lb PR. It took only about 12 weeks of concentrated work on the glute ham raise. The Soviets used it for sprinting, and Fred Hatfield said it contributed to his 1000 lb squat. Matt Dimel implemented glute ham raises as well for his 1010 squat

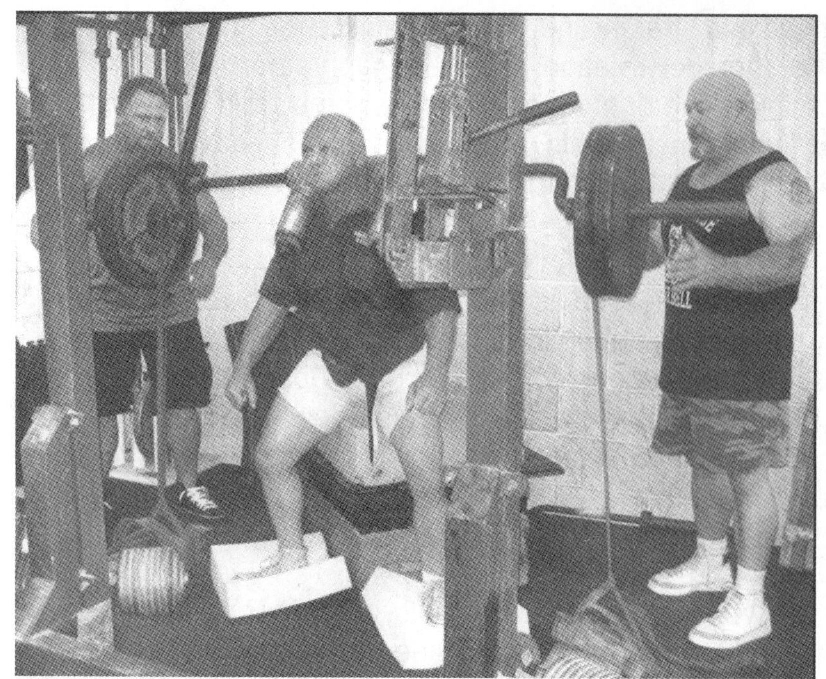

What is the correct foundational work for squatting? Hamstring work plays a large role, as stated above. We do as many different types of good mornings as possible.

All work the hamstrings very hard with the exception of the seated variety.

Of course, a good morning is a compound exercise that also works the spinal erectors and glutes to a greater degree than squatting.

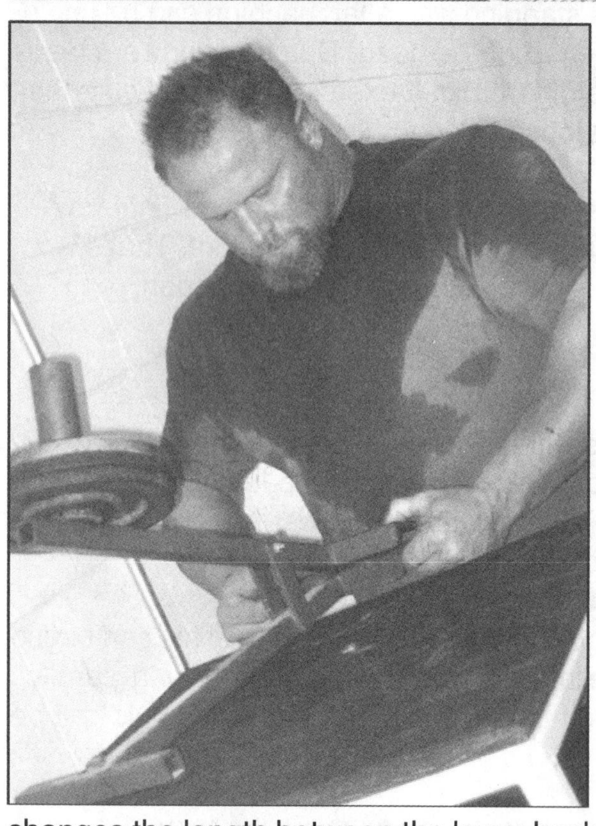

Here are three of our favorite exercises for the hamstring. The reverse hyper machine is tremendous for the hamstrings, outperforming the Romanian deadlift almost 2:1 on an EMG machine. Glute ham raises are great. Someone at Westside is always doing them. A lifter needs to be fairly strong to do one. Pull throughs are effective when one uses a low pulley machine with a single crossover handle. Face away from the machine, grasp the handle between the legs, and walk out a few feet.

Let the machine pull the handle between the legs and squat up and down. It will blow up the hamstrings. All three exercises work the glutes as well. For the back, back raises, good mornings, reverse hyperextensions, and a variety of special squats (safety squat bar, MantaRay, front squat) increase back strength. Many of these squats as well as good mornings can be done with chains, bands, or weight release devices. Using a MantaRay, safety squat bar, or front squat harness changes the length between the lower back and the center of the bar, lengthening it and thus, forcing the spinal erectors to be worked harder than ever.

Because most of the muscles that squat also deadlift, our max effort day for squatting and deadlifting is the same day. We always add lat work on this day. Lat work and shrugs are done next to last. For lat pull-downs, we switch bars and grips quite often, always hitting the lats from different angles. Rowing should be done as well. We do chest supported rows most often, one- arm rows occasionally, and barbell rows sparingly. Barbell and dumbbell shrugs are done as they assist the bench press.

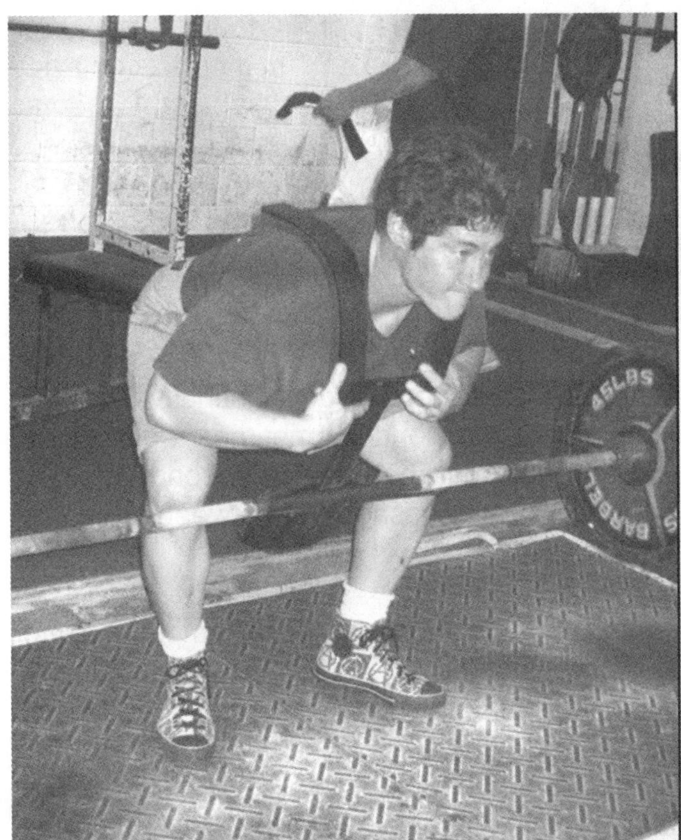

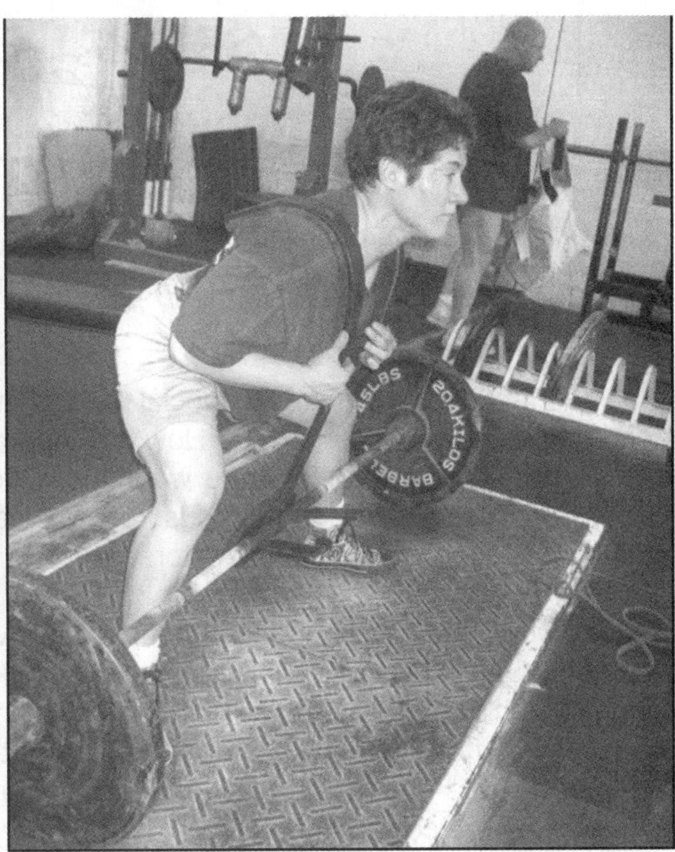

We do a lot of sled dragging, which builds tremendous hip and glute strength. We drag 200 feet at a time, which constitutes a set. Do six sets with weight that does not cause you to lean forward too much. If possible, do them the day after squat and deadlift day. This is active rest, which works as restoration and also raises work capacity. Kneeling squats also build the hips.

When it comes to squatting and deadlifting, the abdominals play a tremendous role. Some at Westside work their abs every day. I don't recommend crunches because they are mostly a waste. When squatting or deadlifting, abdominal work should be completed while straightening the legs. That is why an individual should do lots of leg raises. Start with the legs bent and gradually work into straight leg raises. Also, do a lot of side bends. The obliques do most of the work because of how they attach to the hip and back. Static abdominal work is important, too. Learn how to push out and hold the abs against the belt for the duration of a lift. For sit-ups and leg raises, we often use chains and bands.

Zercher squats work the abs. Hold the bar in the crook of the arms with hands against the chest. Squat while forcing out and expanding the abs. If you are always worried about your waistline, you are in the wrong sport. A strong waistline is big and powerful like any other muscle group.

Remember, after a core exercise such as a squat, bench, deadlift, or good morning, do 3–4 special exercises that pertain to that lift. By choosing correctly, not only will you become stronger but your form will be far better.

Muscle groups such as the pecks, quads, biceps, and all other "showy" muscles develop easily. It's the hips, lower back, hamstrings, and glutes that no one seems to look at that do all the work. Pay most of the attention to the functional muscles, not the "showy" ones. If you want to build a tremendous future, you have to build a solid foundation.

SPECIAL EXERCISES

TRAINING THE MUSCLES

Our special exercises, such as: triceps extensions, lat work, low back work, and abs, are performed in macrocycles every 2–6 weeks. Each macrocycle lasts 2–3 weeks and coordinates with our speed or dynamic method day.

When controlling the amount of special work for a particular muscle group, do it instinctively. Think, does this exercise work for you? How are you responding to the work? Sometimes it is better to divide special work into separate workouts. Often more work can be done in second workouts because rest or restoration methods such as ice, hot tubs, and massage fall between workouts. Many times simple rest acts as restoration.

Special work is raised throughout the first three weeks in an upward wave. For example, if a lifter does glute ham raises for more than three weeks, progress stops. At Westside, we recommend training special work as hard as possible. By doing this, he's able to make further gains after three weeks. The lifter then switches to an exercise that closely mimics the preceding exercise. This is the conjugate method. Westside utilizes this method in all facets of training. Even restoration methods can be constantly switched. Learn to regulate training in this manner to succeed.

Exercises can fall into three categories:

1. general
2. directed
3. sports-specific

General exercises include the reverse hyper machine, glute ham raises, box jumps, inverse curls, lat work, ab work, triceps extensions, and hip extensor/flexor work. Directed exercises include good mornings, belt squats, deadlifts on a box or from a rack, floor presses, rack or board presses, and dumbbell presses. Sports-specific exercises encompass legal depth box squats, close grip bench, wide bench, and deadlifting with the opposite style that you normally use (sumo versus conventional).

At Westside, all three categories are used weekly but not done simultaneously. Why? If a specific type of strength is not trained during a three-week period, a loss in strength of 10% or greater occurs. This is true for agility, coordination, and even flexibility.

Back Exercises

Many lifters train with a bad back, and they often ask me what to do to decrease their chances of getting hurt while squatting or deadlifting. I fractured my fifth lumbar vertebra twice. In 1973, I pulled a 670 deadlift at 181. Shortly thereafter, I broke the vertebra while doing bent over good mornings. In 1983, I broke it again falling off my ice-covered porch. This time, the doctor said he wanted to remove two disks, fuse my back, and take off a bone spur. I declined.

Having successfully come back from those injuries, I have discovered many ways to work around a bad back or prevent our lifters from getting one. In 1973, my knowledge was limited. During 1974, I was on and off crutches for ten months. One of my most important discoveries was chiropractors. Because of my inactivity, my spinal alignment was terrible. I had misgivings about going to a chiropractor, but my doctor wanted me to go in for traction for a couple weeks. I hate hospitals, so finally I broke down and went to a chiropractor. To my surprise, my back was much better after a few adjustments, and I was able to start training again. However, my problem came back, and my back still hurts all the time.

In 1975, my back was still fragile. That's when I started doing reverse hyper extensions. Through the motion of rotating the sacrum in a safe way and the blood pumping action, my back was quickly rehabilitated to the point that I pulled 710 in 1977 at 198. We picked up many exercises as the years passed, and after breaking my fifth lumbar vertebra again in 1983, my rehabilitation was much faster. This time I used acupressure and acupuncture to speed up the healing. I also received oxygen injections directly into the muscle, which helped greatly. Aside from progressive medical help, we have found an array of back and abdominal exercises that have all but eliminated our low back aliments.

When squatting or deadlifting, a successful lift is dependent on keeping the back in a good position. This takes a strong back as well as strong abs. At Westside, we do max effort work for squatting and deadlifting on the same day—Monday. The same muscles work in these two lifts. It saves energy to lump together the special exercises that contribute to both lifts.
Let's talk about the spinal erectors and how to develop them.

Good mornings

Good mornings are often used as a max effort exercise. There are many variations, including bands, chains, and weight releasers to accommodate resistance. The stance can also be varied from having the feet together to standing with them ultra wide or use a lift under the heels like the old Paul Anderson style. Work up to a 1–3 rep max; as assistance exercise, do sets of 5–10 reps.

The following variations of good mornings can be used:

Bent over good mornings: Place the bar on the back in a squat position or slightly lower and bend over, rounding the upper and lower back. It is up to the individual how far to bend over. A lifter with a small waist finds it easier to bend over farther. This builds the erectors, hamstrings, and glutes by extending the legs and back simultaneously. Bent over good mornings with the legs straight build the erectors and increase flexibility in the hamstrings.

Arched back: This style builds static strength in the erectors, which contributes to keeping the back arched while squatting or sumo deadlifting. Lower the bar as far as possible without losing the arch.

Power arched good mornings: Use a very wide stance, a low bar position, and lean, don't bend, forward until the bar is in front of the knees. Heavy weights can be employed. This is not a quarter squat; the bar must be in front of the knees after leaning forward.

Combo squat/good morning: This one is very important for learning to extend all the squat and deadlift muscles. With a moderate stance and the bar held low on the back, bend forward until the back is close to parallel to the floor. Roll the lower back over and descend into a full squat. To stand up, straighten out the legs. This is very effective for building tremendous extension strength as well as tremendous tightness. You feel like your eyes will pop out when you're in the bottom.

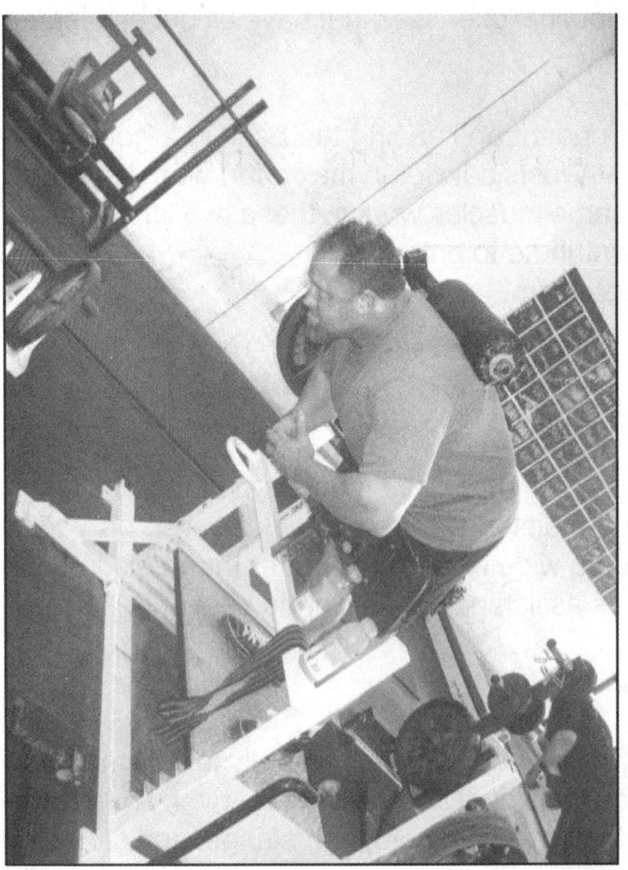

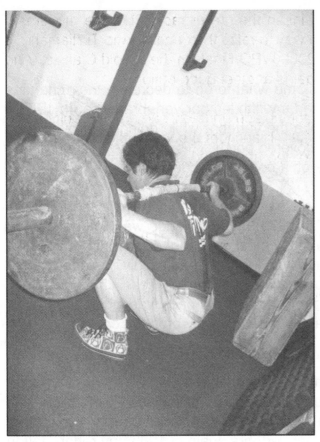

Seated good mornings on a box: Sit on a parallel or above parallel box and bend over. This takes the legs out of the exercise, which is helpful if a lifter is injured or have a large stomach.

Good mornings on floor: Good mornings done while seated on the floor are effective. Sit on the floor with an empty bar across the shoulders. Now, bend forward as far as possible. Breathe normally, or in other words, relax! Don't arch the back to return to the starting position but rather push with the heels. Flexibility increases rapidly.

Suspended good mornings: Suspend the bar on chains in the power rack. Start the movement from the down position, which can be a very effective way to raise the deadlift. Ano Turtiainen did a solid 893 after doing these while preparing for the 2002 WPO Finals in the Arnold Classic. Ano used a cambered bar on these, but the safety squat bar is another good option.

Back attack: We do a lot of work on a good morning machine appropriately named the Back Attack. This machine makes the strictest good morning possible. It anchors the feet with rollers and has an abdominal pad to keep the legs straight. A roller for the upper body makes it comfortable. Of course, we add bands to the weight. With heavy weight, we do 6–10 reps.

Several special barbells can be used for all of the good morning variations mentioned above. The camber bar, buffalo bar, and safety squat bar are the most effective ones. The strength curve can be changed by using the weight release device, flex bands, or chains. Vary the work by using a lot of weight and a little chain, light bar weight and lots of chains, or heavy or light eccentric loading with the weight release. These combinations are known as the contrast method. Caution: Use of the flex bands can make one very sore because of the tremendous eccentric overloading from the tension of the bands, which causes delayed onset of muscle soreness (DOMS). This phenomenon occurs with any type of eccentric stress but especially with the use of flex bands.
Now, let's isolate…

Back raises or hyperextensions
These are done on a special bench where the feet are anchored and the torso is supported while lying face down. The bench can be parallel or at a 45-degree angle. Lower the upper body until the head is close to the floor. Then, raise up to parallel but no higher to avoid hyperextending the back. Perform reps of 3–8 and work up to a new max set whenever possible.

The 1968 Olympic weight lifting champ, Waldemar Bazanowski, was able to do 225 for four reps, so get to work. Back extensions can be done with a rotation or by keeping the upper body shifted on one side, targeting the obliques.

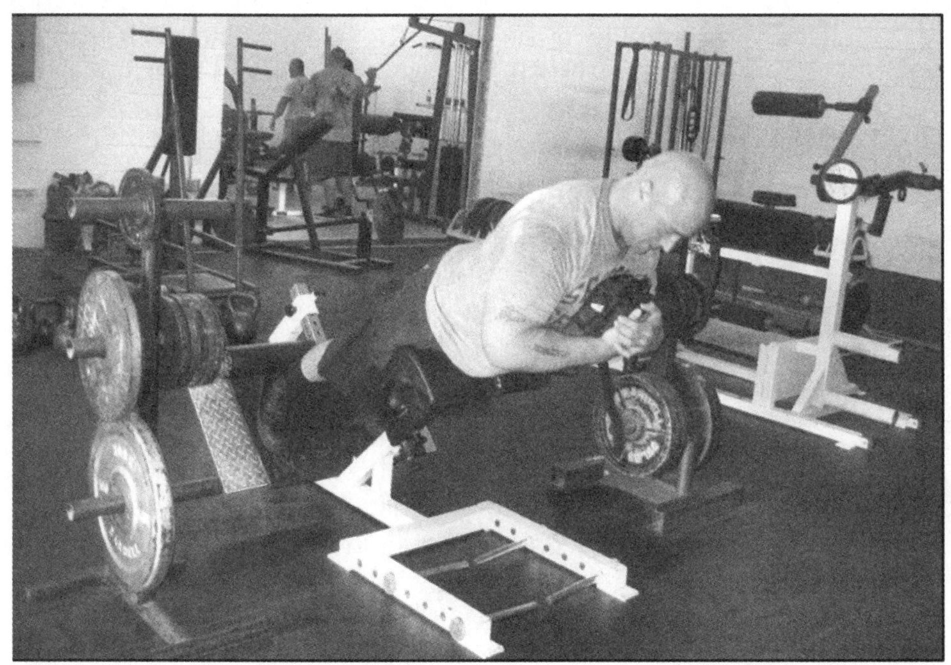

Pull-throughs with straight legs

Pull-throughs with straight legs really hit the lower back. For more variety, stand on a box or do a semi-squat to activate the hamstrings. Pull a low pulley cable through the legs while facing away from the machine. If done with the legs straight, this exercise hits the lower back. Use high reps, sometimes to failure. If done with the legs bent, this works the glutes.

Reverse hyper extensions®

For the mid to the very lowest part of the back, the reverse hyper machine is far superior to any back exercise. Not only does it completely work the low back, but it rotates the sacrum. Also, on every rep when the plates are under the face, it opens the disks and allows spinal fluid to enter, providing restoration as well as strength building.

At Westside, we do many 45-degree reverse hyperextensions. This style dramatically hits not only the lower back but also the hamstrings. They are done very heavy on either squat day or max effort day for the squat and deadlift. Six to ten reps are performed, and the number of sets depends on a lifter's level of physical preparedness. We do 2–6 sets. Reverse hypers are the best exercise for lower back problems that I've ever seen. People with bulging or herniated disks can do them without pain. They rotate the sacrum in a very safe way with virtually no compression on the lower spine. At the same time, they build the glutes and hamstrings.

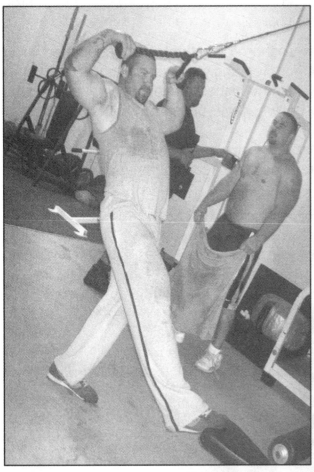

We've been using the reverse hyper machine since 1975. The real secret of this machine is that it tractions the vertebrae while building strength and working as restoration at the same time. We do these at least four times a week—twice heavy and twice light. Chuck Vogelpohl and I use the machine heavy before and after squatting on Friday mornings, and I do them light on Friday evenings. This is repeated on Monday, our max effort day. On Tuesday evenings, Eskil Thomasson and I do heavy again because they traction the back, so they can be done repeatedly throughout the week. The reps range from 8–12 on heavy workouts and 15–30 on light workouts.

Sled dragging

One of the most effective lower back therapies is walking. It is the most natural way to rehabilitate a bad back. Dragging weights has a positive effect on the lower back, and the most effective ways to drag the sled are forward and backward. Sled work can be used like any other exercise for building strength. Dragging the sled trains the glutes, hamstrings, and quads, depending on which style is executed. Read more about sled dragging in the GPP section in this book.

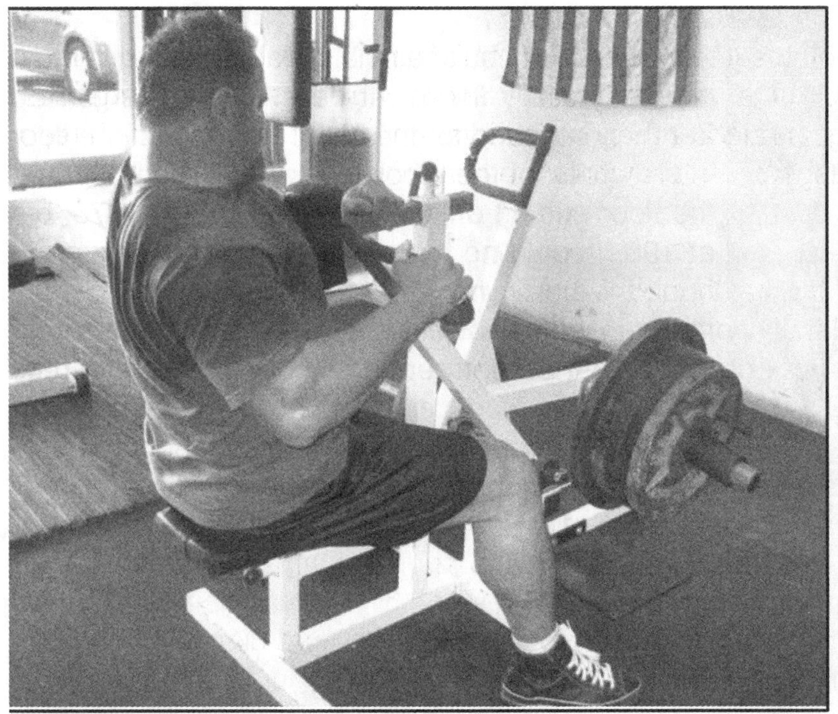

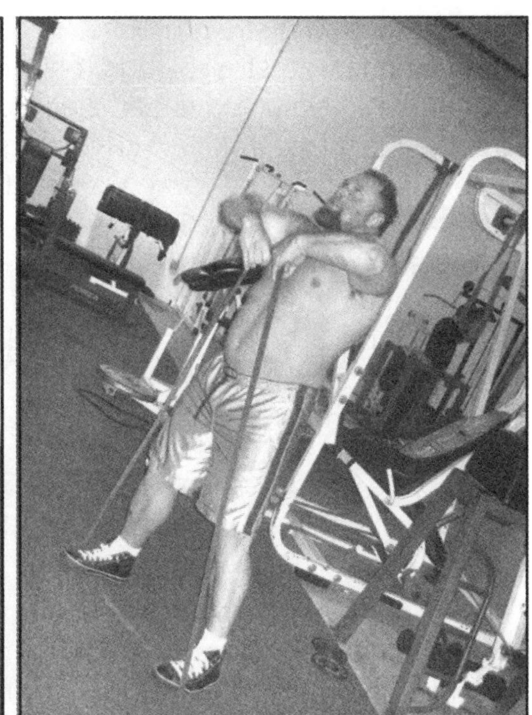

Upper back and lat work

Westside lifters do an enormous amount of upper back work because the upper back plays a large role in all three lifts. For squatting, the farther back the bar sits, the greater the leverage. Notice that I said back on the back, not down.

Upper Back

We perform many upright rows to thicken the traps along with inverted flies with dumbbells and dumbbell power cleans, sometimes very heavy for low reps. We use a machine called the Hurricane, a multipurpose device for an assortment of exercises. These really add mass to the entire upper back. We have a high school discus thrower who does four sets of four reps in the one arm power snatch with a 100-lb dumbbell. By the way, we don't do the Olympic lifts. Rows of all types are done at least three times a week. The guys who only bench do rows just about every workout, which is four times a week. The full powerlifters do even more rows per week. Chest supported rows are a mainstay. Very heavy weights are used by most. Among the rows that are performed are the old-fashion t-bar rows with different handles, wide-bar and V-handle rows, one arm rows across the body, regular barbell rows occasionally with bands, and one arm dumbbells rows.

Lat work

Chins are great either with weight or without. Honestly, we don't do them very often. Everyone does lat pull-downs at Westside, but the Westsider with the strongest lats told me that pull-downs don't help his lat strength as much as rows. This is the majority of our upper back work. We also do a lot of band work and sled work for the upper back. Overhead pressing works the upper back. We do the majority of our overhead work seated. Most articles on deadlifting address upper back work to assist the deadlift. That, of course, is good, but the lower back is injured more often than all the other back muscles combined.

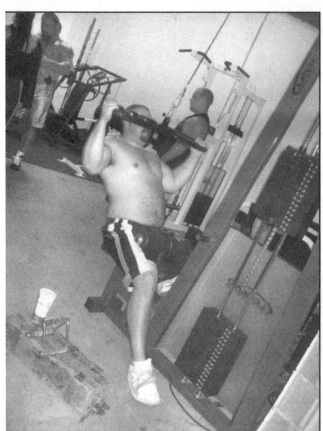

Zercher squats

Zercher squats build all the squat and deadlift muscles, especially the lower back. Their inventor, Ed Zercher, intended for the bar to be lifted off the floor in the crook of the elbows. At 181, I made 320 off the floor and an official deadlift of 670 in 1973, but at 198, I could no longer bend over far enough to hook the bar in my elbows. At that point, I placed the bar on the power rack pins and squatted from there. Bob Burnett reportedly did 390 for five reps in 1967 and made a 675 deadlift at 165 lbs. We now do Zercher squats with a Strongman rack. They can be done for 1–3 reps, but I prefer high reps of 8–12.

Deadlift using the opposite style

Most sumo deadlifters train a lot with conventional style, but how many conventional style lifters use sumo in training? Training the deadlift in the sumo style eliminates a great deal of back trauma. It is also a good way to monitor flexibility. Mariah Liggett trained sumo and pulled conventional at meets, pulling 484 at 132.

Leg Exercises

A tight lower back usually equals tight hamstrings. In addition, a weak back is almost always accompanied by weak hamstrings. When doing any type of squat, occasionally wear shoes with heels because this places more of the work on the quads. Also, squat as deep as possible. Depending on the amount of resistance, the reps are 5–12 per set. All of the above squats can be accomplished holding a barbell or dumbbells. I hope some of the exercises mentioned here can raise your squat and deadlift. Some of the exercises are very old, and some are relatively new, but all are proven to work. It's up to you or your coach to place them where they can do the most good.

Glute ham raise

The glute ham raise is a highly advanced exercise. While kneeling on a padded bench with the feet hanging off the end of the bench, have a partner sit on your ankles to hold you down. Lower slowly without bending at the waist until the chest touches the bench. Now pull yourself back up as if doing a leg curl.

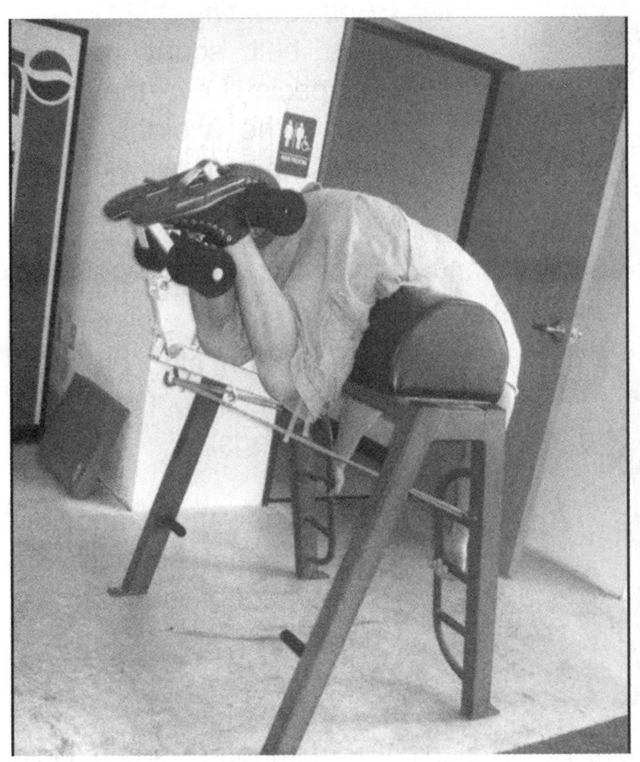

Let me recommend two ways to work up to a full rep. The first is to lower slowly and hold for 3–6 seconds at various points of this movement. This is very taxing on the hamstrings and glutes. It builds the top and mid-portion of the exercise. You can lower all the way down until the chest comes in contact with the bench and then use the hands to assist in the raise until the hamstrings and glutes can curl you up the rest of the way.

The second method is to lower yourself down to elastic bands located midway between the top and bottom positions. This helps reduce body weight while lowering yourself, and it helps spring you back up to a kneeling position. As you get stronger, use fewer or weaker bands until completing a rep unassisted.

The inverse curl is a form of the glute ham raise. The glute ham bench is elevated in the back by about 30 inches. Do a partial leg curl and a back extension at the same time. Hold at the top position (do not push with the toes). This exercise works the hamstrings at the hip and knee insertions simultaneously. A standard leg curl does not do the same.

Dimel deadlifts
Use a shoulder-width stance and grab the bar with the hands outside the legs. First, stand up with the back straight and arched. Maintain this position and drop the bar to just below knee level by squatting down. Quickly return to the top. Do 15–20 reps for two sets. These can be done up to four days a week but only for two weeks at the most. These are named after my dear friend, Matt Dimel. They pushed his 820 squat, which was stalled for over a year, to 1010 in 16 months. The same exercise raised Steve Wilson's deadlift to his all-time best of 865.

Pull-through
The pull-through is a great exercise for the hamstrings. Face away from a low pulley machine. Grab a single handle between the legs. Walk out a few feet and squat down, letting the handle be pulled through the legs as far as possible Use the repetition method. Go to failure on each set. Three or four sets are plenty. This exercise builds the hamstrings where they tie into the glutes.

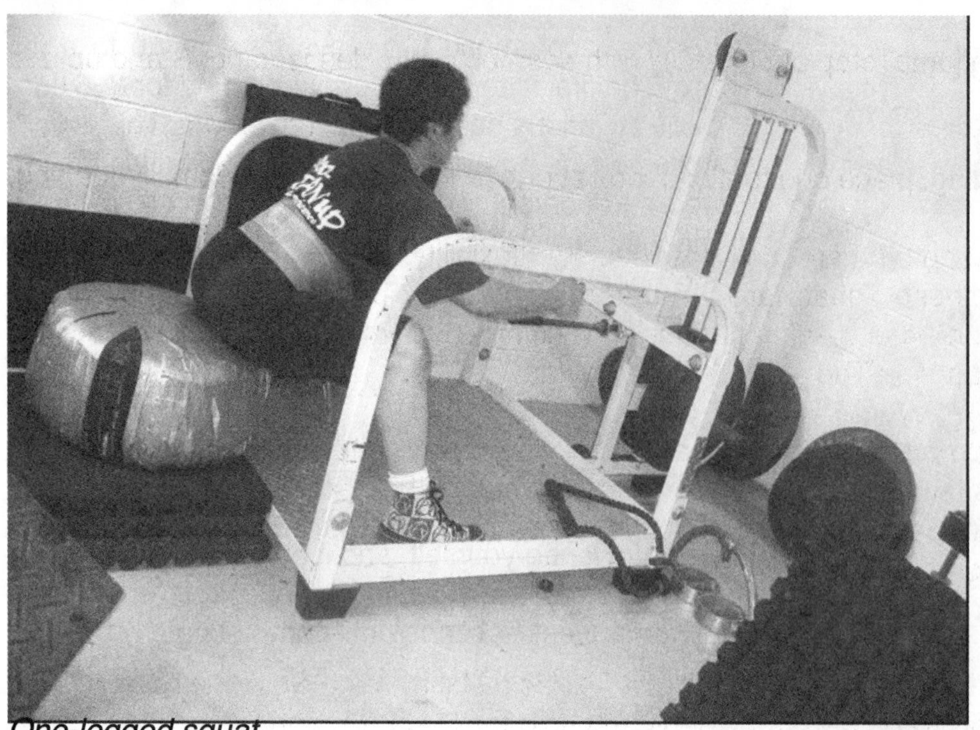

Belt squatting
The belt squat requires a special belt—the squat belt. The weight hangs from the belt, allowing only the lower body to do the work. You may have seen our belt squat machine in our squat video. Belt squats can also be done on an incline. Don't lock out the legs.

Do these with a MantaRay or on a flat surface; the safety squat bar can be used.

One-legged squat
Do these with one leg supported behind you on a bench. This is also called a sprinter's squat. Hold on to a support for a little resistance. The hardest one-legged squat is done by balancing while unassisted.

Leg curls with bands
Do these seated on a bench in front of a power rack. Secure a band to the bottom of the rack, hook the band with the back of the ankles, and pull the feet under the bench.

Deadlifts behind the back
This builds great leg strength for deadlifting. If you have large hamstrings, this exercise may be difficult. Ano, the great Finn, is experimenting with these to get some leg drive back into his deadlift.

Squatting can also be done to develop flexibility. Here are some different types of squats:

Lateral roll squat: Start by squatting down as deep as possible. Roll the body weight to the right leg in a lunge position, shift to the left leg, and stand up. Squat down again and repeat in reverse.

Frog squat: Squat down with the hands over the head; then, place the hands between the legs and touch the floor.

Side-stepping squat: With a jump, step out laterally with both feet while descending. Stand up and repeat.

Uneven squat: While squatting, place one foot on a box about six inches high and do full squatting.

The variety of squats presented here are intended for flexibility and agility, something that most lifters lack. Many of these squats are illustrated in *Twisted Conditioning* by Bud Jeffries (1-866-STRNGER). This book has training tips for powerlifting, Strongman competitions, and no holds-barred fighting such as Vale Tudo, which I'm a big fan.

Other leg developers include pushing cars forward or backward and walking with a heavy wheel-barrow. Jesse Kellum likes this type of training at certain times of the year, and his legs are just about as strong as I've ever seen. Front squats, free squats, or Hindu squats can be done for high reps in the 20–500 rep range.

Wall squats: Jesse Kellum suggested that I try these. This is a static squat. Slide the back against a wall to an angle where you want to work the legs and hold for 15–60 seconds.

Plyometrics and jumping

Paul Anderson was doing jumping exercises in the 1950s. He would jump onto boxes of different heights to build explosive leg power. Norm Schomanski, our great Olympic lifting champion, also did a lot of jumping. He was reputedly able to jump onto a four-foot high bar top at a local tavern. One of the benefits of kinetic energy on the lowering phase is that it produces a phantom loading effect on the landing. I highly suggest an individual do a lot of research on plyometrics before using them in his training because they must be used correctly.

Abdominal Exercises

Abdominal strength is extremely important in preventing back injury. There are many back and abdominal exercises to choose from. These are just a few. Some work for certain individuals better than others. That is precisely why there needs to be many to choose from. The information in our series of articles and this book is the result of experimentation by the Elite powerlifters we have developed over the years. We have a system that teaches a lifter how to teach himself. For example, learn to use the abs correctly while wearing a lifting belt. Push out against the belt because it is very important to push out to the sides or exert outwardly with the obliques. This starts the action of straightening out the legs. Please don't be confused by bodybuilding magazines. Hip flexers/ extensors and abs must work together.

Standing abdominal work

We do a great deal of abdominal work standing up, and why not? When an athlete fights, wrestles, plays ball, and lifts weights, he is standing up, not sitting. Attach a strong strap from the power rack to the front of the belt and lean back until there is no slack in the strap. Now, slide the feet forward until you are leaning backward.

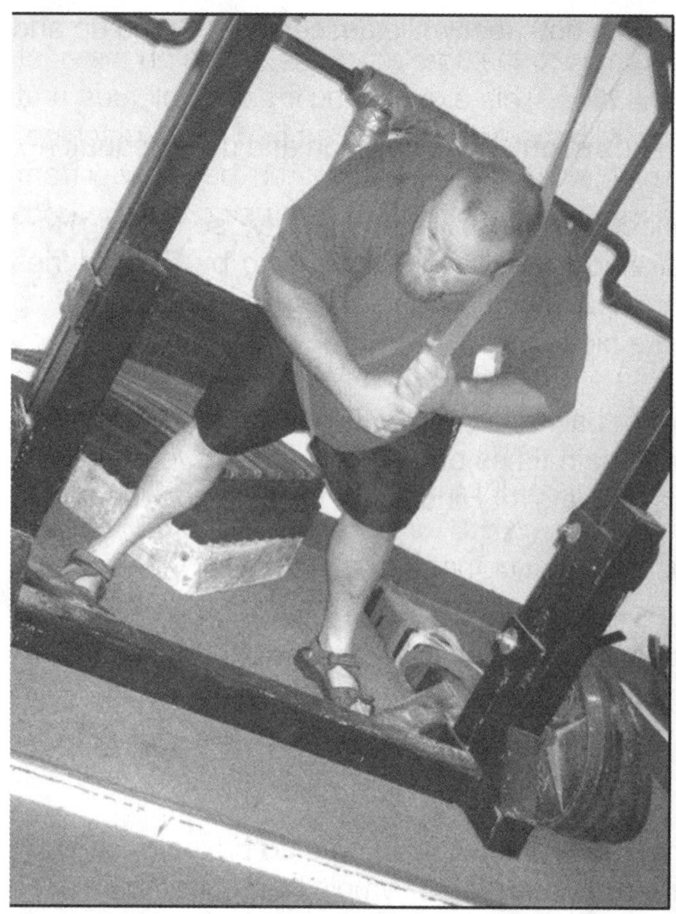

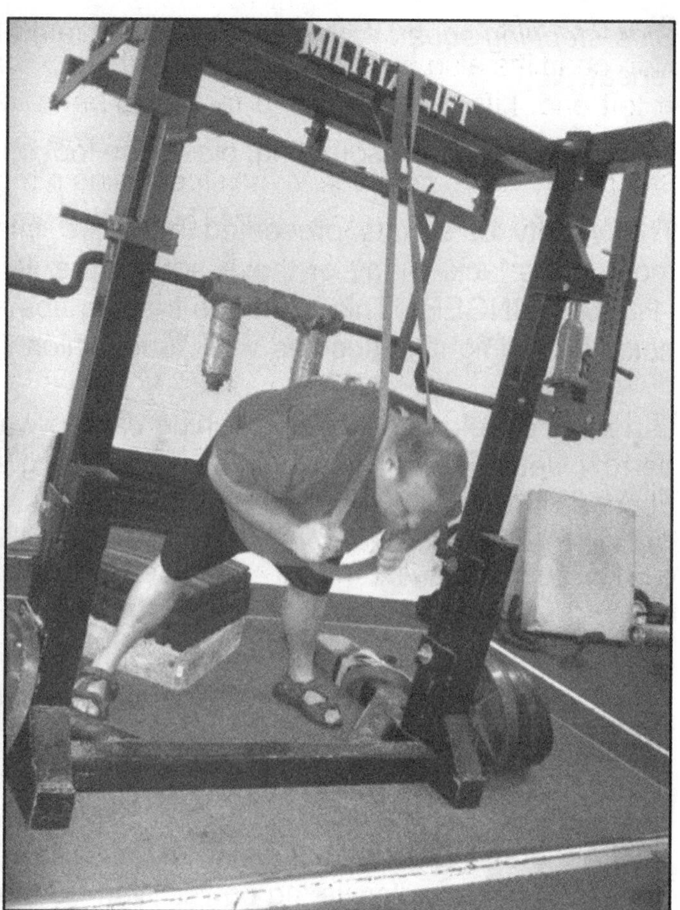

Place the abs in a pre-stretched position. Crunch the abs while holding a medicine ball or cable device behind the head. This works the abs effectively. Hook the strap on the belt to do oblique work. As a bonus, hook the strap to the rear of the belt, and with the body inclined forward, perform deadlifts with a barbell or dumbbells. This is great for the lower back, hamstrings, and glutes.

This is just a partial list of exercises that help fix a bad back, or more importantly, prevent one.

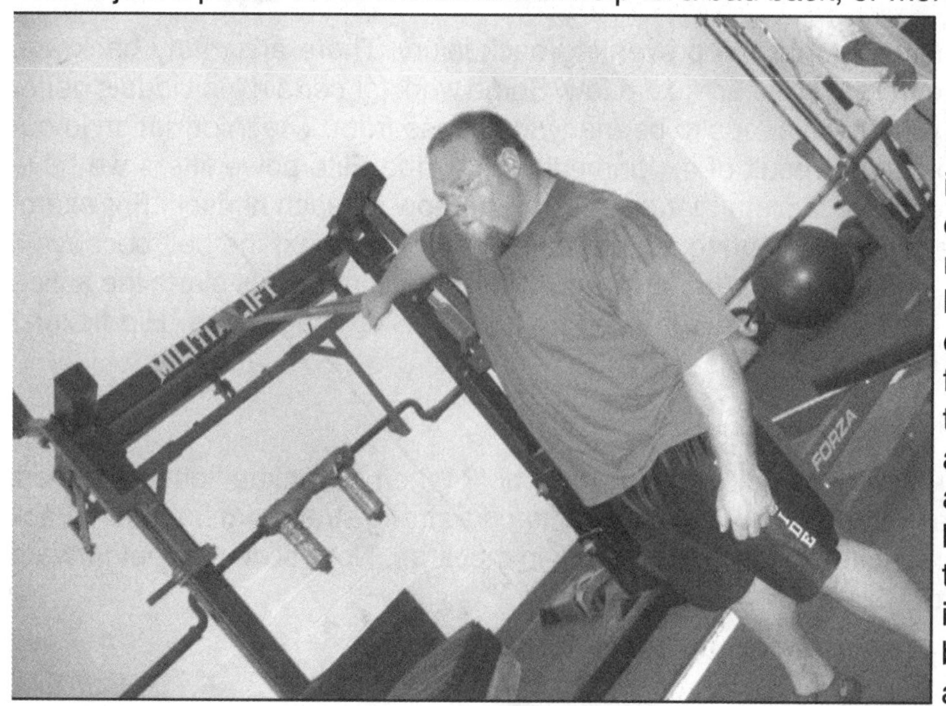

Side bends

In my opinion, the side bend is the most important exercise for the abs. The obliques not only work as stabilizers but are responsible for hip extension when lifting off the floor or out of the bottom of the squat. Learn to push the abs out, expanding them against the power belt. Side bends with a dumbbell at a time are great for this. Holding a dumbbell in the hand, bend to the side and return to a standing position.

Side deadlifts

Side deadlifts also work the abs and obliques. Stand next to the bar, facing the plates on the right or left end. Lift the barbell and try not to bend to the side. This exercise builds the obliques and stability in the glutes. We prefer to do our side bends with the help of an overhead cable machine. Stand with the lat machine to the side. Using a triceps strap held against the neck, bend away from the machine and do a side bend. There appears to be little stress on the spine using this method.

Standing sit-ups with the lat machine

Hold a tricep strap around the back of the neck with the two ends held against the chest while facing away from the machine. Now, bend over as far as possible while pushing out the abs. Most lifters are very weak when first attempting this exercise but be patient. The weight will go up and so will your squat and deadlift. Use light weights for high reps or for a certain length of time. We start our workout by doing 3–5 minutes of this exercise to warm up our abs and lower back. By adding weight, you will realize quickly how weak your abs are. Just compare the weight on the machine to your bodyweight, and it will open your eyes.

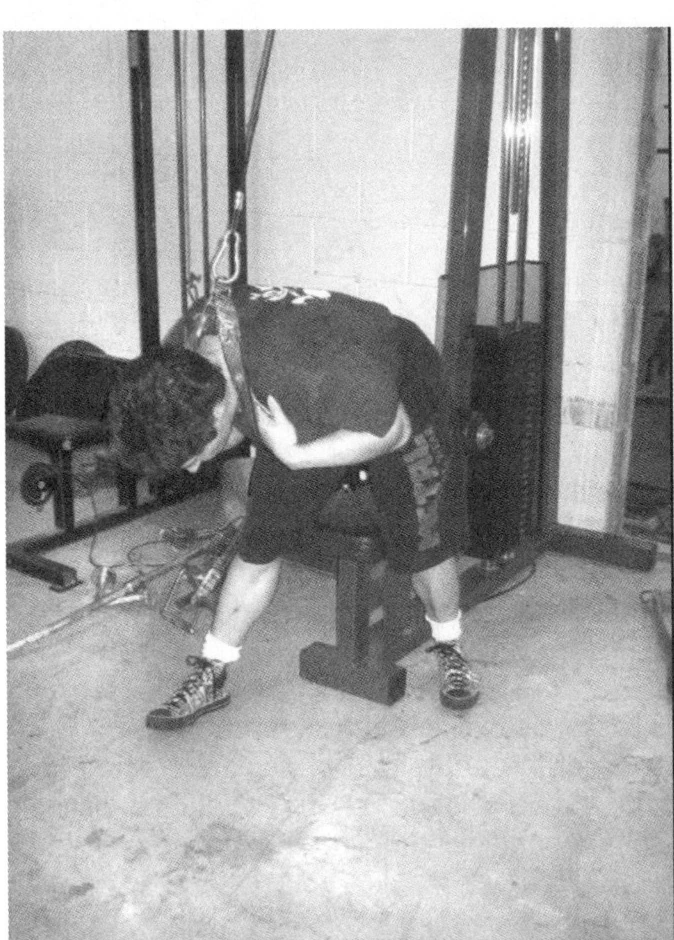

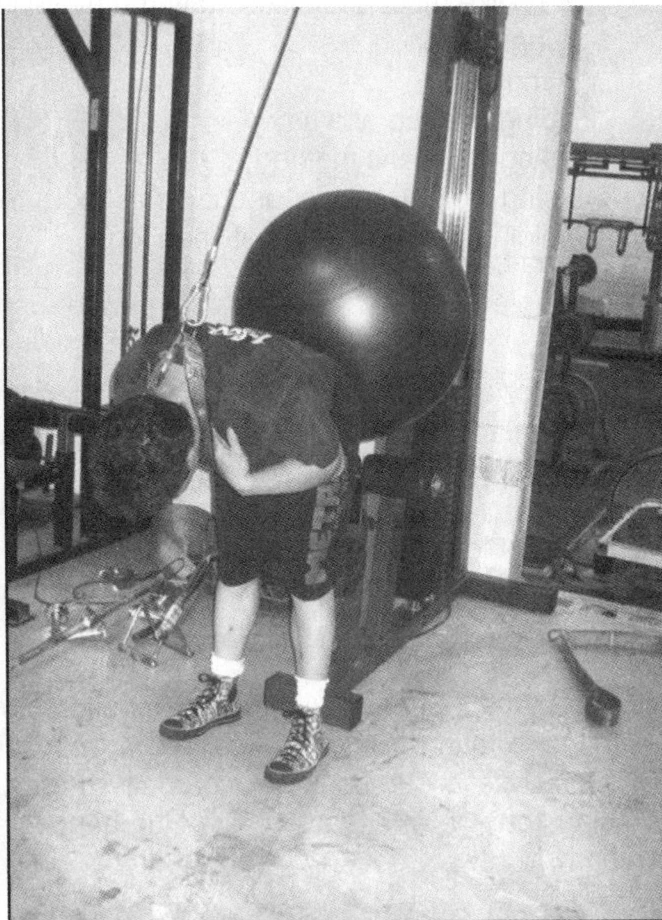

There are several variations of this exercise that we use at Westside. These include the following:

- medicine ball on back
- one leg in front
- different foot stances
- static hold on 2–3 positions for 2–5 seconds
- torso twisted to one side
- legs straight or bent

Leg raises

Leg raises of any kind are good. They are very effective when done hanging from a chin-up bar. To do these, raise the feet until you touch the bar that you are hanging from. These are great for strength and flexibility and are the hardest. Start with lying leg lifts with the legs bent and progress to straight leg lifts. If your shoulders are good, do hanging leg raises. Do them with bent legs until you are strong enough to keep your legs straight. Use weight if possible.

Leg raises, like most exercises, have many variations:

- lying on bench
- hanging
- doing one leg at a time
- using the static method
- using weight, bands, or chains as extra resistance
- holding medicine ball between legs

Landmine

We do a lot of rotational exercises on the landmine. This is a popular exercise for wrestlers and mixed martial arts fighters. If you don't have a landmine, place the end of a 45 lb bar in a corner. Grab the other end (use a handle if possible) and rotate the bar overhead from one hip to the other. For a better workout, superset these with the reverse hyper machine, rows, pull-throughs, good mornings, or lower back exercises. This enables you to rotate the back in four directions and gives you an unbelievable pump. This exercise has pushed up our deadlifts at Westside.

One-arm lifts

Lifts performed standing with one arm build stability. Exercises like one-arm presses or one- arm snatches, rotating from one side to the opposite side of the body train the spinal erectors and obliques. Use a dumbbell or a barbell shorter than standard length or try Pavel Tsatsouline's Russian kettlebells for variety. The Hurricane is also a very efficient tool for torso and upper back strength.

Sit-ups

Many types of sit-ups can be done. A bent leg sit-up is worthless unless you have a very weak back and stomach. Try these variations:

1.Sit-ups while holding a ball or cushion between the thighs realigns the lower back. It also helps to decrease the pressure on the back by increasing abdominal pressure.

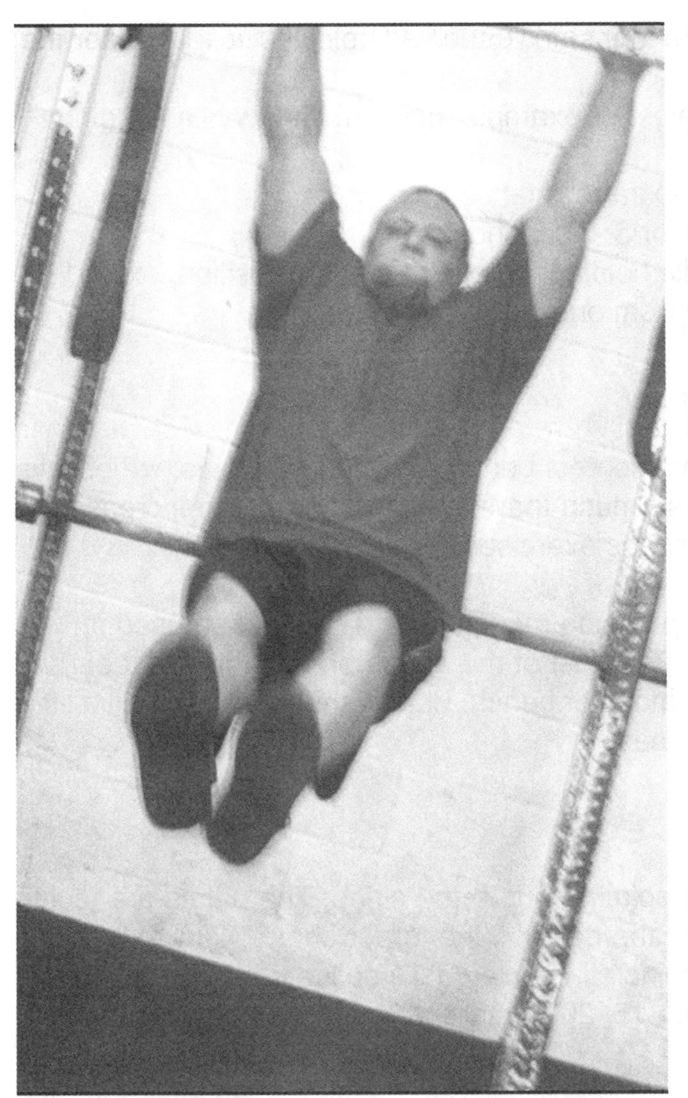
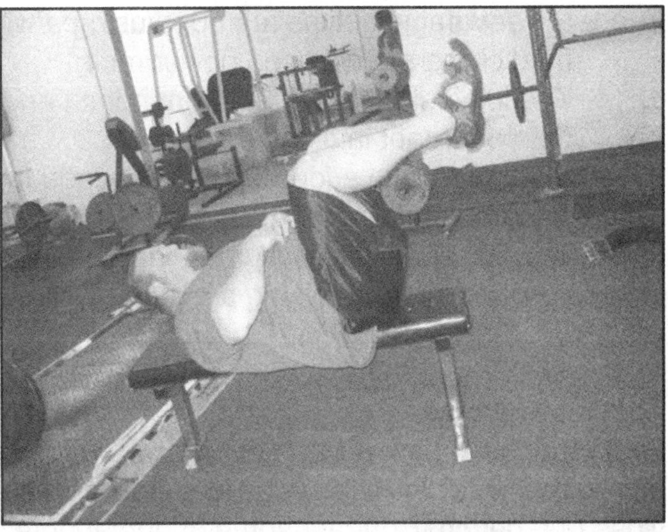
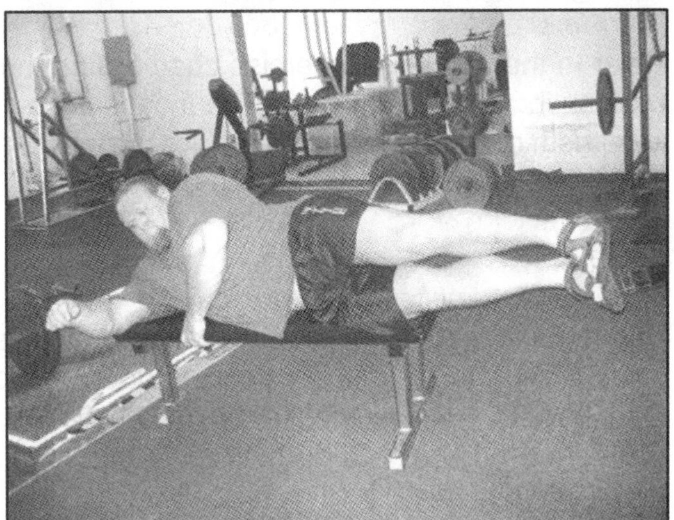
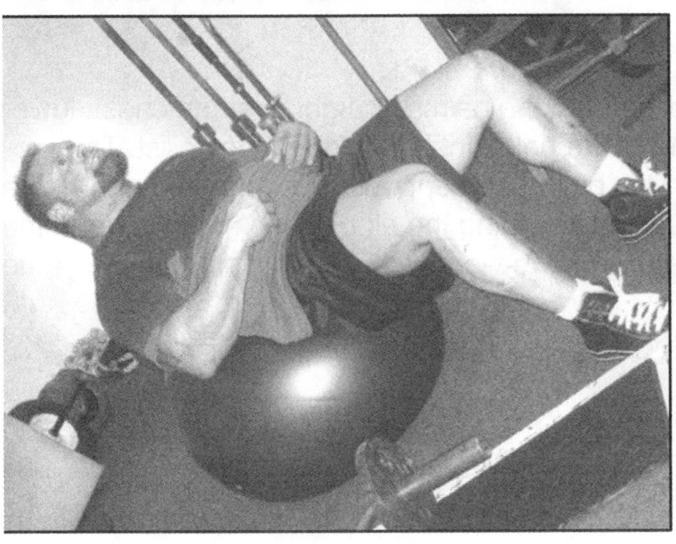
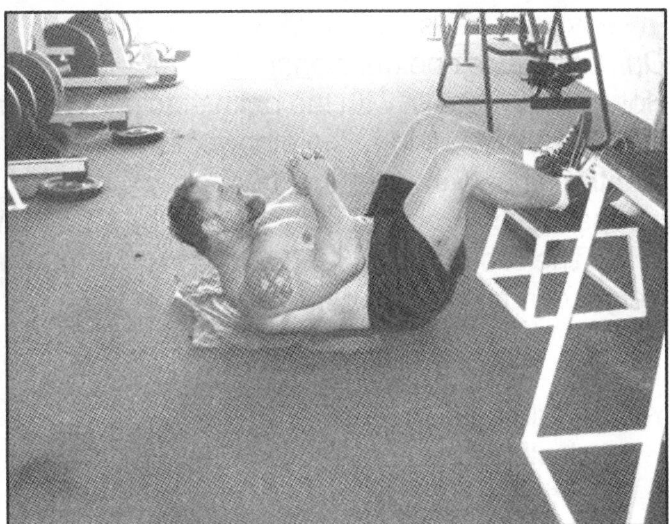

2. Spread eagle sit-ups are done using a wide foot stance such as holding the feet under the bars of the sumo based power rack.
3. Try doing sit-ups with different bench angels. For example, perform them while hanging from your feet in a chin-up bar.
4. Do sit-ups with added weight or bands for extra resistance.
5. Use the static method; stay in the position for 3–5 seconds.
6. The Russian twist is a great variation. While holding the abs in a static position, extend your arms while holding a plate and rotate from one side to the other.

Triceps exercises

Everyone thinks that a close grip bench will raise a contest bench press. At Westside, we believe this is very true. In fact, we believe it to be true so much that we find new ways to increase the close grip bench. Here are some of our favorite triceps exercises.

Refer to the max effort exercise chart to find the pressing movements. They can be used for rep work such as a 3–5 rep max. The triceps account for most of the bench press progress. Learn to train them correctly because they are the key to a monster bench. Bench shirt or shirtless, if a lifter doesn't become stronger, his bench will never increase.

Flared arm dumbbell extensions

One method is to do extensions with the elbows pointing out to the sides. The palms are facing forward and the thumbs are pointing down. Touch the bells on the upper chest. Now, extend the dumbbells to arms' length, keeping the bells touching all the way. This builds tremendous lockout strength. Start light and do high reps, for example 15–20 to start, and increase slowly. This is a tough one but very effective.

Dumbbell triceps extensions

Hold the dumbbells with the palms facing each other. With the palms straight over the chest, lower the bells by bending at the elbows. Lower one end of the bells until they touch the chest. Then rotate the elbows upward and back over the head. This builds tremendous tension at the part of the triceps that connects at the inside of the elbow. Without dropping the elbows too much, extend the bells. The rep range is 6–12 and about 60 total reps seem to work well. Multiple sets on the same weight can be executed, or work up on each set.

You can do these in several ways:

- incline
- decline
- lying on the floor
- flat bench
- standing
- mini-band behind the back for extra resistance

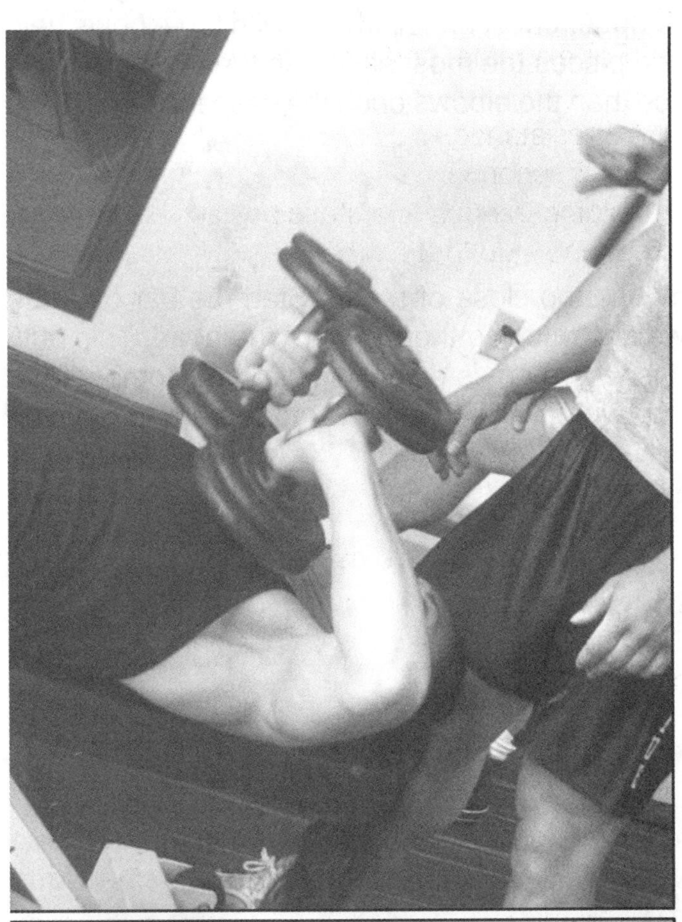

Exercises with bands

- Choke a band on top of the power rack and do band push-downs for high reps.
- Do triceps extensions with the band behind the head.
- Loop a band over the lat bar and do push-downs.

JM press

Another exercise that is popular is the JM press. It is done with a close grip, lowering the bar in a straight line down toward the upper chest and stopping about six inches above the chest. The elbows are at a 45-degress angle from the body, thereby taking the delts out of the lift and leaving the triceps to do most of the work. I refer to these as JM presses in honor of JM Blakley, who first demonstrated them for us. He is very dedicated to powerlifting and has traveled all over the United States and

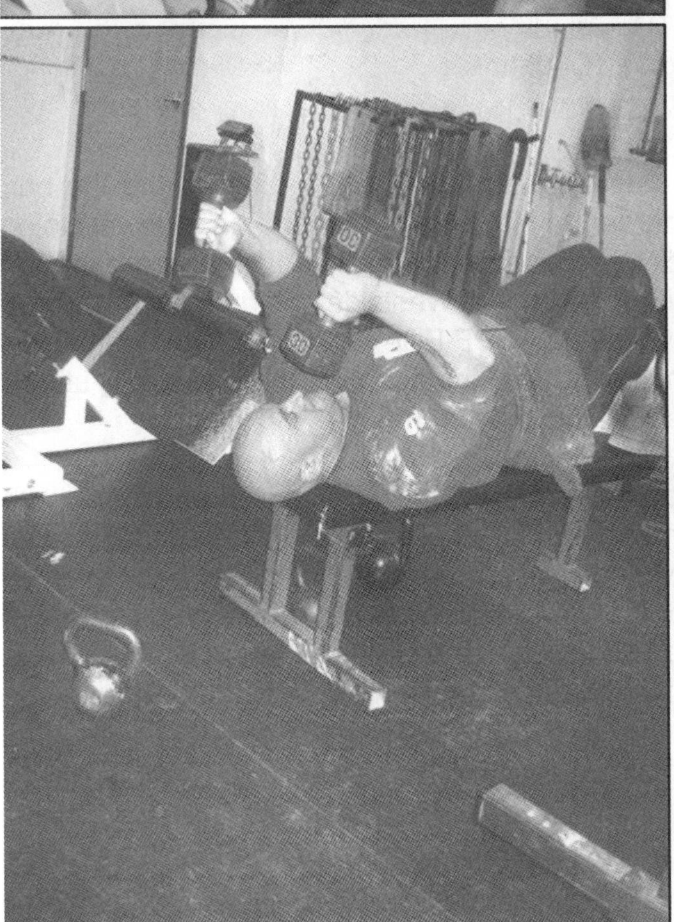

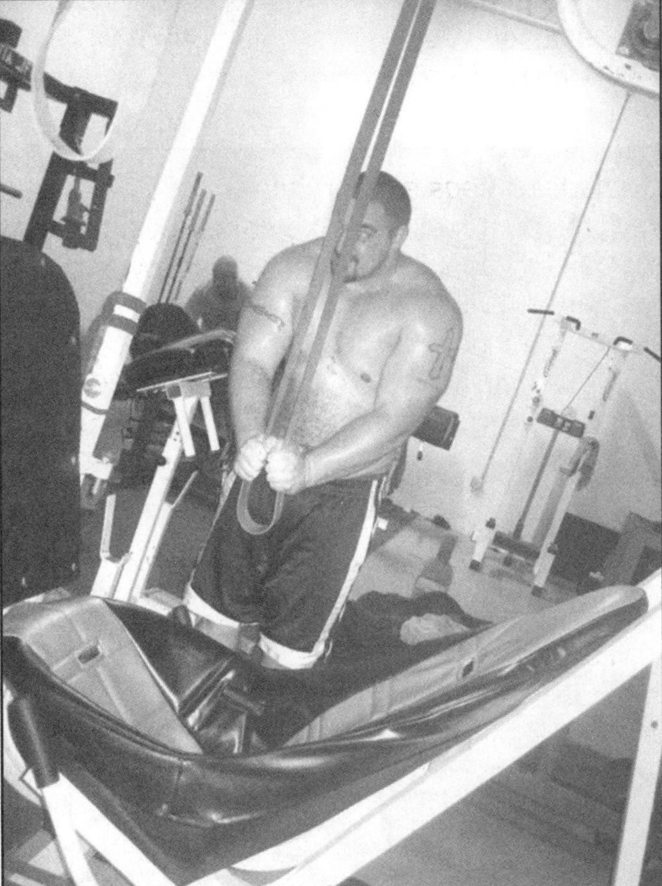

overseas to compete. I'm honored that he represents us with such passion and dignity. Use a close grip and lower the bar straight down over the upper chest or collarbone with the elbows held in a normal position. This reduces the delt work and places the most stress on the triceps. This is accomplished by having the hands closer to the face than the elbows once the descent starts. Stop the bar at your worst possible leverage point.

Straight bar triceps extensions

Remember to hold in the elbows tightly, and don't use too close of a grip. Start the bar over the lower chest. Lower it in an arch, raising the elbows and pushing them toward the head. This puts the most of the work around the elbows, and that is where one's extension strength comes from. This is strength building, not bodybuilding. Work up with five rep sets. We don't want to develop the lateral head of triceps.

There are several variations of this exercise:

- incline
- decline
- lying on the floor
- flat bench
- use mini-bands
- implement chains

For barbell extensions, the bar can be lowered to the:

- forehead
- nose
- chin
- throat

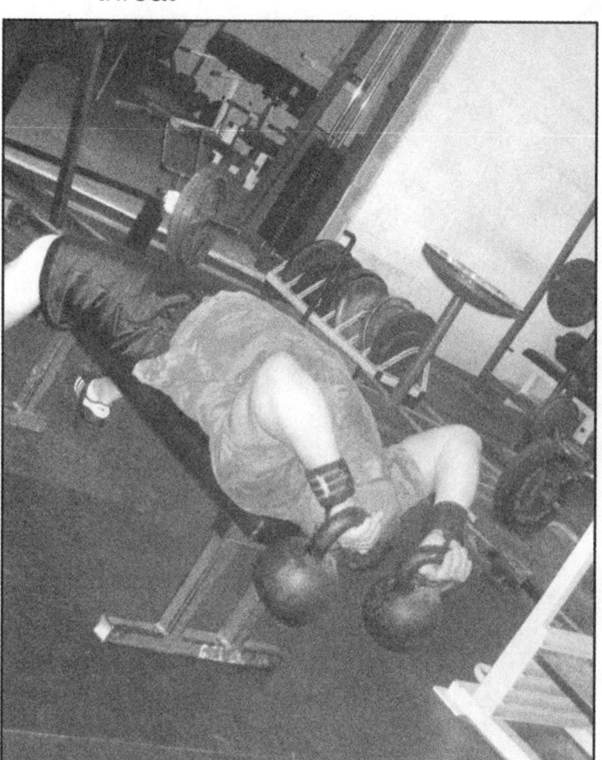

The closer to the throat that a lifter lowers the bar, the harder he hits the area around his elbows. Doing special exercises like the ones listed here has kept our lifters healthy at Westside and greatly contributed to my totaling USPF Elite for a span of over 24 years even after several injuries. Like me, there may still be hope for anyone who tries.

I hope you can see how all this works together with our rack pulls, band pulls, and all the special squats that we do. There are a vast number of back exercises for the upper and lower back that complement the three power lifts. One of the above exercises could be the difference between success and failure.

PLYOMETRICS AND POWERLIFTING

Plyometrics were developed by Yuri Verkhoshansky in 1958 after he watched a triple jumper train. He was astonished by the energetic rebounding after each landing in the triple jump. That energetic response was the basis of plyometrics. Plyometrics have proven vital in the training of explosive as well as absolute strength.

Yuri Verkhoshansky is referred to as the father of plyometrics. His work on shock training is well-documented from the early 1970s. Exercises consisted of depth jumps, plyometrics, bounding, and medicine ball work, leading to a few special devices. What is shock training? It's a system of impulsive actions of the shortest duration of time, beginning at the end of an eccentric phase and the beginning of the concentric or overcoming phase. It is a process of a fast stretch followed by a voluntary action.

At near Earth, the speed of gravity is 9.8 meters per second. When an athlete drops off a box to the floor then immediately rebounds, the energy is kinetic energy. This kinetic energy is transferred into the soft tissue and connective tissue of the body. One should be able to squat two times his bodyweight before attempting to use plyometrics. A 300 lb man may not safely land from a high altitude drop of the same magnitude as a 150 lb man. Why? It's dangerous. Kinetic energy increases when mass or velocity is increased: KE = / mv. From this equation, it is evident that increasing the velocity of an object has a greater effect on the kinetic energy than increasing the mass of an object. As velocity increases, the kinetic energy becomes exponentially greater.

Velocity can be increased through the use of bands. If an athlete merely drops off a box and lands on a surface, he is moving at 9.8 meters/second. The kinetic energy is proportional to his mass and speed. Two different masses fall at the same speed, but a larger mass has more force upon landing and an even greater force when acceleration is added by attaching bands with a great amount of tension at both the top and bottom of the landing.

Newton's second law states that force = mass x acceleration. We conducted a study at Westside to measure the effect of bands. We found that when box squatting with weight only, the eccentric phase was approximately 1.6 seconds with 550 lbs on the bar. However, when using a large amount of bands and a small amount of weight, the eccentric phase was 0.52 seconds, three times faster. Here, a virtual force occurs (i.e. a force that is present but not recognized).

For example, a certain thickness of ice can support a 50 lb ball without breaking. If the ball is dropped from a distance, moving at 9.8 meters/second, it breaks the ice on landing. Although it still weighs the same, it had acceleration in the second case. This is the case when squatting with bands. When we land on the box, a virtual force occurs due to acceleration.

When power development is discussed in the United States, the Olympic lifts come to mind. However, jumping and plyometrics are used in Europe where they are much more sophisticated in their training methods. The greatest amount of power is developed with lighter loads. I recommend that everyone, except for the lightest lifters (165 lbs and below), only jump on boxes for explosive power. First, if a lifter jumps, he must avoid detraining by doing small loads of jumping, first to condition himself for more directed work toward improving his sport. He must choose the right amount of jumps per week and per month leading into

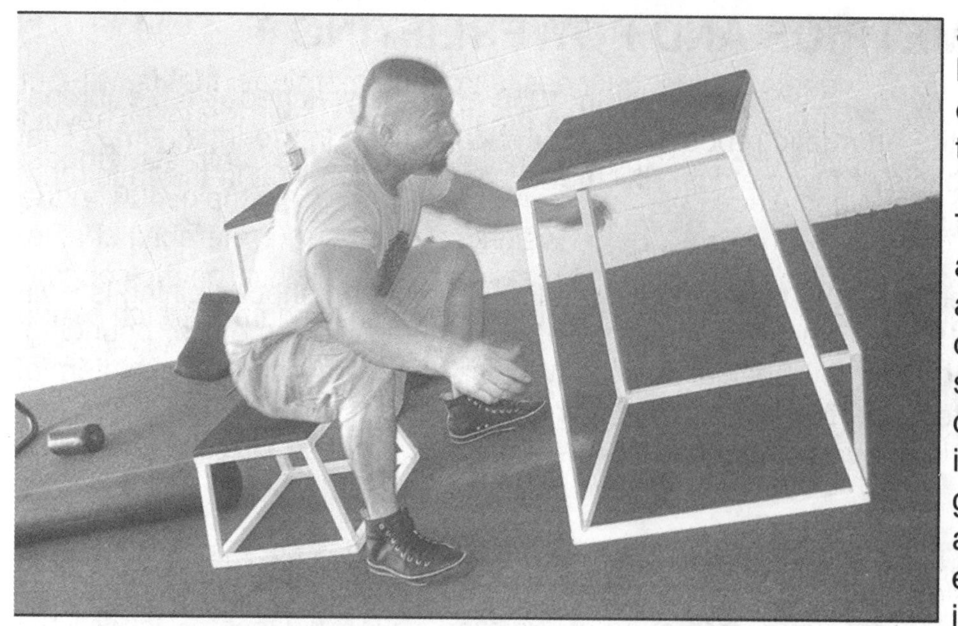

a yearly plan. Most importantly, he must choose a jumping exercise that is specific to his training.

There is no eccentric phase in a depth jump. By definition, in an eccentric action, the muscle must be active during the stretching phase. The energy created by the body dropping is gravitational potential energy. When the body lands on a surface, it becomes kinetic energy, which is transferred in the body as a stretch reflex. It is essential that explosive strength play a large role in training because it isn't only a means of developing absolute strength but also a method of raising physical fitness that is directed toward solving a specific-sports task. Of course, many sports combine jumping as part of the sport itself such as in ball games and gymnastics. Here, jumping, or plyometrics, aids greatly in raising GPP. In sports like powerlifting, explosive strength can be developed with the reactive or contrast method, which includes the use of weight releasers, bands, or chains or by special means such as: jumping onto a box of a designated height or standard plyometrics, which refers to depth jumps, altitude jumps, or bounding drills on one foot or both. The reason for including these exercises is to develop powerful legs and hips.

It is important to direct a series of work to closely duplicate a specific sport, which in our case is the squat, deadlift, and bench. Two types of training methods are used to develop explosive strength. The first is the use of a barbell with special attachments such as: bands, chains, weight releasers, or a combination of all three. The second method involves jumping exercises. Jumping exercises and/or plyometrics cause the fastest rate of explosive strength because as resistance is lessened, the motion time becomes shorter.

This is caused by a sudden eccentric stretch of the muscles and connective tissue preceding a voluntary effort. Of course, the faster the eccentric phase, the faster the concentric phase through an increase in kinetic energy. How can this be accomplished with a barbell? Explosive strength can be developed by using moderate resistance with maximum speed. This is the dynamic method. Two simple training methods to accompany the dynamic method are the box squat for squatting and pulling strength and the floor press with dumbbells or a barbell. For both exercises, after the eccentric phase, many of the muscles are in a relaxed state.

This is followed by any explosive concentric motion. This increases the rate of force development (RFD). We also find that maximum concentric work also increases the RFD. With the use of extremely heavy weights, bar velocity may be slow, but nevertheless, overcoming a large load dynamically causes a fast RFD.

The Practice of Plyometrics at Westside

At Westside, we do quite a lot of concentric squats, benches, and good mornings, that is, without an eccentric phase. I believe this would help weight lifters greatly in the United States. They lift their weights fast enough but can't move world class poundage. Let's look at the contrast methods. We load a barbell with 80% of a 1RM and place 20% on weight releasers. For example, 400 on the bar at the top equals 320 lbs of bar weight and 80 lbs on weight releasers or (preferably) chains. After the eccentric phase, the 20% is released from the bar making the load lighter on the concentric phase and building explosive strength. A more advanced method is to use jump-stretch bands on the bar, using a moderate amount of bands to increase the lowering phase. This added acceleration downward increases kinetic energy. A light amount of bands plus a light weight (40–60% of a 1RM) causes an over-speed eccentric phase and accommodates resistance in both the yielding and the overcoming phases.

A third method is box squatting. Always use a box when doing dynamic day squats. Learn to box squat properly (i.e. the Westside way). Box squatting allows a lifter to overcome a load concentrically after a static phase where some muscle groups are relaxed. This produces a higher RFD than all other types of squatting. Note to track and field trainers: At top sprint speed, 5–6 times bodyweight is being imposed on the runner, many times causing stress fractures. At no time have I seen stress fractures from box squatting, nor is it possible to use 5–6 times body weight.

A fourth method is to attach two sets of bands to the bar. After performing the first rep, re-track the bar. Have your training partners remove a set of bands and immediately do a second rep. One more method is the lightened method. Hook strong bands in a power rack or Monolift at the top. Next, place a loaded bar in the bands. It should be lightened by 20% of the max at the bottom. For example, a 750 lb squatter would first load the bar to 150 and then add weight. Train with 50–60% of the 1RM, representing the weight at completion, for explosive strength. A 750 squatter would use 375–450 for 10 sets of two reps with short rest intervals (no more than 60 seconds). The lightened method works well for floor press as well as regular benching, power cleans, high pulls, and push press or jerk in front or behind the neck with a barbell or dumbbells.

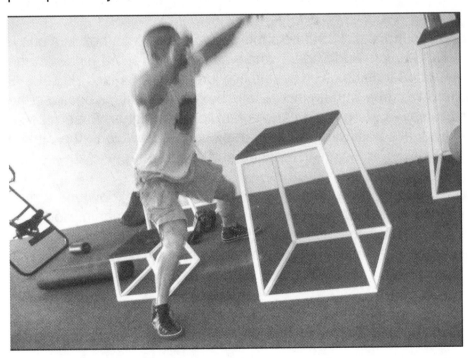

It is advantageous to use bands for the over-speed eccentric phase. For upper body explosive strength, use jump-stretch bands to enhance the eccentric phase during ballistic benching. Lower the bar as fast as possible and catch it before it touches the chest. Reverse to the concentric phase as fast as possible.

How can explosive strength be trained in the deadlift? Use the lightened method. Attach bands at the top of the rack to reduce 135 lbs to zero at the start. Next, stand on a platform that does not permit the plates to hit the floor. Take the bar off a set of pins and lower until the bar is nine inches off the floor.

Reverse and pull explosively to completion. This works much like a hang clean and serves the same purpose. By using the lightened method, a lifter can get an explosive start. It works great for both explosive and absolute strength. This brings me to a question that I was asked recently at a seminar—why is the box squat superior to the power clean? It's simple. The box squat has an eccentric phase while a power clean does not. The eccentric phase utilizes the property of kinetic energy adding to the stretch reflex. Most lifters can hang clean more than an actual power clean for the same reason. Remember, the squat weight can easily exceed clean weights and is more beneficial when done with the same speed. Absolute explosive power causes a much greater increase in power with respect to time by nature of a lighter load, most often bodyweight i.e. (jumping).

At Westside Barbell, we use the dynamic method throughout the year. Its purpose is not to build maximal strength but to improve the rate of force development and explosive strength. Of course, the lighter the load is, the faster the rate of force development.

Start by doing basic jumps. Drop down and flex quickly to start a stretch reflex. Jump on boxes of different heights. We like to have two jumping days per week: moderate jumps on Wednesday (no less than 12 and no more than 24 jumps at about 70% of the height of the box used on Sunday) and maximum jump day. For example, if a lifter's max jumps are on a 30-inch box, use a 21-inch box on the light jump day. For those who use a 40-inch box, the light day would call for a 28-inch box.

Coming from a box squat only background, John Stafford's top day was a 44-inch box at a bodyweight of 285. A friend and former Olympian, Jud Logan, who was the U.S. record holder in the hammer, normally worked on a 44- or 48-inch box. His best is five jumps on a 54-inch box at 285 body weight. His increase in the throws came with an increase in box height. This is because the greater speed with which a person leaves the ground causes him to jump higher. First, muscular force becomes equal to an individual's bodyweight. When it exceeds bodyweight, the athlete jumps upward and accelerates until maximum height is reached and speed returns to zero.

If a person is extremely slow to start a load, here is a drill that works well. Kneel down on a gym mat with the hips relaxed. Then jump to the feet. When this is mastered this, kneel again. However, this time place a bar on the back and do the same. Next, kneel down with the bar held across the lap and jump into a power clean. For the last stage, kneel down and jump into a power snatch. This greatly increases reactive time.

For specializing in pulling or squatting, my favorite method of jumping is done like this. Squat down onto a low box about 10-inches high. Relax and then jump onto a box about 20-inches high. After a warm up, hold weight or use a weight vest. I have never had strong front legs, but I have seen amazing results with this exercise even at 55-years-old. Eighteen jumps are adequate for a great workout.

Jud Logan advised me to do the heavy jumping on Sunday, the day before max effort day for the squat and deadlift, to eliminate delayed onset of muscle soreness (DOMS). This has paid off for me. After all, Jud gained his knowledge from the former East Germans.

Remember these points for jumping:

- Get in shape to jump
- Specialize
- Plan your jump loads
- Land on the middle of the box
- Keep all reps at maximal velocity

In the late 1960s, isometrics were used not only by the Soviets but also here in the United States by the York Barbell team. They were very effective but were overused because they didn't mix in other types of resistance. Plyometrics are overused and misunderstood in most cases. They should be just a small part of training for explosive strength.

Most children jump rope, a simple form of plyometrics. Yes, it is very important to develop power quickly, but it is also important to maintain power for sports such as football, wrestling, and some running events. All ball players run quickly and slowly and have quick changes in direction. This is very taxing on the central nervous system. If an athlete wants to become more explosive, he must raise maximum strength.

At Westside, it is common to see Chester Stafford jump onto a 35-inch box with a pair of 70 lb dumbbells at a body weight of 290, or Andre Henry at 460 jump onto a 20-inch box wearing an 160 lb weight vest. Neither man had a previous plyometric background. Phil Harrington, the world record holder in the squat at 900 at a body weight of 181, can also jump onto a 50 inch box. As his squat increased, so did his box jump. We have a thrower who trains with us occasionally. He can do a kneeling jump squat with 255.

When Jud Logan, the Olympic hammer thrower, failed to increase, he employed box jumps to push his throws to new lengths. He had a 440 power clean and a back squat of about 770. His box jump was an incredible 55 inches at 285 body weight. Jud was already strong and used box jumps for quickness, increasing his throws just like Westside uses the jumps to increase our squat and deadlift.

In the book *Explosive Power and Jumping Ability* for All Sports by T. Starzynski and H. Sozanski, Olympic lifting is never discussed. Starzinski coached two Olympic gold medalists, and Sozanski is a coach and professor, specializing in problems of training for jumping ability. Seated barbell presses off the floor are illustrated in their book.

There are much better exercises than the standard Olympic lifts. Here are some examples:

- Kneeling squats (after kneeling down with the heels touching the glutes, jump into a full squat)
- Kneeling power cleans (the next progression is the kneeling power snatch)
- Kneeling split snatch and kneeling power snatch
- Straight leg power clean and snatch and clean
- Power snatch while sitting with the bar across the legs

We concentrate on box squatting and use the contract and reactive methods. Thomas Kurz stated in The Science of Sports Training that to develop explosive strength, explosive efforts can be used such as: jumps, shot put, or jerking dumbbells or a barbell. "But it is easiest and safest to increase it by increasing maximal strength."

Wide stance squat works the quads to the same degree as a close stance squat but with the bonus of using more hip, glute, and hamstring muscles. Anyone who tries to squat as much as possible soon learns that a wide stance produces greater results. This was proven at a test at Ball State University. Did you know almost all college and high school football teams do power cleans and power snatches, yet they are not used in the NFL combines?

Did you know that there is a deceleration phase when lifting barbells? For this reason, you must use jump-stretch bands or chains. They accommodate resistance. When joint angles become more favorable such as at lockout, you can lift considerably more weight. With barbell weight,

the bar can be too heavy at the start to generate sufficient acceleration to complete the lift. The bar can also be too light, and as it nears completion, it slows down causing a deceleration. The bands also can be used as a contrast method. As the bar descends, the band tension decreases. As one rises concentrically, the bands increase the load, causing a contrasting load difference. The contrast and reactive methods must be used for the development of speed-strength and explosive power.

Explosive Leg Strength

When most people look at Westside training protocols, they automatically think of powerlifting. The truth is the Westside system is used in track and field and in football at all levels. I am very proud to have a picture of Johnny Parker of the Patriots and Kent Johnston of the Packers on the Super Bowl field when they played each other in 1997. They both had spent a week at Westside, learning to implement some of our methods in their programs. Johnny Parker is now with the 49ers and recently spent another week with the Westside guys.
Five major rugby teams from Europe have visited us and have had great results. Professional boxers, MMA fighters, wrestlers, and others have used our system. Why? If nothing else, it was to produce stronger and more explosive leg strength.

Absolute strength controls all strength gains. An analysis of Hill's equation shows that the speed of movement is dependent on absolute muscular strength: $v = Ft/m$. This can be found in *Fundamentals of Special Strength—Training in Sport* (Verkhoshansky 1986). Thomas Kurz in *Science of Sports Training* reported many ways to become more explosive, but the simplest is to increase absolute strength.

A lifter must constantly raise his work capacity. This is a must for jumping and squatting. Bompa (1996) states it can take four years to perform high-intensity plyometrics. Many books talk about methods and theories but not results. I love to read those books, too, but more importantly, I love increasing results.

How does someone build explosive leg strength? This can be accomplished through the reactive method, jumping off hard and soft surfaces, over-speed eccentrics, box squatting (which causes a virtual force effect), and accommodating resistance. There are two major components of explosive power—a fast rate of force development and increasing velocity. This applies to light objects such as: a shot put or a heavy object like a max deadlift. Common sense and science tell us that speed of movement is controlled by the amount of external resistance used. Light weights look fast, but can light weight alone move a 320 lb lineman backward? No. Lifting light weight always produces a deceleration phase.

We have extremely strong squatters at Westside: 1141 at SHW, 1118 at 275, 1025 at 220, 905 at 181, and 575 by a female at 148. The latter four are world records. We are also very explosive: 50-inch box jumps, a box jump of 35 inches holding a pair of 70 lb dumbbells at 290, and a jump from a kneeling position to the feet with 255 lbs on the back at a bodyweight of 255. How is this done? The dynamic method is essential. This does not increase maximal strength but will increase the rate of force development and explosive strength. Here, box squatting is used for all squats. The box makes it possible to break the eccentric/concentric chain. The box height is just below parallel, and the interval method is used, and the rest between sets is 45–75 seconds. A three-week pendulum wave is used.

The percents used are 75, 80, and 85% of a max box squat record. Then, we wave back to 75% in the fourth week. As noted in Managing the Training of Weightlifters (Laputin and Oleshko), almost 50% of all lifts are at this percent for the snatch and clean/jerk and, for us, the squat. To accommodate resistance, jump-stretch bands must be attached to the bar. A large load of bands eliminate bar deceleration. They also increase the speed in the eccentric phase. An increase in velocity has an exponential effect on kinetic energy.

We conducted a test on Matt Smith, a SHW who at the time had a 930 squat. Matt box squatted 550, consisting of all barbell weight in roughly 0.9 seconds both eccentrically and concentrically. Then, jump-stretch bands were attached to the bar in addition to the weight. The realized weight was 750 lbs at the top and 550 on the box. Because the bands pull the bar downward, the eccentric phase decreased to 0.5 seconds. The concentric phase was the same—0.5 seconds. How did Matt do this with the added 200 lbs of band tension? Over-speed eccentrics. Matt has now squatted an official 1141 lbs. How's that for results?

Not only did the bands increase kinetic energy, but the actual collision that occurred when contacting the box also produced kinetic energy. The same process happens when a sprinter comes in contact with the track at full speed.

Speed-Strength. For speed-strength work, 75% of the total load should be from bands and 25% from weight. The concentric speed should be 1.0–1.3 meters/second. This works regardless of strength level.

Strength-Speed. For strength-speed, the ratio of weight to band tension is 50/50. The bar speed will be about 0.4–0.5 meters/second. After the bands are removed is where one becomes incredibly powerful. Using a large amount of bands creates an over-speed eccentric phase, causing tremendous reversal strength. Note: Band strength must be great at the bottom of the lift.

To become more explosive, an individual must constantly become stronger. This is exemplified by the famous weight lifter, Naim Suleymanoglu. His best clean/jerk was about 407 in comparison to his front squat of 518. Weight lifters are very explosive. However, to become more explosive, Naim became very strong, having a surplus of 20% in the front squat to his clean/jerk.

Another example is the throwing events. The object being thrown is constant in weight, yet the thrower is always trying to become faster and stronger. My friend, Jud Logan, a four-time Olympian in the hammer throw, was very strong and very explosive. His stats were as follows:

478 raw bench, 770 squat, 550 x 5 and 600 x 1 in the front squat, and 440 power clean. Like myself, in the 1980s, his top strength grew, but his throws stagnated. Some of his East German friends suggested he push his box jumps up. As he improved to five jumps on a 52-inch box and a single jump on a 56-inch box at about 275 body weight, his throws began increasing. I experienced the same type of progress after I started to use the dynamic method in 1983.

Not only does concentric speed have to be increased but so does the eccentric phase, which is the most important, as has already been discussed. Speed has to do with external resistance. That may be why Olympic lifts are popular for building explosive strength. If an athlete does jumping, Olympic lifts are not needed. Many coaches argue with me, but I've done it their way. They haven't tried my way. At a Beat training center in Cincinatti, Ohio, Matt Weiderman trained James Taylor, a professional football player, to jump onto a 59-inch box at 6' 2" and 205. Taylor also ran a 4.33 40-yard, and his best box squat was 550, and he moved 315 at 0.8 meters/second.

John Harper can jump on a 51-inch box at 270, and he is ranked eleventh nationally in the discus. One end of the spectrum is moving very heavy weights very slowly. The other end is to move the body as quickly as possible. How? Jumping! A 42-inch box jump is the minimum height to reach an adequate amount of explosive power. We use the optimal number of jumps based on a maximum jump.

We use the formula as presented in Prilepin's lift table. For example, if an individual's best jump is 40 inches, a 75% jump would be 30 inches, 80% 32 inches, and 85% 34 inches. When doing jumps in the 80% range, do 15 jumps per workout. This also holds for jumping with dumbbells, ankle weights, or a weighted vest, or a combination of any of the above.
At Westside, we do many squats and jumps off of soft surfaces. This causes the muscles to do more of the work and doesn't limit it to the ligaments and tendons. In two out of three workouts, we step down off the box onto other boxes. On the third workout and the highest box, we do a depth jump down onto a soft gym mat. We don't do an immediate jump upon landing; we just stick it with legs slightly bent landing on the balls of the feet.

Our goal is to jump as high as possible, and therefore, squat as much as possible. We do it the same way—off a box. We duplicate the same procedure as box squatting. Before jumping onto a box, we first sit on a box, relax, and then jump, producing a much greater effort. The forces that produce movement are external, internal, and reactive strengths. This was established by Bernstein (Verkhoshansky 1986). When lowering onto a box, a greater amount of kinetic energy is expressed because mass as well as speed contribute to kinetic energy. Landing on the biggest part of the lower body yields an increase in kinetic energy. In addition, by lifting the feet and slamming them on the floor, an over-speed eccentric phase occurs. This combination effectively increases jumping power. I have had veteran NFL linemen long jump their best in 1–2 sessions.

The stretch (eccentric) and shortening (concentric) phases cause reversible muscular action. If a lifter does very heavy slow squats with the aid of over-speed eccentrics by using bands with weight and move the fastest with no resistance (box jumps), the sky's the limit. Remember, explosive strength is somewhere between strength and speed. By using these two elements, desired results can be reached.

Using the Virtual Force Swing

When doing pure plyometrics such as dropping from a prescribed height, the speed of descent is about 9.8 meters/second or the speed of gravity near earth. With depth jumps, there is an immediate rebound, causing a powerful stretch reflex produced from the kinetic energy of the dropping phase.

We do not use depth drops. Rather, we implement a swing. It is much like the one in Figure 6.12 in the book Zatsiorsky's Science and Practice of Strength Training. That swing can be changed by increasing the mass and range of motion. Our virtual force swing does the same thing. In addition, we can adjust the amount of speed desired. It is designed to convert potential energy into kinetic energy. We know through physics that increasing the mass is not as effective as increasing the velocity in order to increase kinetic energy.

When inanimate objects such as pool balls collide, no kinetic energy is lost. This reaction is referred to as perfectly elastic. However, in humans, it is somewhat different because of the inhibition of myotactic reflex receptors. Mechanical efficiency (ME) has been studied for years. In studies by Margaria (1968), Kaneko (1984), and Acra and Komi (1986), they show that the velocity of shortening or stretching influences the value of ME. It is also known that the stretch- shortening cycle causes very different loading conditions with different ME (Strength and Power in Sport by Komi). Having said this, it is easy to see why the virtual force swing (patent pending 2004) is so effective.

Potential energy of the tendons and soft muscle tissue can be released two ways. If it is done slowly, the energy is released slowly. If it's done quickly with a short amortization phase, it produces a high level of power. Just imagine the advantage of a swing where it is possible to adjust mass and velocity.

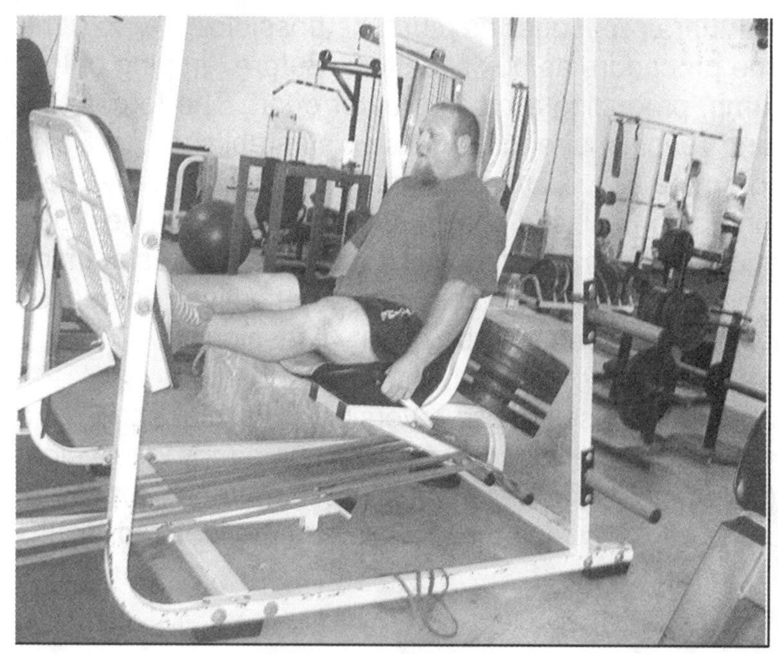

Much is known about the eccentric phase. It causes most muscular soreness or delayed onset muscular soreness. This soreness can reduce dynamic strength and damage the myofibrils and connective tissue (Friden 1983). Eccentric work can generate much higher forces due to the tension generating capacity of the connective tissue. This can create an increase in tensile strength of the tendons and other elastic components of the muscle complex (Garrett 1986). When high velocity eccentric work is introduced progressively, it enables the connective tissue to resist high impact forces that accompany high impact activities such as jumping, running, and depth jumps.

High speed or over-speed eccentrics are vital to superior training and results. When squatting or benching during the eccentric phase, a lifter invariably descends slower as the weight grows heavier. This isn't conducive to speed-strength. It's as simple as this—if lowering a barbell slowly is right then plyometrics are wrong. However, we know that's not true. Remember our experiment with over- speed eccentrics, using a high percentage of band tension versus a lower percentage of bar weight? The same is true for the virtual force swing. Using a large amount of bands to increase velocity and adding weight plates to change mass produce a very positive training effect. Increasing velocity has a much greater effect 2on kinetic energy than increasing mass.

Much is known about the eccentric phase. It causes most muscular soreness or delayed onset muscular soreness. This soreness can reduce dynamic strength and damage the myofibrils and connective tissue (Friden 1983). Eccentric work can generate much higher forces due to the tension generating capacity of the connective tissue. This can create an increase in tensile strength of the tendons and other elastic components of the muscle complex (Garrett 1986). When high velocity eccentric work is introduced progressively, it enables the connective tissue to resist high impact forces that accompany high impact activities such as jumping, running, and depth jumps.

High speed or over-speed eccentrics are vital to superior training and results. When squatting or benching during the eccentric phase, a lifter invariably descends slower as the weight grows heavier. This isn't conducive to speed-strength. It's as simple as this—if lowering a barbell slowly is right then plyometrics are wrong. However, we know that's not true. Remember our experiment with over- speed eccentrics, using a high percentage of band tension versus a lower percentage of bar weight? The same is true for the virtual force swing. Using a large amount of bands to increase velocity and adding weight plates to change mass produce a very positive training effect. Increasing velocity has a much greater effect 2on kinetic energy than increasing mas

Part 4

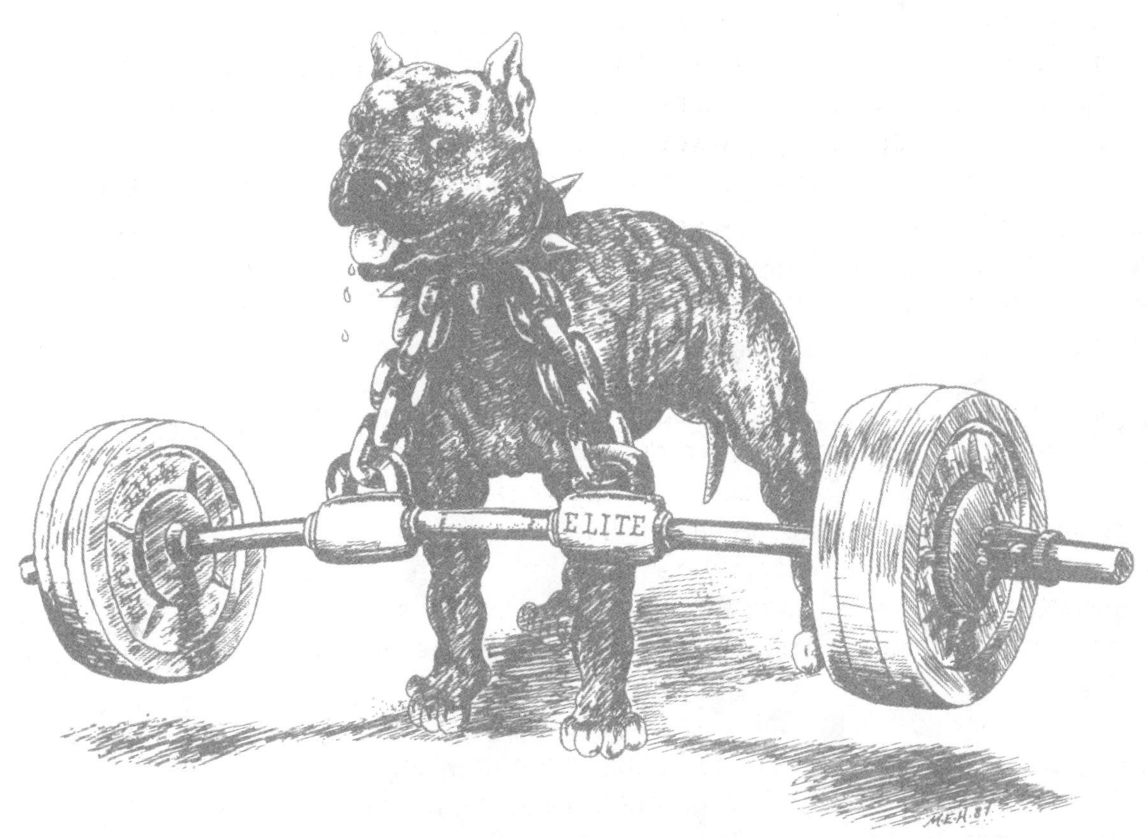

WESTSIDE BARBELL™

MISINFORMATION ON STRENGTH TRAINING

Every time I pick up a Powerlifting USA, I see some miracle squat program, calling for squatting 3–4 times a week. This is ridiculous, to say the least, and impractical for the full powerlifter. Those four times a week programs are intended for sports like track and field and rugby or sports for conditioning, not powerlifting. It would kill a bench press, and how would one do deadlifting workouts during this time? If a lifter had bad form, this type of training would make it worse. If the lifter had a muscle group that's lagging, he would have an injury before long. If you want to learn to box, why don't you box four times a week with Mike Tyson. Right, you would land in the hospital for sure.

The U.S. Approach

I am fascinated whenever my pit bull, Jackie, chases his tail. Round and round he goes, going nowhere fast until he finally realizes that he's right back where he started. I will give him credit. At least he knows he's going nowhere fast. My dog attended obedience school for four weeks, so maybe he has an advantage over his human counterparts, doctorates in exercise physiology in schools that are still teaching progressive gradual overload.

I recently read an article written by a U.S. author with a doctorate. He described a yearly plan consisting of four phases. The first phase was designed to increase muscle mass (i.e. hypertrophy) and the training base. A point that must be made is that after the end of phase one, an individual's muscle size started to diminish by 10–15% causing, in a sense, a detraining effect in as little as two weeks. The stronger the lifter, the faster this happens. For example, work lats or abs intensely for 2–3 weeks. This does not make much sense to me, and I hope it doesn't make sense to you either. Raising muscle mass or raising GPP is not only a yearly goal but a multi-year goal. It can be accomplished by incorporating a dynamic day on which just one of a variety of special strengths is refined and a maximal effort day that occurs 72 hours later using several sets of well thought out exercises for the particular muscle groups that need strengthening. This can also be accomplished by doing extra workouts during the week.

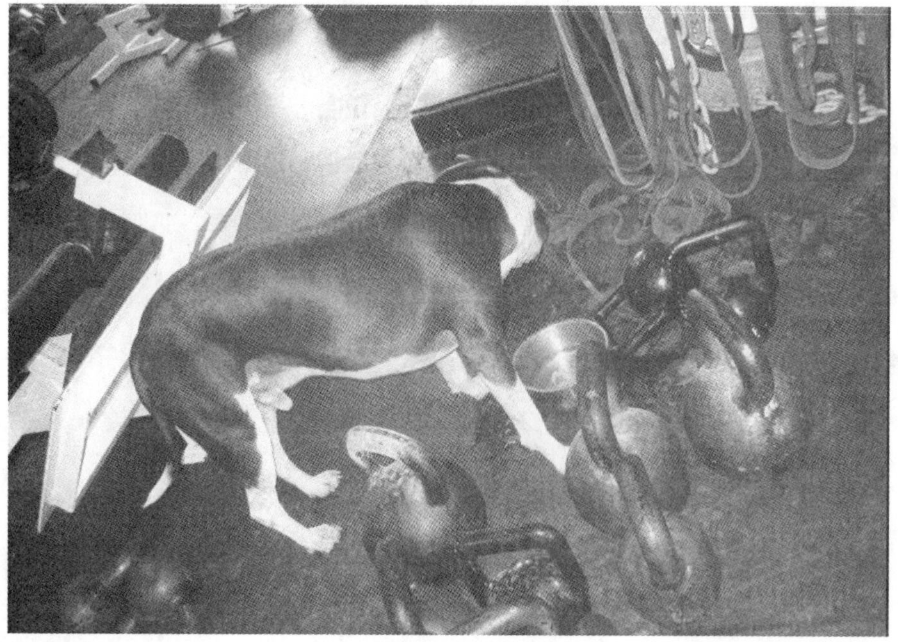

What's wrong with the progressive overload system commonly used in the United States? Recall what I said about the force-velocity curve. In the early stages of the progressive overload system, the weights are too light—too light even for velocity work. This can be illustrated by throwing a whiffle ball. No matter how hard it's thrown, it just doesn't go very far as compared to, say, a baseball. The weight of the baseball is more compatible with applying velocity and force. It's true that muscle hypertrophy is accomplished during this phase, but we are trying to achieve muscle strength, not size. As the weeks continue in the progressive overload system, the weights reach the 65–82.5% range. For a while, a lifter is achieving maximum velocity provided that he is trying to do so. However, as the weights grow heavier, the force factor comes into play. Slowly but surely, he loses that important factor—velocity. With the progressive overload system, it isn't possible to maintain max force and velocity simultaneously.

An additional negative effect occurs with progressive overload. A lifter has lowered his volume to the point that it can no longer support the work needed to produce positive results at meet time. He may be at his strongest 2–3 weeks before the meet and fall on his face more times than not when it counts. A lifter must train at 90% and above for maximum muscle recruitment, but this can only be done for a six-week period before training efficiency decreases dramatically.

For max strength, weights from 30–100% + of a one rep max are used, which causes a restricted blood supply resulting in a hard muscle contraction, thus providing a strength gain. The extra workouts that use weight or resistance less than 30% affect restoration by increasing circulation. Ten extra workouts a week is a normal load. Doing special exercises for the classical lifts increase strength and perfect form. Concentrate on only the muscle groups that aid in raising the lift or total. For example, don't squat but do special exercises for squatting such as: glute ham raises, pull-throughs, reverse hypers, or belt squats plus abdominal work. Also, do exercises for flexibility. In place of benching, do triceps extensions with a bar, dumbbells, or bands; delt raises; lats; upper lock; and external rotation work. With this method, a lifter never stops building muscle mass. Switch exercises that work the same muscles (the conjugate method). This allows one to constantly build muscle mass, GPP, and SPP. According to the article I was reading, phase two is the pre-competitive phase.

The author now states that one must raise top strength or absolute strength. During this phase, the lifter concerns himself with raising his squat, deadlift, and bench press using all major exercises, rack work, good mornings, etc.

Let's look at an alternative method—the maximal effort method. This incorporates the conjugate method, using special exercises that closely resemble the classical lifts. Examples are squatting with special devices such as: the MantaRay or cambered bar, concentric work, good mornings, or deadlifts using the contrast or reactive method. The weights are always 100% plus, depending on a lifter's level of preparedness (i.e. how close one is to top lifting form), which incidentally should never drop below 90% of his all-time records. The maximal effort method is calculated much like the Bulgarian system, meaning that he should always be doing the most possible even when far from contest time. As you can clearly see, this method allows you to lift your current max every week of the year, not just for a few weeks near one or two contests during the year.

Well, so far the doctorates from the U.S. advocate building muscle mass and then allowing it to disappear after ceasing the hypertrophy phase. This is not training but detraining. The same happens after phase two. However, the Westside method allows one to become larger, more muscular, and stronger all year long. The doctorate's classes are now learning phase three for explosive strength. This phase again lasts about six weeks, and its main goal is to increase bar speed. The weight here reaches 60–85% of a one rep max, and they add in plyometrics. Then, they move into the peaking or contest phase. Here, they recommend going from high reps, light weights or high volume, and low intensity to heavy weights and low reps, which results in lower volume but high intensity. Controlling volume and intensity is very important. When a lifter does sets with 70, 75, 80 and then 85% for doubles, it is impossible for him to understand what task is the goal. How do you determine if you are lifting with the same effectiveness at each percentage? If the weights are moving at the same max rate of acceleration, all is well. However, when the weights are raised that high, this isn't possible. Rule of thumb— train at intensities of 60%, 70%, 80%, or 90–100% +.

Prilepin's studies of more than 100 Olympic, national, and European champions showed that there is an optimal number of reps at certain percent ranges. If an individual uses one percent per workout, the task is easier to realize. Lighter weights are implemented for explosive and speed strength (60–80%) and weights of 90% or more for strength-speed. It is not advisable to train for two types of strength in one workout. It is done for multiple sets—one rep pulls, two reps for the squat, and three reps in the bench.

For speed-strength, use a pendulum wave:

- Week 1: 60%
- Week 2: 65%.
- Week 3: 70%
- Week 4: 60%
- Week 5: 65%
- Week 6: 70%

Then, drop back to 60% in week seven. This is a pendulum wave. This kind of wave is used because a lifter can't increase in speed or top strength after three weeks of increasing the weight. If he continues to increase the weight, the bar speed suffers dramatically, which must not happen. What about absolute strength? Three days separate the dynamic workout and the max effort day. This is because the major muscle groups recuperate in 72 hours. The max effort workout is performed with the conjugate method, allowing an individual to lift weights of 100% + each week. This is possible by switching exercises each week. Here are some examples.

The squat and the deadlift day:

- Week 1: ten-inch low box with the MantaRay
- Week 2: bent over good mornings
- Week 3: 12-inch low box with the safety squat bar

For the bench press:

- Week 1: 3-board press
- Week 2: floor press
- Week 3: lightened band press

There are many core exercises to choose from. For the Olympic lifter:

- Week 1: snatch grip high pulls
- Week 2: straight leg power cleans
- Week 3: cleans from above the knee

This method of training allows a lifter to work on weak areas often overlooked by doing the classical lifts. It also perfects form and coordination. This type of training also enables an individual to perform extra workouts for strength, restoration, and flexibility.

The Bodybuilding Approach—Hit or Miss?

Many readers may not realize that I am involved in the training of professional football teams, college football and basketball teams. For example, the Kansas City Jayhawks and Utah Utes are heavily influenced by our training as it relates to speed-strength. Two of the professional football teams are the Green Bay Packers and the New England Patriots. Not a bad group to be associated with, huh? I also talk to a head strength coach who has been affiliated with a winning tradition in the NFL. He told me, although he was ashamed to admit it, that he has linemen coming into the league who can't vertical jump 19 inches or squat 300 lbs. He related to me that these players are from "high intensity training" (H.I.T.) schools and that this type of weight program is making his job next to impossible.

While I was at their camp, a professional lineman told me that when he was placed on the HIT program in college, his team was the top fifth school his senior year. He thought he was strong until the combines. When he got only 12 repetitions with 225 pounds, he was embarrassed. He was picked by a professional team that utilizes our training and who has an excellent strength coach. In two years, this lineman did 17 reps with 315 lbs. He made a remark that machines and HIT were useless. This got back to his old college team, who immediately banned him for life from their weight room. Gee, what a pity.

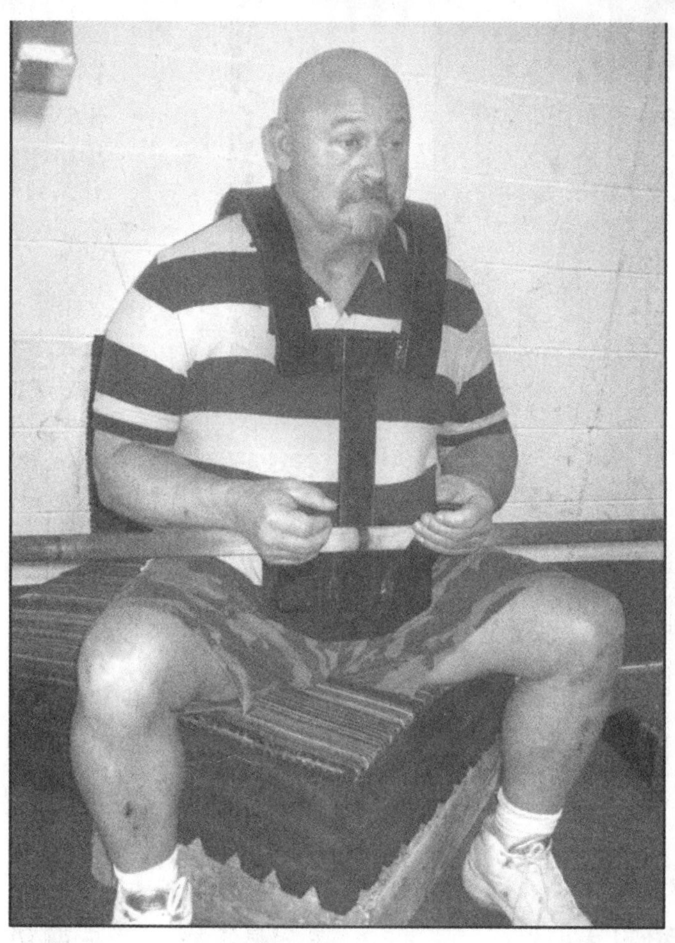

At Westside, we thought we would do some research on HIT. Dave Tate and I looked into this, I must say, misguided method. What is their viewpoint? Where was their research taken from? Why is it loved by some and despised by others?

First, let's look at the concept of intensity. Apparently, HIT views it as a feeling like a pump, a term bodybuilders made popular. Is it a scientific term? No. Is a bodybuilder quick or explosive? No. If you know a converted bodybuilder who powerlifts, he almost always lifts well under what he appears to be able to do. Why? He has trained only the muscle, not the central nervous system. That is why smaller ball players are almost always faster and many times stronger based on percent of bodyweight. Bodybuilders develop no reversal strength or starting or accelerating strength. Any sport coach will tell you that acceleration is paramount in sports.

As Prilepin suggested, in order to achieve the proper intensity, one should use the rep/ set scheme shown in the table to ensure the greatest development of speed and strength. He discovered that if seven or more reps were performed at 70%, the bar speed slowed and power decreased. The same holds true when using 80–90%. Once one goes above the rep range shown, the bar slows, which translates to less power. Doing fewer or more lifts than Prilepin suggests causes a decrease in training effect.

Along the same parameters are the findings of Dr. Tamas Ajan and Professor Lazar Baroga. They describe the zones of intensity as follows: 30–50% is low intensity for speed-oriented sports; 50–85% is medium intensity for force-oriented sports such as weightlifting; 85–95% is high intensity for weightlifting and other sports; and 100% and above is maximum and over maximum intensity for the development of absolute strength.

Most authors who have studied strength as a physical quality examine it in four forms:

- absolute
- speed
- explosive
- strength endurance

The latter, strength endurance, is basically all the HIT program can possibly build. Strength endurance is characterized by a combination of great strength and significant endurance. It is needed by athletes who must compete for a prolonged period of time (3–4 hours) without diminished work capacity. Well, HIT may increase endurance, but it does not promote great strength. In fact, it eliminates it completely by neglecting the other three elements of strength- absolute, speed, and explosive.

Dave Caster showed me an interesting paper, Strength, Power and Speed in Shot Put Training by Dr. Poprawski, director of the Sport High Performance Institute in Toronto and former coach of world shot put champion, Edward Sarul. First, Poprawski realized the importance of intensity zones as described by Prilepin and the importance of using one weight percentage per workout.

For example, weights of 50–75% are used for training speed and power. Much like our training, this training is based on a true max of, let's say, 500, 600, or 700 lbs. Poprawski realized that a shot put always weighs 16 lbs. Therefore, he found that it was best to use one weight for a particular workout and focus on increasing bar velocity rather than heavier weight to increase power. What was the key element for success? Speed, speed, and more speed.

Sarul was tested against other superior throwers, and while some could lift more weight, he was far ahead in tests of bar speed during the snatch and squats of 1–3 reps. His advantage in speed and the development of power was directly achieved by increasing bar speed while the others fell behind from lifting too slowly. What does this tell us? Fast is good and slow is second team. HIT proponents use a lot of machines; this is truly a mistake because no stability can be developed. Most machines work on the peak contraction theory. Let's look at the pec machine. If an individual loads a pec machine to the max, starting the movement requires a max effort, which is very difficult and dangerous. Yet at the finish, where the most weight can be lifted because of accommodating resistance, machines show his downfall.

More importantly, let's consider the strength curve. Take the case of two 700 lb deadlifters. A lifter may blast the weight off the floor to near lockout and then fight the last 3–4 inches. The second may have difficulty starting the bar off the floor, pick up speed, and lockout easily. What does this illustrate? In the real world of strength, these two lifters have quite different strength curves. If these same two lifters were to use a machine, only one would receive any benefit from that machine because the machine has a predetermined strength curve. That's a 50% chance the machine won't work for him. Also, a machine does not build stability. The only good thing about a facility full of machines is that the instructor could be a moron, and it won't make any difference. For some reason, HIT proponents think that explosive weight training is dangerous. One should know that explosive weight training should only be done after warming up past 25% of a one rep max. Look at the percent charts by Ajan and Baroga and then start at 30%. Don't push super light weights explosively until reaching 30%. If you're going to criticize something, you should understand it first.

Finally, I ask is anything more dangerous than football itself? HIT proponents also think that if an athlete exercises slowly, he won't become slow. Have they heard of exercise specificity? A sprinter must practice sprinting to be successful. A long distance runner must learn to conserve himself to run a long distance. If a marathon runner started to sprint at the beginning, he would run out of gas long before the end of the race. If an individual works slowly, he becomes slow, and he will be watching the fast kids play while he develops splinters in his butt. Remember that external force is directly responsible for speed. A boxer may appear very fast with eight-ounce boxing gloves, but hand him a pair of 100 lb dumbbells and he can hardly move his hands at all.

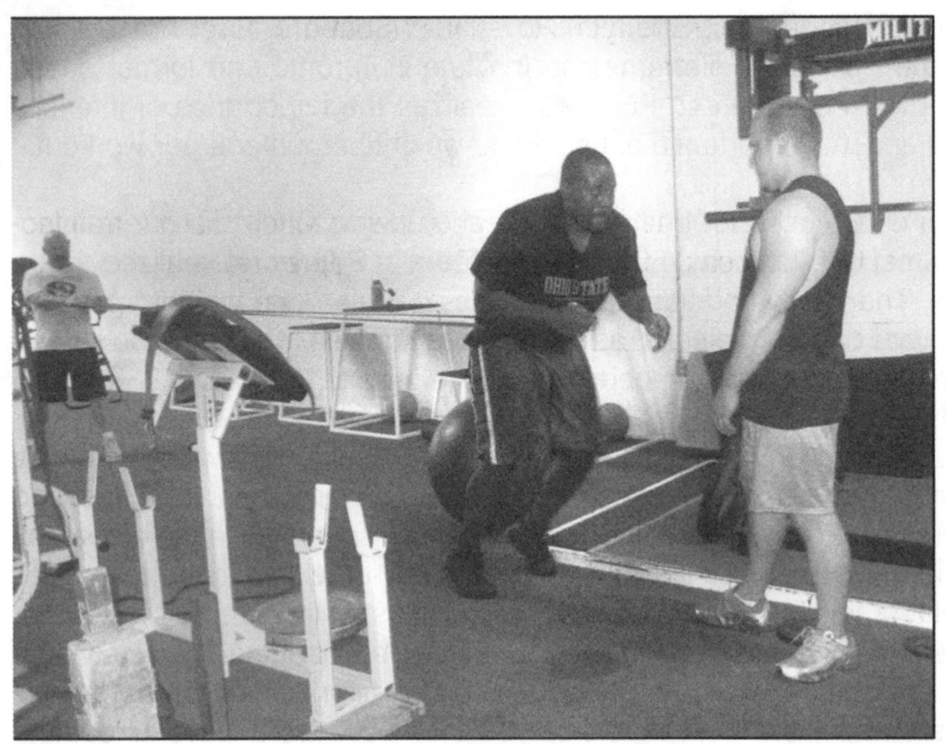

Although I am not a proponent of the Olympic lifts, they certainly have a place in weight training. However, I must say the term "quick lift" applies only to the snatch and clean and jerk when sub-maximal weights are used. With max weights, they are no quicker than any other lift. That's why we devote one workout a week to the dynamic method with weights close to 60% of a 1RM max for multiple sets of 2–3 reps with short rest periods. We duplicate almost exactly the play time and rest time of football.

HIT advises working to failure, especially in the concentric phase, and sometimes up to 10–15 seconds. They call this an isometric rep. Well, if a person was to exercise for that length of time, which is much longer than a football play, it would be of absolutely no benefit. A good friend of mine was at a football conference and watched a demonstration in the deadlift for reps. The person did 20–25 reps with 425 lbs. Wow, what an effort! But did he recover in 35 seconds, the time period the football game requires? Absolutely not!

Wouldn't it be more beneficial to exercise for 7–8 seconds and repeat a set of weights? That's how the game is played, right? A workout like that described above is fine for a two-week minicycle, but not for any longer. A professional boxer trains for a three-minute round using training intervals of three minutes and a rest time of one minute. Football should do the same. Active work should duplicate a play and rest cycle. The friend I am referring to is a coach who is a two- time all American. Using our program, he currently has over 68 men who can power clean 300 lbs or more out of 90. I give credit to the recruiters for teams who use HIT. They pick skilled people who can sometimes survive HIT, but the linemen can't survive. If you watch the Heisman Trophy winner who was on the HIT program as a college athlete and is drafted by a professional team that uses HIT, invariably he is nonproductive or injury prone.

Guys, if you want to play for pay, check out the weight facility. If there are more machines than weights and you're not in the snack room, think twice before entering. The truth is the HIT philosophy comes from companies that sell machines. Even Arthur Jones realized that doing one set to failure was a mistake and retracted his statements years ago. It was merely a ploy to run as many customers through a facility as possible. It was later popularized by Mike Mentzer, a successful bodybuilder in the late 1970s and early 1980s. His claim to fame was the one-set- to-failure system. He was, I might add, the only one to use it successfully. It's not a good idea to try to be the exception to the rule. Instead, follow the accepted methods of weight training by working on the many types of strength that are needed in a sport. Just remember what Bill Starr said—only the strong will survive.

Misinformation on Bands

Bands and chains have been around for years. The fact is most people could not use them effectively to fully utilize their true benefits. This includes both powerlifters and doctorates at major universities. Marquette University ran a study and concluded that there was no value in using bands or chains. I have listed the amount of bands needed to develop specific types of strength such as strength-speed and speed-strength. I tested only subjects who squat at least 850 lbs (20 in total). I doubt any university in the United States could match that. If one does not have an Elite group of subjects, how can a valid study be conducted?

Some studies used only 10% band weight to accommodate resistance at the top. What about the bottom tension rate? That is where the process must begin (i.e. virtual force, which is force that is in effect although not in actual fact).

Academic researchers seem concerned only with accommodating resistance or simply making the lift harder at the top. They have stated that it is useless because one is stronger at the top. If no eccentric phase is used, this would be true because of the relationship between force and posture. However, in the real world, a lifter must first lower himself to just below parallel during the eccentric phase and then rise concentrically to completion. Seldom do we miss at the bottom but rather from just above parallel to near completion. At least this is what I see in the hundreds of meets and training episodes I have witnessed. To prove this, near maximal or maximal lifts must be performed. This is why extremely strong lifters or athletes must be experimental subjects.

If colleges and universities are going to conduct studies on the effects of bands and chains, why not contact Westside Barbell and do it correctly and obtain valid results that can be passed along to grad students? We welcome any PhDs in exercise physiology to observe Westside in action. We would especially like Jeff Voleck, PhD., to witness box squatting done the correct way as taught by Westside. I also invite Rafael Escamilla, PhD., to investigate the various and correct methods for utilizing chains for the right purpose—to increase explosive strength. I will even send Westside's reactive method tape or special strength tape to any university to study, free of charge, if requested. Discover why strength athletes such as powerlifters must consider speed- strength work in order to succeed. All of the testing performed at universities made a significant mistake. They neglected to use a large amount of band tension at the bottom of the squat. Also, they didn't use a box. The tension should not be reduced completely by band shrinkage. Tension must be strong at the bottom as well.

Recommended reading

This is Louie´s favorite book list for training information. These are the most important books where Louie gets his training information and uses it successfully on his lifters with world known results:

Books That Lou Recommends

A Program of Multi-Year Training in Weightlifting by AS Medvedyev
A System of Multi-Year Training in Weightlifting by AS Medvedyev
Adaptation in Sports Training by Atko Viro
Basic Physics by Karl F. Kuhn
Beyond Stretching Russian Flexibility Breakthroughs by Pavel Tsatsouline
Circuit Training for All Sports by Manfred Scholich, PhD
European Perspectives on Exercise and Sport Psychology by Stuart J. H. Biddle
Explosive Power & Strength by Donald A. Chu, PhD
Explosive Power and Jumping Ability by Tadeusz Starzynski/Henry K Sozanski, PhD
Facts and Fallacies of Fitness by Dr. Mel Siff
Fitness and Strength Training for All Sports by Jurgen Hartmann, PhD
Fundamentals of Special Strength Training in Sports by YV Verkhoshansky
Manage the Training of Weightlifters by Nikolai Petrovich Laputin/Valentin Grigoryevich Oleshko
Periodization Theory and Methodology of Training by Tudor O. Bompa
Periodization Training for Sports by Tudor O. Bompa
Power Training for Sport by Tudor O. Bompa
Programming and Organization of Training by YV Verkhoshansky
Science and Practice of Strength Training by Vladimir Zatsiorsky
Science of Sports Training by Thomas Kurz
Secrets of Soviet Sports Fitness and Training by Michael Yessis, PhD
Serious Strength Training by Tudor O. Bompa
Soviet Training and Recovery Methods by Rick Brunner/Ben Tabachnik
Sports Conditioning and Weight Training by WM J Stone/WM A Kroll
Sports Restoration and Massage by Dr. Mel Siff/Michael Yessis, PhD
Strength and Power in Sport by PV Komi
Strength Speed and Endurance for Athletes Jurgen Hartmann, PhD
Strong Together by Walter Gain/Jurgen Hartmann, PhD
Supertraining by Dr. Mel
The Naked Warrior by Pavel Tsatsouline
The Training of the Weightlifter by RA Roman
The World Atlas of Exercises for Track and Field by Andrzej
Theory and Methodology of Training by Tudor O. Bompa
Training for Warriors by Martin Rooney
Warm-Up and Preparation for Athletes of All Sports by Zoltan TEnke/Andy Higgins
Weightlifting and Age by LS Dvorkin
Weightlifting Year Book, 1980, 83, 85, Fizkultura I Sport Publishers
Weightlifting Year Book, 1981, Fizkultura I Sport Publishers

THOUGHTS ON EQUIPMENT

Personal gear

I made the top ten in the United States in 1972 in Powerlifting News. At that time, they kept track only of the top ten, and this was without equipment. In 1973, I made a 1655 total at 181, again without gear—a 605 squat, a 380 bench, and a 670 deadlift. At the time, 1605 was Elite, but it was later adjusted to 1643. In 1980, at the YMCA Nationals, I made the top ten in the bench press with a 480, and this was done without a bench shirt. Then, with the introduction of power gear, from four-inch belts to squat and deadlift suits, and of course, the bench shirt, I totaled Elite in five weight classes through the years from the 181s to the 275s. In the 2002 rankings, my bench press was sixth at 575 in the 220 weight class. However, I experienced many setbacks before 2002. I broke my fifth lumbar vertebra in 1973 and again in 1983, and I tore my right bicep in the USPF Senior Nationals in 1979. Six months later, I was lucky and won the YMCA Nationals and pulled a 705 deadlift, which was 33 lbs more than the weight with which I tore my bicep. As luck would have it, I tore two small holes in my lower abs and sustained a partial tear of a pelvic tendon (this still bothers me today).

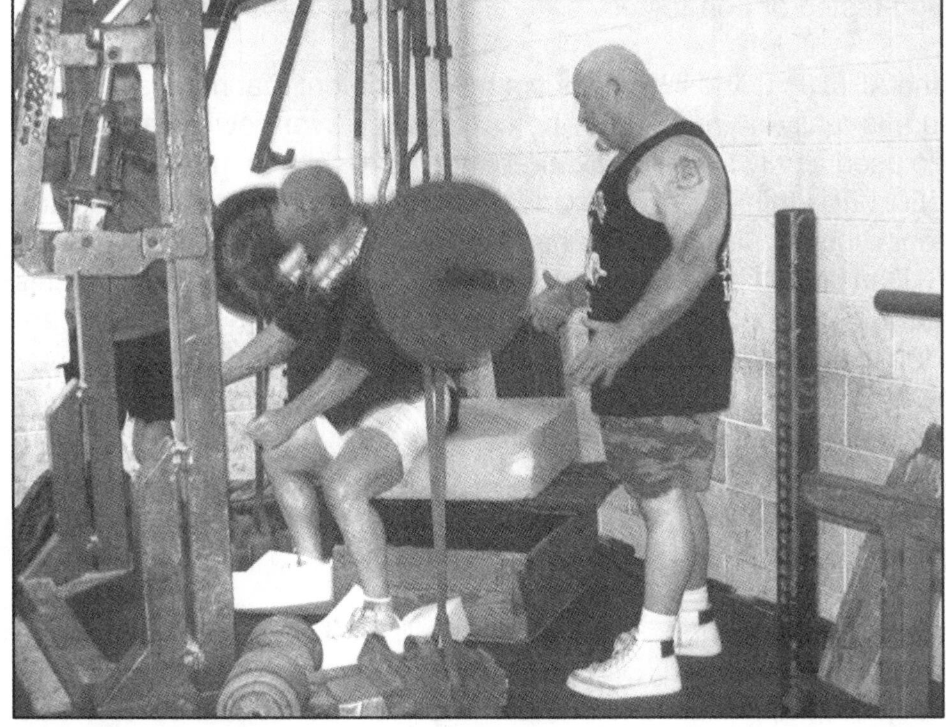

I finally made my first 2000 total in 1987 at the YMCA Nationals in Columbus. My left knee had been bothering me for about a year. I had a heavy workload for the next five years. While training for the APF Seniors in Pittsburgh, I suffered a complete patella tendon rupture of the left knee. I went in for a second minor surgery 14 weeks later and nearly died from a reaction to anesthesia. A tracheotomy was performed and chest tubes were inserted after I stopped breathing for four minutes. The chest tubes severed nerves in my ribcage, causing sever shoulder pain to this day. I was seriously thinking about giving up lifting, but I trained hard and made a 680 below parallel box squat (there were no Monolifts at the time) with no knee wraps and without the straps up on the suit. Before this, my best squat was 821 at 242.

Meanwhile, Kenny Patterson benched 728 at 22-years-old in 1995 at 275 and was ranked the best pound-for-pound bencher. But in 1997, he still had not broken that record. We were doing a bench workout, and I said, "Damn, Kenny, I'll squat 700 again before you break that bench record." He said, "Old man, you will never have 700 on you back again." Well, I can thank Kenny Patterson because he brought me out of retirement at that moment. I competed seven times in the next 11 full meets and some push/pull meets. My best bench was 530 at 242 in 1992. I broke my bench record several times, ending up with 600 lbs (a dream come true for me). I also squatted over 800 in 1997. This was important for me because no one 50 years or older had made a 600 bench. I also squatted 900 and 920 at 52-years-old and had a 2100 total. I was not pleased because, as usual, I could not put my best lifts together, which were a 920 squat, a 580 bench, and a 710 deadlift at 235. After squatting 810, I recall telling Jesse Kellum that I could do 900. He said, "Buddy, why don't you?" So, I did. He was a big help just being himself.

Chuck Vogelpohl also helped me greatly, always pushing me to the limit along with all my Westside training partners. Ambition, determination, and my powerlifting friends from around the world helped as well. But none of this could have happened if powerlifting gear had not evolved to the point where it is today. I went from no knee wraps to Ace bandages to horse wraps to the Canadian wraps such as the TP5000 wraps to today's best—Frantz, Inzer, Titan, and Crain. They also have their brand of suits and bench shirts. Choose from polyester, denim, or canvas. Each federation has its own rules so take your pick. This is the USA, and you have the right to lift in any federation that you choose whether it is drug-tested or non-tested.

At Westside we lift primarily in the APF, IPA, and WPO. It's not the equipment that makes a champion but rather one's mind. There is really no reason for the controversy over power gear. When Fred Boldt came to Westside, he used a poly shirt. It took three months for him to master a double denim. In his first meet, he did 450, but within a year, he made 540 in the same shirt. Where did the 90 lbs come from? Training. People come to Westside all the time to train and learn, and most walk out the door with an all-time PR. Don't lie, dudes. You all would love to lift more. The simple fact is a lot of lifters can't master the gear. For bench shirts, Bill Crawford has the golden hand. For canvas squat suits, Ernie Frantz is the man. At Westside, we have the greatest collection of benchers. Four men have held the all-time biggest bench in six weight classes, and I believe another will be added soon. Our lifters have evolved right along with the sport. Chuck's squat of 1025 was done in a double ply squat suit in keeping with WPO rules. The bench records were done in double ply shirts. Nothing has changed since powerlifting began. Everyone looks for an edge. That's simply sport. I remember 20 years ago some knee wraps had a rubber lining.

Bill Kazmaier had a pair of shoes that were supposed to be worth $1000. In 1979 at the North American Championships in Canada, Fred Hatfield (Dr. Squat) showed up at the equipment check with a pair of knee wraps make of jock strap waist bands. The IPF referee looked at them and said he couldn't wear them. They were twice as thick as normal wraps. Fred won the argument and proceeded to break Ron Collins's world record squat. He also had the squat rack pulled out of his way instead of walking the weight out. Was he cheating or innovative? Being a lifter, I thought he was innovative. Every lifter should take advantage of people like Dr. Squat who pave the way to bigger numbers. Is the use of squat and deadlift bars cheating? No. That's progress. When people see a boxing match, they want their man to knock out the opponent. Someone told me, "You have to have the right size fish." I think equipment is the same. Dave "Zippy" Tate said he felt that the only regulation on power gear should be for novices, for example, up to a Master total. Then, somewhat stronger suits could be used by those between Master and Elite.

Only the strongest and the bravest would use unlimited gear. That's right, I said the bravest. I have seen many lifters stop progressing because they were scared. That's right, they're scared, and they won't admit to it. They hate those who dare to break today's records. Look at what's happening today. It's embarrassing what raw lifters are lifting compared to the lifts in the early 1970s. Remember my 181 total of 1655. Jack Barnes held the top spot at 1745. At this time, Larry Pacifico was doing 1900 at 198. I saw Larry do a 530 bench at 198 in Cincinnati, and eight weeks later in Dayton, he benched 590 at 228. These lifts were done in full meets with a one and a half hour weigh in. Don't think for one minute that today's raw lifter would bench over 600 or squat in the 800s just by putting on gear. Powerlifting is years behind other sports as far as equipment is concerned, including swimming, track, football, and even bowling. However, the gear is getting better in every powerlifting federation including the IPF.

As race cars go faster, the rules call for more safety equipment to keep the drivers safe. The racing association made recommendations for a better safety belt harness after Dale Earnhardt's death. In powerlifting, when new innovations come about, we're cheating? This doesn't make sense. I don't know a single strong man who complains about better gear. It's not easy to learn how to use bench shirts and squat suits. Matt, a 275 from Ball State University, had just made a 479 bench PR but could not master his new bench shirt. During a visit to Westside, he made a 530 bench in 45 minutes with plenty to spare. His shirt is 100% legal; he just needed to learn how to use it.

I notice that the people who bad mouth the top powerlifters are invisible at power meets. I have to attend the APF Nationals, IPF Nationals, the World Cup, and the WPO semifinals and finals at the Arnold Classic not to mention the WPO Bash for Cash, and I never see these guys. I know for a fact that the great lifters at these meets would never give them a second look. After all, what have they done? Until the end of time, people will seek out a way to win. That's human nature.

Why not use what's available? Most use computers today, not an ink quill. I read a lot and suggest to you a book—A Sport's Odyssey by Dr. Judd Biasiotto (2001). It has been advertised in Powerlifting USA. Dr. Judd is opposed to modern lifting gear, and his opinion on drug use is the same. His goal was to total 1400 at 132. You can read how he used hypnosis, biofeedback, mind control, and just about everything a cybernetics lab can offer. He was a man of positive thinking. See how long his power career lasted. And, oh yes, how that quest for a 1400 total turned out. He eventually squatted 603 at an AD-FPA meet in 1989. If hypnosis works that well, give me two bottles of it. I invite Dr. Judd to Westside to see what modern lifting is like.

How to Use Bench Press Shirt

There's always a lot of talk today about the bench shirt. In the beginning, everyone welcomed it on the scene. Unfortunately, bench shirts provided only a small increase over one's raw bench record. That was the 1980s. In the late 1990s, shirts became much stronger. As the shirts got better, the bench records started to move up little by little. Working with Inzer Advance Designs, Kenny Patterson helped refine the denim shirt. They developed the radical cut shirt. The records then started going up and up. Todd Brock had a 480 bench and was stuck. After wearing an Inzer radical cut shirt, he skyrocketed to 540 in the same weight class. Then, Phil Guarino had the insight to cut the back of the shirt, making it an opened back version. What an innovation that was! I helped him warm up at the Bash for Cash, one of Kieran Kidder's meets in Daytona some years ago. After Phil warmed up, he amazed me with a 661; I knew he had a great idea. Vanessa Schwenker, a 132 lb woman, had a 260 bench. We went to a bench meet and somehow the back of her shirt tore completely. She didn't have a backup shirt and had to use the torn one. She benched 290, a PR. We felt lucky. When she got back home, she had the shirt sewn back together, but meet after meet, she never made more than 260. She eventually retired, and it wasn't until a year later that we realized it was the open backed shirt that increased her bench.

Now, we know that the open backed shirts are the best. Just look at the big money meets and see what they're wearing. Looking back, I am amazed how Phil mastered that shirt. Like a fast race car, these shirts are hard to master. I took Todd for a ride in my 1960 corvette, and it made him sick. At the time, the car went 10.70 seconds in the quarter mile with about 475 horsepower. It seemed faster but not for long. I got bored and added nitrous to the 355 Chevy. It went 9.40 in the quarter mile with 800 hp. Again, that seemed slow to me, so I put a 404 motor in and soon made an 8.60 pass. My reflexes were matching the car's horsepower, now about 1000. You guessed it. I got bored again, so a 598 on nitrous was added. It went 7.90, 175 mph. What's the point of all of this?

Had I started with a 7.9 car, I would be dead, and Todd would be real sick. My reflexes would not have matched the strength of the car. That same thing happens with lifters. They try shirts much stronger than they are. Oh yes, and there are people who think the shirt is doing everything. They're wrong. At Westside, we have held the all-time best in the bench at 132, 198, 220, 242, 275, and 308 at one time or another. Why don't the rest of us put on shirts and bench the same? We were not strong enough. You've got to have the right size bait for a particular size fish. The same is true for bench shirts. How do you master a bench shirt? Most lifters don't know how to use one correctly.

Dan Cummings visited from Iowa and trained with Becca Swanson. He stayed a week. His best was 600. On max effort day, I saw him work out, and I felt he was closer to a 700 bench. He disagreed with me. The next workout, we worked with him, and in a span of 45 minutes, he made 665. Not bad, huh? I did a seminar in Tennessee for my good friends Tony Hutson and Brent Tracy. We worked with eight guys, and seven got new PRs. Here's how we did it using Brent's workouts as an example.

Brent's best was 528 at 198. First, he warmed up to 315 off his chest. Next, with the 4-board press, he did 365x1, 405x1, and 455x1 without a shirt. Then, he did a 3-board press with his shirt with 495x1. Then, he did a 2-board press with 515x1. Next, he did 530 off his chest and then 545 off his chest for a second PR. I know this all sounds too good to be true, but it's true. The trick is each time you go to 4-boards, raise your head and lower the bar as far down your torso as possible. With 3-boards, raise your head and shoulders if necessary in order to touch the board and go even lower down your torso. With 2-boards, raise your head and start lowering the bar as low as possible by rolling the shoulders up like a sit-up. Each time you go to fewer boards, pull the shirt a little lower off the shoulders. This, of course, makes the shirt a bit stronger. As you increase the weight, raise your head and shoulders and keep your eyes on the bar until it touches the chest. This enables you to touch the chest with a lighter weight than thought possible and at the same time lift a lot more weight. Now that the secret's out, we're all even, right? I just told you how to kick our ass. If you don't do it, it's your problem, fool.

At the 2003 Arnold Classic, Fred Boldt warmed up as I just described. He did 405 off his chest, skipped the 4-boards, put on a shirt, and did 495 on 3-boards. Then he did 530 on two boards and went on to the stage and did a 540 opener. He did 551 on his second attempt. After Markus Schick made a 567 world record, Fred took 1 kg more and pressed it only to have it turned down for a technicality. Not bad for a 165 who is 5ft 9in tall, benching in front of a crowd of thousands. I hope this information helps you break your bench record and have a better understanding of how to use legal equipment.

Coaching Equipment – The Tendo Unit

Have you ever wondered how you measure up to other athletes or lifters? Are you quick with light loads? What about heavy loads? How explosive are you when jumping or bounding? These are just a few very important questions that need to be addressed. Let's look at a device that can do just that. It's the Tendo velocity measuring device. It measures the speed of a lift in meters per second or the actual wattage produced by an athlete. For sprinting, you can determine the quickness of the athlete. Quickness is the ability to perform high speed movements with no significant external resistance or great energy, meaning simply how fast one reacts to a stimulus. Some drills for sprinting are one leg bounding for either stride length or frequency, bounding over hurdles, box jumping, or plyometrics. By attaching the Tendo unit to the athlete, the speed being developed can be measured. The Tendo unit can also measure the velocity with which one throws a medicine ball of different weights. While beginners gain explosive strength as well as maximal strength from jumping, the same exercises will not produce the same results for the advanced athlete. Barbells must be incorporated into the training.

The Tendo unit can be attached to a bar to measure how fast one can move a light weight for speed-strength and near maximal weights as well. By using a determined amount of rubber bands on the bar, you can regulate the bar speed to simulate explosive speed or even strength-speed work. The more bands used, the slower the bar speed becomes, representing near maximal or maximal loading. If you do not become faster, you will not become stronger. Also, if you do not become stronger, you will cease to become faster. The Tendo unit can determine this. When the yearly plan calls for a general preparation microcycle or a sport-specific microcycle with different activities or weights plus jumping, the Tendo unit can help log important data from month to month or year to year. It can help determine how many jumps per set or the total volume of jumps for the optimal jump loading. This provides valuable information to the coach and athlete. The Tendo unit can regulate the intensity zone at which an athlete can best perform as well as when to wave into a different loading zone. Training is individual. Introverts need a slower pace of exercise; whereas, extroverts require more stimulation, or more exercises of variable intensity. The Tendo unit could dictate when it's time to switch exercises.

Many times exercises are performed in a fatigued state to simulate a contest environment. The Tendo unit can regulate the amount of sets or reps before a decreased training value distorts progress. The Tendo device can be used by hockey players when hitting a regular or heavier puck or to determine what weight is optimal for a baseball player's bat, and it could be used for all types of strength development, not only for vertical but also for lateral movement. A shot putter can track his speed with the Tendo unit with shots, ranging from 7–12 kg. A hammer thrower can be tested with short, standard, and long wires to determine his quickness with each. This tells the coach which types of strength the athlete needs improvement on. In powerlifting or weightlifting, top velocity while lifting weights is essential, especially with the five classical lifts. The amount of weight determines just how fast the particular load moves.
The Tendo unit can measure the speed of any load up to 100% max lifts. Does an individual lifter squat 700 lbs mostly by speed-strength or strength-speed? This can be determined by doing squats with a high percentage of bands, roughly 65% with 35% bar weight. This type of squat is very slow, allowing for no momentum. This produces strength-speed. For speed-strength, 40% of the total weight is bar and plates. At the top, bands add 25%, making the top weight 65% of a 1RM. At the bottom, the band tension adds 10% to the bar, making the weight at the bottom 50%. The bands accommodate resistance as they reduce the deceleration phase of the barbell. Remember, any motion that has acceleration also has a deceleration phase. While pressing, pulling, or squatting, the acceleration of the bar depends on the net force acting on the bar. This changes as external resistance is increased or decreased. With the Tendo unit, the bar velocity can be checked at any bar speed, whether for speed-strength, strength-speed, or near maximal weights of 90–97% of a 1RM.

The Tendo unit is used primarily to control bar speed for the development of special strengths. As an experiment in the bench, Karen Sizemore, an official 450 bencher, was tested with a variety of weights. Her power output was measured with each weight:

Weight (lbs)	Power output (watts)
45	270
95	379
135	474
145	453
155	459

Karen's normal training weight was 135 for nine sets of three reps. As noted, 135 lbs resulted in the highest power production. A band was attached to Karen's bar, adding 45 extra pounds at the chest to equal 180 lbs. The bands added an additional 85 lbs at the top to equal 220 at lockout. The Tendo unit proved we were using the correct weight for her speed work.

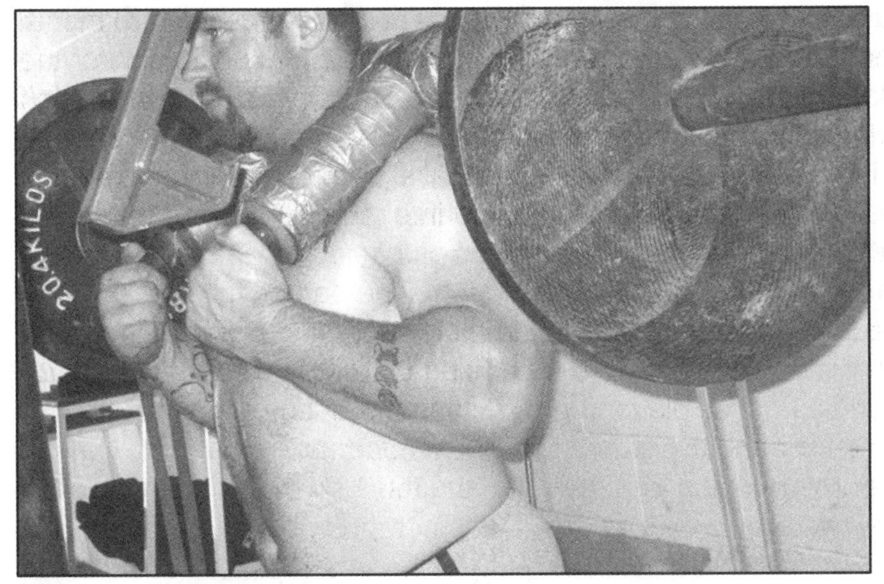

What if the objective is to raise a training weight for speed-strength? Fred Boldt has made official benches of 450, 480, and 495 at 165. His bar speed was 68–72 meters/second with 185. We increased his training weight to 195. Fred's bar velocity remained the same, which produced an official 540 bench at 163. Without the Tendo unit, we could only guess what weight to use as his strength was raised. Fred also copied the same band tension as Karen. It may be surprising to many, but if you look only at Karen's chart, you can see that weights can be too light or, of course, too heavy to produce much force. The Tendo unit has many applications in sport. Sometimes what appears to be the truth is not.

At Westside, we do many lifts in the lightened method to increase speed. In track, the athlete runs down a track inclined four degrees or runs while being pulled back by an elastic cord. A rower can row a lighter boat. Throwers can use lighter shots, hammers, or disks. All of these movements can be measured by the Tendo unit. Training is based on a particular sport but must be controlled individually by the athlete. These are just some applications that the coach or athlete can use to determine optimal training loads to increase progress. It works while doing general, directed, or sport-specific exercises, which highly trained athletes must do year round. The Tendo unit is a great tool for anyone whose goal is to reach the top.

Gym Equipment

There are franchises, and there are gyms. Westside Barbell is definitely a gym. What's the difference? A franchise is a place where they sell baggy pants, T-shirts, protein powder, and a whole bunch of junk you don't need. You can't make noise (don't even think about cursing), and chalk is forbidden. They have lots of mirrors (all you weirdos who look in them for hours…you know who you are) and bodybuilding magazines featuring lots of girls and lots of bull. What does a gym have that's so important?

First, someone must be able to instruct the team and teach others to do the same. This coach must know proper technique in not only the three competitive lifts but also the special core exercises for all three lifts in addition to assistant exercises. He must be able to recognize why a lifter may have a form problem. Is it a mental mistake or a lack of strength in a particular muscle group? Or is the lifter emotionally not up to the task of handling the load? What exercises would help a lifter overcome a plateau? Can he recognize different personalities? An introvert can survive on less exercise and is easily satisfied with even mediocre equipment. This person may not even need reading material. An extrovert, on the other hand, will always seek out more exercises and books, always asking how to be better. If the lifter is timid about taking new weights or fails at meets, does the coach know how this can be fixed?

Second, the entire gym must always strive to improve at meets as well as in the gym. In other words, there must be rivalries within the gym at all times. On one Friday, Paul Childress was visiting and squatted with Chuck Vogelpohl and Mike Ruggiera. What a sight it was to see three 1000 lb squatters going at it together. The following week, there were six 275s squatting in the morning group, the weakest one with a 2100 total. Talk about pecking order. No one is the king at Westside at least not for very long. That keeps everyone on his toes and working hard. If someone has a bad attitude, he must go. Everyone can't be a world champ. If someone looks down on the other lifters or won't go to meets to help his teammates, he's kicked to the curb. One bad attitude can destroy a gym. Everyone must believe in the system no matter what it is. Teamwork is essential. This could mean pushing your training partner or letting him know he is slacking off. He may not like it, but you have to tell him. At Westside, treat me as an equal (i.e. I get no respect). A new lifter came to the gym and was going to load my plates for me. I asked him if he respected me in the gym. He said he did. I then told him that if he ever respected me in the gym again, I would kick him out. From that day on, he treated me like everyone else.

My job is to bring a new guy in the gym and then try to run him out by pushing him to the limit. The morning crew, with whom I train, is always trying to kill me, pushing me to the limit every workout. This is how it should be.

Third, what equipment does a gym need? It should have chains and jump stretch bands for squatting and benching plus a deadlift platform for the bands. If it can afford it, the gym should have a Monolift. Don't buy junk. If the budget is low, obtain a power rack with one-inch hole spacing for deadlift and bench lockouts. It is a must. As far as bars, every gym should have a bench bar, a squat bar, and a deadlift bar. It also needs a good, solid bench. At Westside Barbell, we always bench inside power racks. Depending on the budget, a safety squat bar, MantaRay, and a couple of different cambered bars really make training more versatile. I believe every gym should have a pulling sled. It makes the posterior chain stronger as well as builds GPP. For sports, it helps prevent hip, ankle, and knee injuries. It is also great for the upper body when pulled with the arms. We do a lot of work on our stationary sled. This is a resistance sled much like a dog slat mill used for conditioning dogs, but it has attachments that work like pulling a weighted sled. Bands fit around the ankles, which build the hip extensors and flexors.

Jason Burns, an ex-Cincinnati Bengal, said that had he used this sled, he would probably still be playing. Westside also has dumbbells up to 175, a stability ball, sturdy boxes for box squatting, and platforms for deadlifting. If an athlete is interested in increasing the squat and deadlift, a calf/ ham/ glute bench is needed.

At Westside, we live on calf/ham/glute raises and inverse curls. They push the squat and deadlift up fast. As long as the weights and reps are regulated, they will continue to raise both the squat and deadlift indefinitely. An exercise that has benefited Westside greatly is the land mine. Wrestlers have done this exercise forever. A bar is placed in the corner. The lifter picks it up and twists it left and right, working the obliques, abs, and low back. The combination of the land mine and roller reverse hyper machine has brought about an increase in the deadlifts recently at Westside. We also have an assortment of rowing handles.

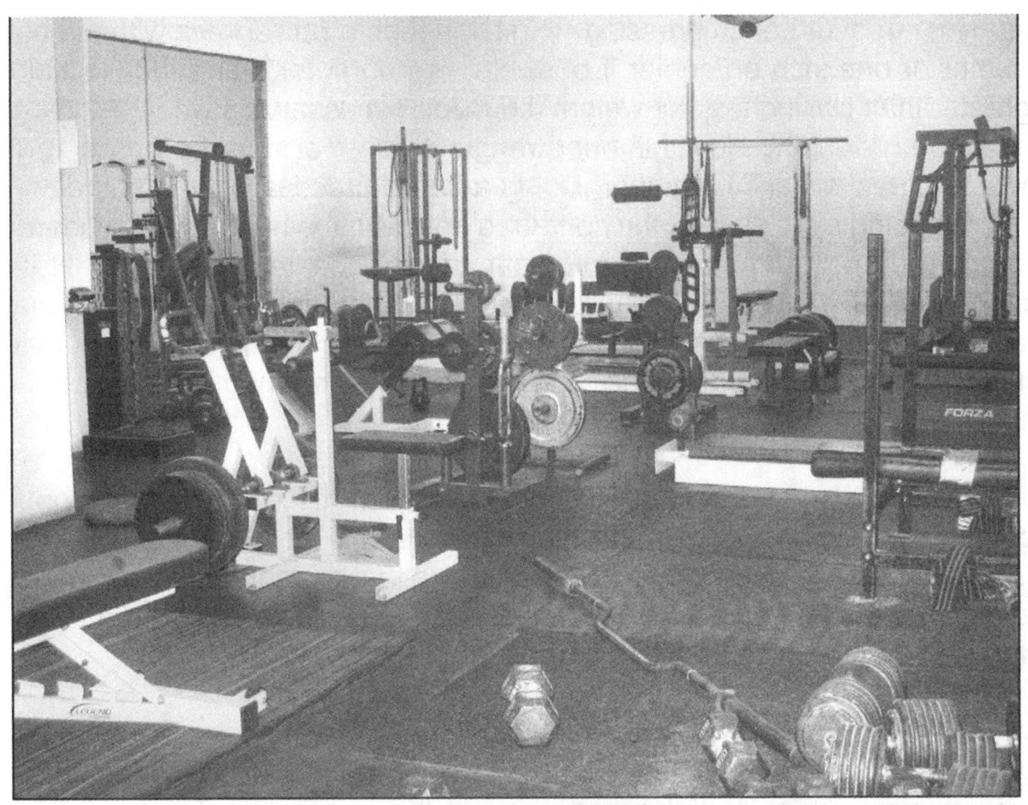

I believe the calf/ham/glute, the land mine, and reverse hyper machine are essential for any hard-core gym. The roller model of the reverse hyper machine isolates the lower back like nothing I have ever seen. When the weight is under the face, the sacrum is rotated maximally. At the same time, it works as restoration by tractioning the back. The reverse hyper machine out-performs Romanian deadlifts almost two to one for low back and hamstrings, as tested by EMG. Although the glutes were not tested in the study, they are hit hard by the machine. Some people report a 100 lb gain in the deadlift and squat from using this machine. However, it's the restoration that the reverse hyper provides that makes the difference. To be successful, combine the old and the new—wisdom and innovation.

Attitude. Everyone must have the same goal, which is to get stronger. We don't care if you are trying a 300 bench press for a PR or a 600 PR. What about equipment? Machines are a waste. They work on the theory of peak contraction, which simply means starting at the weakest point. This is stupid and very dangerous. Machines build no stability. Also, how can one machine work for two people if one is strong at the bottom of a lift and his partner is stronger at the top? It's impossible.

I want to say something here about high intensity training (HIT). Many football teams are using the HIT system. Well, my friends, intensity isn't a feeling but rather a division of "percent of a one rep max" zones. Doing one set to failure does little for speed-strength. If you have a player do 20 reps with a barbell to complete failure, how long does it take him to do a second set? Under 35 seconds, I hope, because that's how long a football player gets to rest between plays. I was talking to an NFL strength coach recently who said that college programs using HIT are sending him linemen that can't vertical jump 19 inches or squat 300 lbs! Chuck Vogelpohl's brother, who trains with us, is a center and weighs 305 at 20-years-old. He has a vertical jump of 31 inches.

What does a gym need for bench pressing? First, it needs a power rack with pin holes every two inches on center or one inch on center if possible, like ours, for doing rack lockouts. If the hole spacing is greater than two inches, the weight reduction necessary between using one set of holes and the next is too great to work within our strength curve. For board presses, a gym needs 2-, 3-, and 4-boards glued or nailed together. Doing a board press is not the same thing as doing a rack press. When doing a rack press, the contact is only with the hands. When board pressing, the weight is transferred through the boards into your chest, shoulders, and arms. Heavy dumbbells are necessary. If a lifter wants to bench more than 600, he needs dumbbells up to at least 175. If he wants reversal strength and who doesn't, the contrast method is a must. For example, sleds and parachutes, which sprinters use, that break away while running help create the over-speed effect.

Explosive and accelerating strength can be developed with the aid of weight strippers or the release device. By lowering extra weight on the releasers and then concentrically raising a lesser load, explosive strength can be increased. Using chains that are connected to the bar, we can create a deloading effect on the eccentric phase through the chains piling on the floor. This process duplicates the strength curve as it relates to the bottom of the lift.

Reloading of the chains concentrically again helps to maximize the complete range of joint motion, effectively accommodating resistance. Flex bands work much like chains because they unload tension upon lowering with a regaining of tension in the concentric phase. A greater amount of reversal strength can be obtained not by lowering a heavier weight, which leads to a decrease in reversal strength, but by a moderate increase in downward velocity. This is kinetic energy, which can be transferred to the storage and reuse of elastic energy, for the concentric phase. This was discussed by Zatsiorsky in *Science and Practice of Strength Training.*

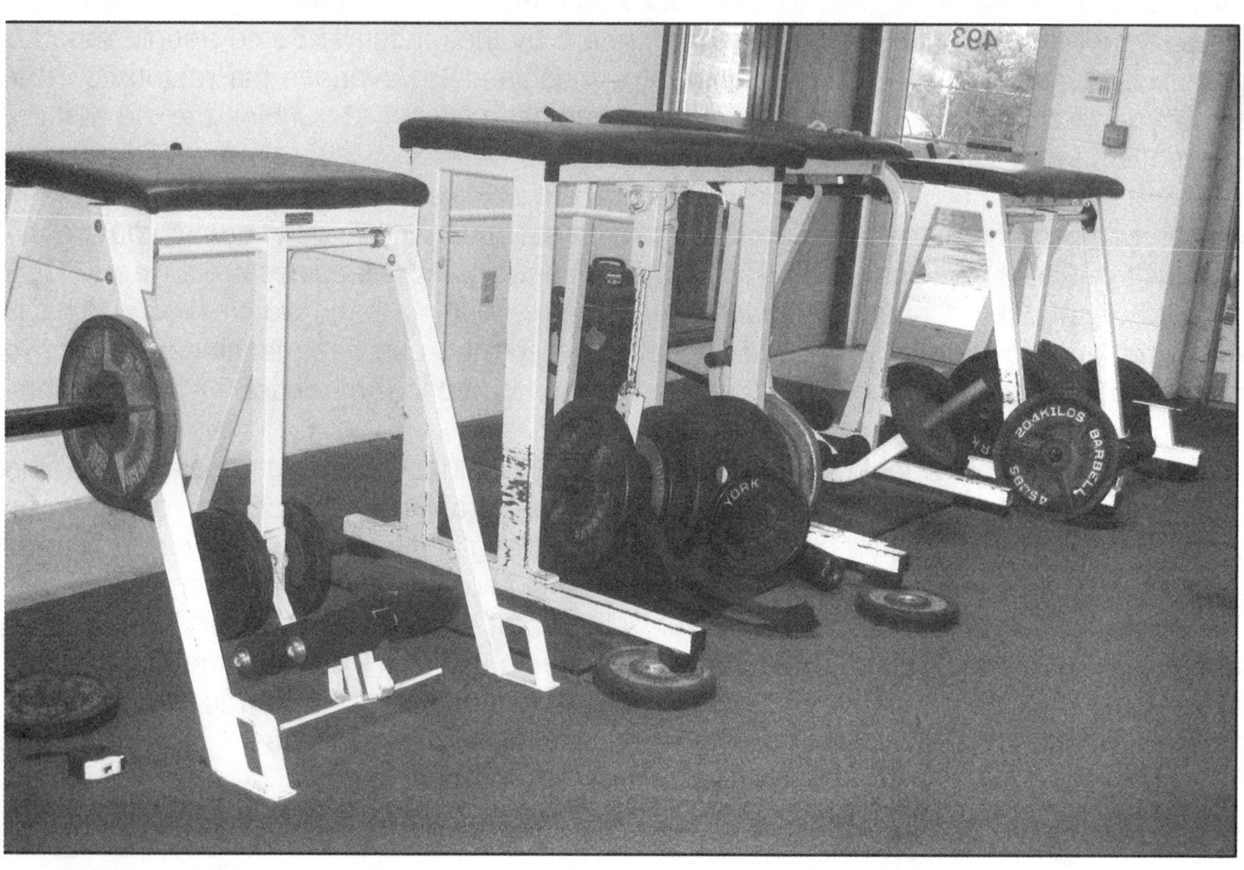

A great piece of equipment is a McDonald cambered bar. An advanced bencher, may have to place a 2x6 or two, 2x6s on his chest to reduce the stretching from five inches to 2–3 inches. A seven-foot EZ curl bar can also be a great benefit. A set of rings resembling gymnastic rings to do push-ups and pull-ups with from a variety of angles is tremendous for building extra muscle.

For squatting and deadlifting, again weight releasers, chains, and bands should be emplyed extensively on max effort day and speed day. An assortment of boxes to squat off of is vital. Also, a MantaRay, a safety squat bar, and for most powerlifters, a front squat harness are needed to change body leverage artificially.

If a lifter is weak on one or all of these devices, this is precisely why they will work. For example, Don Damron used the safety squat bar for a mini-cycle, and his squat and deadlift jumped about 20 lbs every time. A lifter needs many weapons in his arsenal to increase his lifts as well as to prevent boredom. Another bar that we use quite often is the Buffalo Bar by Ironmind. It is very strong and cambered, enabling one good mornings to be completed easily.

Don't forget to include bands, chains, and weight releasers, which affect leverage in different ways. Use lots of chains and a light bar weight or do just the opposite—a light amount of chain and a heavy bar weight. The Russians did a lot of slow lowering with 80%, taking about six seconds and raising up 60% very explosively with the use of weight releasers. Belt squats are the perfect way to work the lower body without trauma on the spine. They are also very therapeutic. If an individual suffers from a back injury, he can still build his lower body with belt squats. This exercise can realign the vertebrae by its traction properties.

A glute ham bench is an absolute must. The hamstring is the muscle group that can make or break squat and deadlift progress. Five women at Westside have squatted or deadlifted 500 pounds or more, and every one of them laid a heavy foundation on a glute ham machine. Doris Simmons made a 341 squat and 349 deadlift at 105 a long time ago, and Amy Weisberger has moved her numbers from a 445 squat and 430 deadlift at 123 to 590 and 500 at 148.

A reverse hyper builds the glutes, hamstrings, and lower back like nothing else. There are many men who merely increase the weight on this exercise near a meet. Billy Masters, who squats 900 lbs, does just that. The reverse hyper is very therapeutic for the low back because it rotates the sacrum on each rep.

A pulling sled will do unbelievable things for one's squat and deadlift. Jim Voronin was stuck at a 683 deadlift forever. We advised him to stop deadlifting and start dragging a weighted sled. In four months, he did a 750 deadlift!

WESTSIDE BARBELL STATISTICS

These are the up-to-date numbers our lifters have achieved. All lifts were performed in sanctioned contests conditions, and most of them are in the APF, WPO, and IPA. This list is under everlasting construction. The numbers are from 21st February 2013 and have already expired in some part at the time of this book's publication.

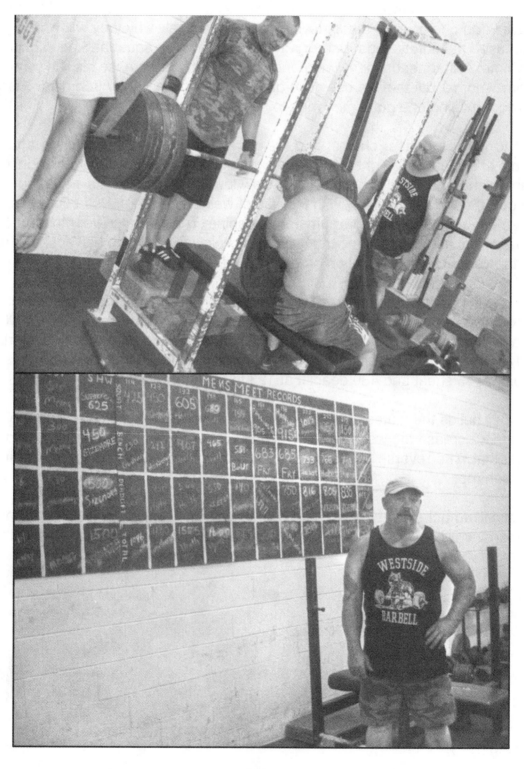

WESTSIDE BARBELL

Top 10 Totals

Rank	Last Name	Name	Total	Wt Class	Weight	Coefficient
1	Hoff	Dave	2960	308	279	1535.6
2	Hoff	Dave	2921	275	275	1521.8
3	Roberts	AJ	2855	308	304	1448.5
4	Panora	Greg	2630	242	242	1410.9
5	Hoff	Dave	2600	242	241	1397.76
6	Anderson	Jake	2755	308	305	1395.6
7	Coker	Jason	2360	198	196	1384.1
8	Panora	Greg	2620	275	262	1383
9	Vogelpohl	Chuck	2605	275	264	1372.8
10	Hammock	Shane	2695	308	304	1361.7

Top 10 Squats

Rank	Last Name	First Name	Total	Wt Class	Body Weight	Coefficient
1	Hoff	Dave	1200	308	279	622.56
2	Hoff	Dave	1190	275	275	619.99
3	Roberts	AJ	1205	308	304	609.2
4	Vogelpohl	Chuck	1150	275	264	606.4
5	Coker	Jason	1000	198	196	586.5
6	Bolognone	Tony	1150	308	300	583.9
7	Alhazov	Vlad	1155	shw	341	579.5
8	Anderson	Jake	1140	308	303	576.95
9	Panora	Greg	1060	242	242	568.6
10	Vogelpohl	Chuck	1025	220	220	567.8

Top 10 Benches

Rank	Last Name	First Name	Total	Wt Class	Body Weight	Coefficient
1	Hoff	Dave	965	308	279	500.6
2	Hoff	Dave	959	275	275	499.6
3	Coker	Jason	830	198	198	485.7
4	Coker	Jason	840	220	205	481.6
5	Coker	Jason	850	242	227	465.37
6	Fry	Jason	750	181	181	464.4
7	Roberts	AJ	905	308	304	457.02
8	Roberts	AJ	910	SHW	312	457
9	Fry	Jason	770	198	198	450.68
10	Halbert	George	766	198	198	449.8

Top 10 Deadlifts

Rank	Last Name	First Name	Total	Wt Class	Body Weight	Coefficient
1	Vogelpohl	Chuck	816	220	220	452.06
2	Edwards	Luke	840	275	265	442.6
3	Vogelpohl	Chuck	835	275	265	439.62
4	Heath	Doug	540	132	132.25	438.9
5	Chorpenning	Jeff	750	198	198.5	438.8
6	Panora	Greg	815	242	242	437.2
7	Vogelpohl	Chuck	805	242	234	437.03
8	Hoff	Dave	825	242	262	435.8
9	Edwards	Luke	810	242	240	435.5
10	Heath	Doug	457	114	114.5	434.8

WESTSIDE BARBELL

64 Members total 2000 or more

2900 CLUB

Rank	Last Name	First Name	Lift	Wt Class
1	Hoff	Dave	2960	308

2800 CLUB

Rank	Last Name	First Name	Lift	Wt Class
1	Roberts	AJ	2855	308

2700 CLUB

Rank	Last Name	First Name	Lift	Wt Class
1	Anderson	Jake	2755	308
2	Bolognone	Tony	2705	SHW

2600 CLUB

Rank	Last Name	First Name	Lift	Wt Class
1	Hammock	Shane	2695	308
2	Smith	Matt	2672	SHW
3	Panora	Greg	2630	242
4	Vogelpohl	Chuck	2605	275

2500 CLUB

Rank	Last Name	First	Lift	Wt Class
1	Connolly	Josh	2590	SHW
2	Harold	Tim	2560	SHW
3	Alhazov	Vlad	2545	SHW
4	Brown	Mike	2518	308
5	Ruggiera	Mike	2510	shw
6	Lily	Brandon	2505	308
	Stafford	John	2502	275

2400 CLUB

Rank	Last Name	First Name	Lift	Wt Class
1	Wenning	Matt	2465	308
2	Edwards	Luke	2465	308
3	Cole	Zack	2455	308
4	Holdsworth	J.L	2437	275
5	Lilly	Brandon	2430	308
6	Myers	Jeremiah	2400	275

2300 CLUB

Rank	Last Name	First Name	Lift	Wt Class
1	Bayles	Joe	2380	242
2	Wendler	Jim	2375	275
3	Coker	Jason	2360	198
4	Fusner	Rob	2357	308
5	Douglas	Rich	2350	275
6	Gutridge	Josh	2325	SHW
7	Hudak	Zack	2305	275
8	Pacifico	Jimmie	2300	220
9	Dimel	Matt	2300	SHW

2200 CLUB

Rank	Last Name	First Name	Lift	Wt Class
1	Lenigar	Matt	2295	308
2	Waddle	Tom	2260	308
3	Harrington	Phil	2250	198
4	Shakleford	John "Shack"	2250	275
5	Henery	Andre	2225	SHW
6	Nutter	Shawn	2210	242
7	Obradovic	Jerry	2210	275
8	Tate	Dave	2205	308
9	Ritchey	Jimmy	2200	275

2100 CLUB

Rank	Last Name	First Name	Lift	Wt Class
1	Burrows	Mark	2160	275
2	Ramsey	Will	2155	308
3	Johnson	Nate	2140	275
4	Smith	Matt 2	2125	275
5	Patterson	Kenny	2115	220
6	Brock	Todd	2115	275
7	Beach	Tony	2105	308
8	Mendoza	Phil	2105	SHW
9	Jester	Joe	2100	220
10	Simmons	Louie	2100	242

2000 CLUB

Rank	Last Name	First Name	Lift	Wt Class
1	McCoy	Joe	2090	220
2	Paulucci	Tom	2080	275
3	Willoughby	Jerry	2070	SHW
4	Ramos	Tony	2060	181
5	Hayes	Bill	2060	SHW
6	Moore	Bill	2045	SHW
7	Forby	Tim	2035	308
8	Gutridge	Josh	2035	SHW
9	Amato	Joe	2033	275
10	Cole	Zach	2030	275
11	Madjar	Matt	2025	275
12	Reitter	Gabe	2020	242
13	Youngs	Bob	2010	275
14	Johnson	Nate	2005	275
15	Kelly	Brian	2000	220
16	Thomasson	Eskil	2000	242
17	Conkley	James	2000	275
18	Blanton	Mike	2000	275

70 Members squat 800 or more

1200 CLUB

Rank	Last Name	First Name	Lift	Wt class
1	Roberts	AJ	1205	308
2	Hoff	Dave	1200	308

1100 CLUB

Rank	Last Name	First Name	Lift	Wt class
1	Smith	Matt	1160	SHW
2	Alvazov	Vlad	1155	SHW
3	Vogelpohl	Chuck	1150	275
4	Bolognone	Tony	1150	308
5	Anderson	Jake	1140	308

1000 CLUB

Rank	Last Name	First Name	Lift	Wt class
1	Brown	Mike	1074	308
2	Panora	Greg	1060	242
3	Wenning	Matt	1055	275
4	Hammock	Shane	1050	308
5	Ruggiera	Mike	1050	348
6	Cole	Zach	1040	308
7	Edwards	Luke	1025	242
8	Connelly	Josh	1020	SHW
9	Dimel	Matt	1010	SHW
10	Lily	Brandon	1005	308
11	Harold	Tim	1005	SHW
12	Coker	Jason	1000	198
13	Wendler	Jim	1000	275

900 CLUB

Rank	Last Name	First Name	Lift	Wt class
1	Harrington	Phil	960	220
2	Church	Shane	960	242
3	Meyers	Jeriamiah	950	275
4	Waddle	Tom	950	308
5	Stafford	John	946	275
6	Pacifico	Jimmie	945	220
7	Tate	Dave	935	308
8	Bayles	Joe	925	242
9	Burrows	Mark	925	275
10	Simmons	Louie	920	242
11	Henry	Andre	920	SHW
12	Shackelford	John	905	275
13	Fusner	Rob	905	308
14	Holdsworth	JL	903	275
15	Hudak	Zack	903	275
16	Nutter	Shawn	900	242
17	Douglas	Richard	900	275

Rank	Last Name	First Name	Lift	Wt class
18	Madjar	Matt	900	275
19	Ramsey	Will	900	308
20	Lenigar	Matt	900	308
21	Guttridge	Josh	900	SHW

800 CLUB

Rank	Last Name	First Name	Lift	Wt class
1	Mendoza	Phil	881	SHW
2	Ritchey	Jimmy	875	275
3	Jester	Joe	870	220
4	Amato	Joe	865	275
5	Smith 2	Matt	850	242
6	Brock	Todd	850	275
7	Willoughby	Jerry	850	SHW
8	Thomasson	Eskil	840	242
9	Douglas	Rich	840	275
10	Youngs	Bob	840	308
11	Beach	Tony	830	308
12	McCoy	Joe	825	220
12	Blanton	mike	825	275
13	Patterson	Kenny	821	220
14	Brown	John	820	220
15	Reitter	Gabe	820	242
16	Ramos	Tony	815	181
17	Hayes	Bill	815	SHW
18	Hawkins	Matt	810	220
19	Obradovic	Jerry	810	275
20	Forby	Tim	810	308
21	Moore	Bill	805	SHW
22	Chorpenning	Jeff	804	198
23	Coleman	Arnold	804	198
24	Bishop	Brad	800	220
25	Trotter	Rick	800	242
26	Henderson	Shawn	800	275

Rank	Last Name	First Name	Lift	Wt class
27	Johnson	Nate	800	275
28	Snyder	John	800	275
29	Damron	Don	800	308
30	Boggia	Bart	800	308

74 Members bench 600 or more

900 CLUB

Rank	Last Name	First Name	Lift	Wt class
1	Hoff	David	965	308
2	Roberts	AJ	910	shw

800 CLUB

Rank	Last Name	First Name	Lift	Wt class
1	Hammock	Shane	865	308
2	Bolognone	Tony	865	SHW
3	Wolfe	Mike	859	SHW
4	Coker	Jason	850	220
5	Bell	Travis	835	275
6	Anderson	Jake	830	308
7	Panora	Greg	820	275
8	Lily	Brandon	810	308

700 CLUB

Rank	Last Name	First Name	Lift	Wt class
1	Wenning	Matt	785	308
2	Holdsworth	JL	775	308
3	Connelly	Josh	770	SHW
4	Halbert	George	766	241
5	Welch	Drex	765	308
6	Keyes	Paul	755	308
7	Martinez	John	750	308

Rank	Last Name	First Name	Lift	Wt class
8	Fletcher	Travis	750	shw
9	Smith	Matt	749	SHW
10	Fry	Jason	740	220
11	Vickory	Scott	740	308
12	Stafford	John	738	275
13	Fusner	Rob	735	308
14	Brown	Mike	735	308
15	Patterson	Kenny	728	275
16	Pacifico	Jimmy	725	220
17	Gutridge	Josh	725	SHW
18	Argabright	Kevin	720	SHW
19	Mann	Roger	720	275
20	Bayles	Joe	705	275
21	Harold	Tim	715	SHW
22	Blakely	J.M.	710	308
23	Obradovic	Jerry	705	275
24	Schakleford	John	705	275
25	Meyers	Jeremiah	700	275
26	Edwards	Luke	700	275
27	Winters	Nick	700	SHW

650 CLUB

07/12/2011

Rank	Last Name	First Name	Lift	Wt class
1	Boldt	Fred	685	198
2	Douglas	Rich	680	275
3	Senter	Marlon	675	220
4	Cole	Zack	675	275
5	Wendler	Jim	675	275
6	Ruggiera	Mike	675	348
7	Lenigar	Matt	665	308
8	Hudak	Zack	661	275
9	Richie	Jimmy	660	275
10	Kuck	David	650	242
11	Conkley	James	650	275
12	Tate	Mickey	650	308

600 CLUB

Rank	Last Name	First Name	Lift	Wt class
1	Kelly	Brian	640	220
2	Burrows	Mark	640	275
3	Ramsey	Will	639	308
4	Vogelpohl	Chuck	635	275
5	Boggia	Bart	635	308
6	Jester	JOE	630	220
7	Harrington	Phil	625	198
8	Beversdorf	Dave	625	275
9	Brown	John	620	220
10	Brock	Todd	620	275
11	Hoff	Aaron	610	275
12	Adams	Jeff	605	220
13	Swanger	Adam	605	242
14	Johnson	Nate	605	275
15	Ramsey	Will	605	308
16	Tate	Dave	605	308
17	Henry	Andre	605	SHW
18	Brown	Matt	600	220
19		Seth	600	220
20	Swauger	Adam	600	220
21	Kelly	Brian	600	220
22	Shortland	Chad	600	242
23	Simmons	Louie	600	275
24	Beach	Tony	600	275
25	Henderson	H	600	275
26	Forby	Tim	600	308

20 Members deadlift 800 or more

800 CLUB

Rank	Last Name	First Name	Lift	Wt Class
1	Anderson	Jake	860	308
2	Harold	Tim	855	SHW
3	Smith	Matt	850	SHW
4	Edwards	Luke	840	275
5	Vogelpohl	Chuck	835	275
6	Stafford	John	832	275
7	Hoff	Dave	825	275
8	Dimel	Matt	821	SHW
9	Ruggiera	Mike	821	SHW
10	Panora	Greg	815	242
11	Roberts	Aj	815	308
12	Obradovic	Jerry	810	308
13	Alhazov	Vlad	805	SHW
14	Meyers	Jeremiah	805	275
15	Hammock	Shane	805	308
16	Holdsworth	JL	804	275
17	Brown	Mike	804	308
18	Paulucci	Tom	800	275
19	Douglas	Rich	800	275
20	Connelly	Josh	800	SHW

Westside Exercise Index

These sample lists show how much variation there is and the possibilities that exist to change training based on an individual's needs. Many exercises can be mixed together such as: board presses with bands, chains, or both.

Variation is one of the most important keys to constant progress. Without that, your lifts will stall or even regress. The most common way to vary training is to change the max effort exercise each week. Variation can be used for speed in waves for each power lift. It has brought great results at Westside

Westside Squat and Deadlift Exercise Index:

Good morning styles:

- regular
- bent over
- arched back
- standing on ramp
- from chains (concentric)
- foot stance

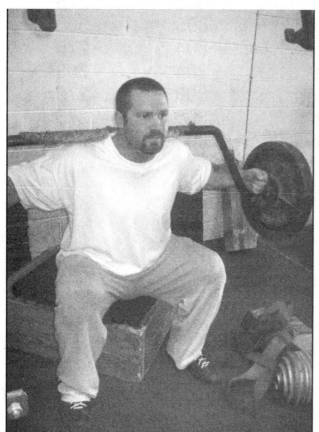

Box squat styles:
- low box
- high box
- soft box (hassock or foam)
- foot stance
- from chains (concentric)

Resistance variables on squats and good mornings:
- chains
- reverse band
- bands from floor
- bands and chains together
- straight weight
- weight releasers

Different bars and tools to use on squats and good mornings:

- straight bar
- cambered squat bar
- safety squat bar
- buffalo bar
- MantaRay
- Dave Drapers top squat
- front squat harness

Deadlift styles:

- regular
- box or platform
- sumo
- conventional
- rack pulls
- snatch grip
- hack deadlifts

Resistance variables on deadlift:

- chains
- reverse band
- band platform
- straight weight

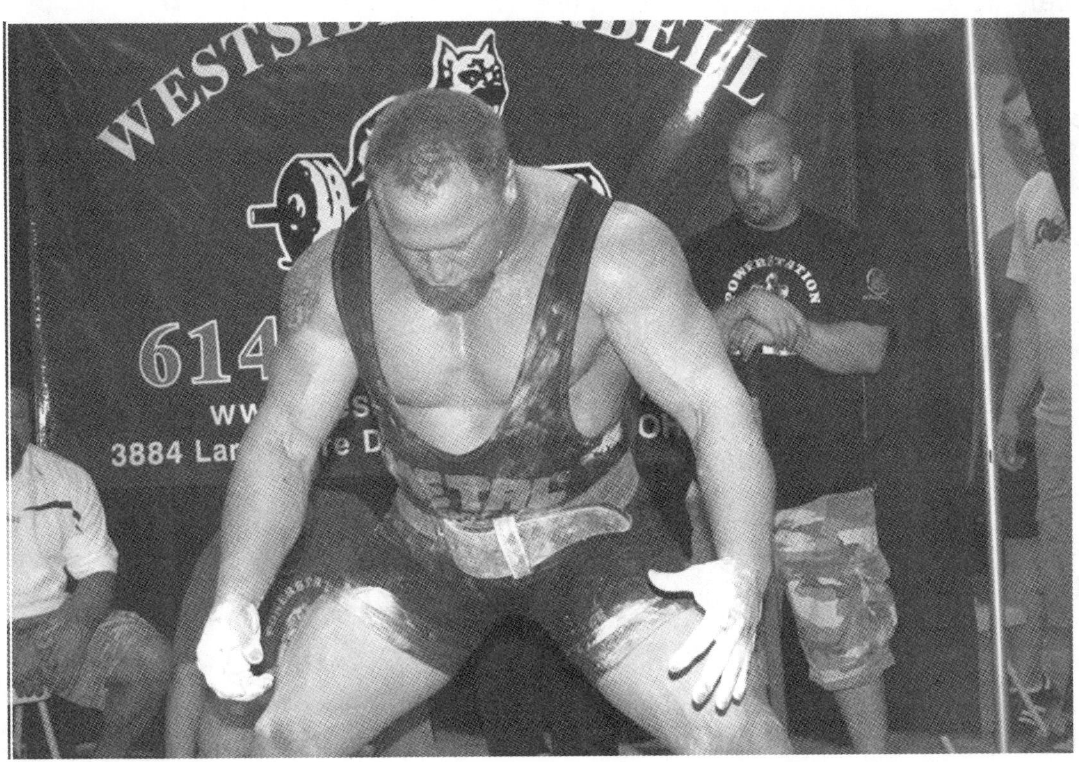

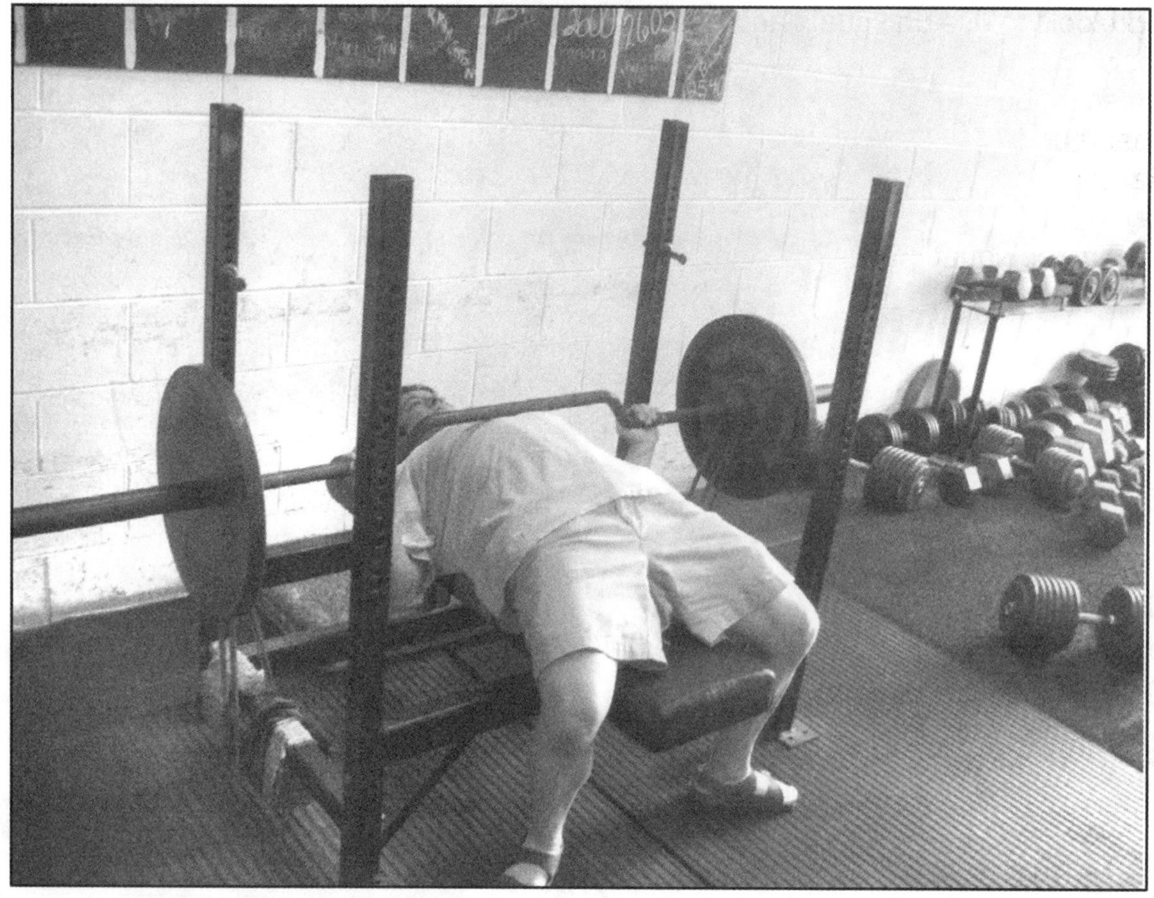

Different bars to use on deadlift:

- deadlift bar
- standard power bar
- thick bars, squat bar, Apollo's axle
- trap bar

Westside Bench Press Exercise Index

Floor press:

- chains
- bands
- reverse bands
- football bar
- fat bar

Board press:

- 1-, 2-, 3-boards
- 3-, 4-, 5-boards
- chains
- bands
- fat bar

Regular bench press:
- chains
- bands
- reverse bands
- all special bars
- incline
- decline

Repetition work:
- dumbbells
- arch bar
- football bar
- buffalo bar
- incline
- decline
- floor
- stability ball

Resistance variables on the bench:
- chains
- reverse band
- bands from floor
- bands and chains together
- straight weight
- weight releasers

Different bars and tools to use on the bench press:
- straight bar
- cambered bar
- freak bar
- buffalo bar
- football bar
- fat bars
- foam
- stability ball

The number of exercises comes up to the hundreds at least, depending on how much variation and how many tools a lifter has in his gym. Choose exercises based on weak points or sticking points, lack of speed on big weights, ability to use equipment, or anything else that may hold progress back. Pick right and progress will be constant.

PLYOMETRICS AND POWERLIFTING
The Practice of Plyometrics at Westside
Explosive Leg Strength
Using the Virtual Force Swing

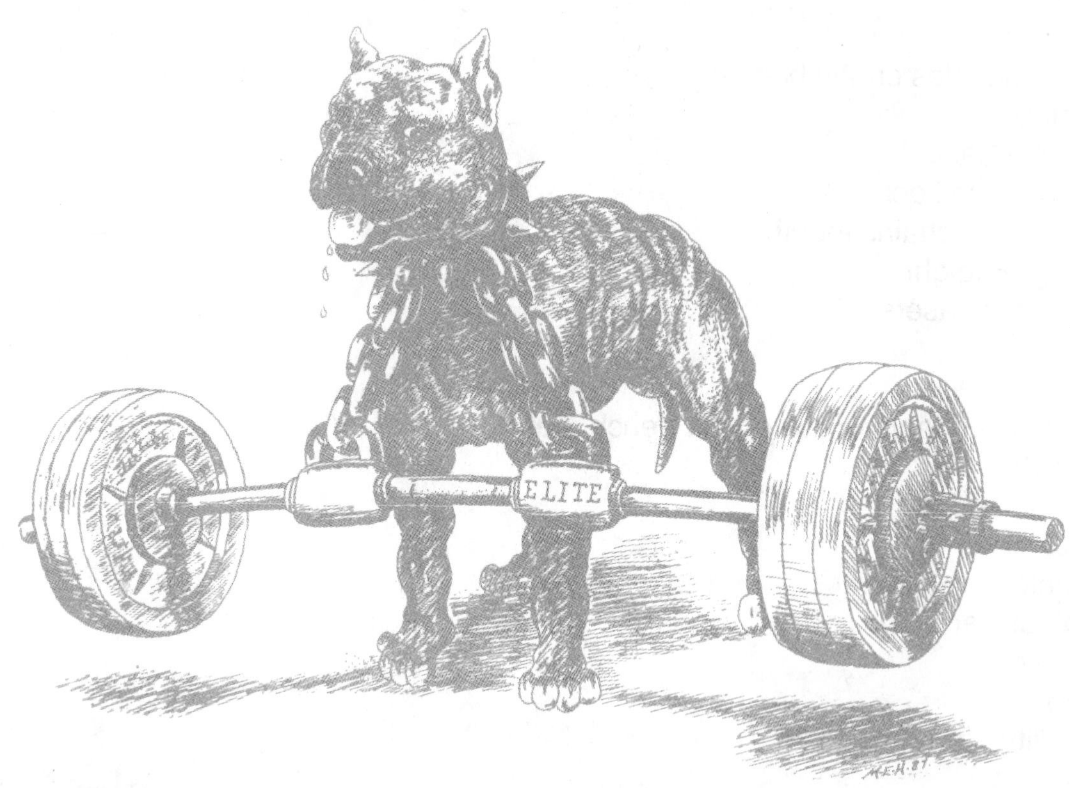

WESTSIDE BARBELL™